THE COUMADIN® COOKBOOK

A COMPLETE GUIDE *to* HEALTHY MEALS *when* TAKING COUMADIN®

SECOND EDITION

RENE DESMARAIS, M.D.
GREG GOLDEN, RCS
GAIL BEYNON

THE COUMADIN® COOKBOOK

A COMPLETE GUIDE *to* HEALTHY MEALS *when* TAKING COUMADIN®

Second Edition

RENE DESMARAIS, MD
GREG GOLDEN, RCS
GAIL BEYNON

Marsh Publishing Company
Salisbury, Maryland

COUMADIN® is a registered trademark of
The Du Pont Merck Pharmaceutical Company

THE COUMADIN® COOKBOOK
A COMPLETE GUIDE *to* HEALTHY MEALS *when* TAKING COUMADIN®
By: RENE DESMARAIS, MD, GREG GOLDEN, RCS and GAIL BEYNON

Published by:
MARSH PUBLISHING COMPANY
PO BOX 1597, SALISBURY, MD 21802-1597 USA

Copyright © 1998 by René Desmarais, MD,
Greg Golden, RCS and Gail Beynon

First edition printed June 1998
Second edition printed December 2000

Printed in the United States of America by
René Desmarais, MD, Greg Golden, RCS and Gail Beynon

ISBN # 0-9664308-1-6

DISCLAIMERS

The use of COUMADIN®, an anticoagulant, is associated with some risk of morbidity and mortality. Although it is hoped that the use of this book will help some patients to regulate, more easily, their dose of COUMADIN® and their prothrombin time/INR, the authors can not and do not make any guarantee regarding these potential benefits. Also, the authors can not and do not guarantee any reduction in the risk associated with the use of COUMADIN®. The risks of anticoagulation with COUMADIN® will not be eliminated by the use of this book and, therefore, the authors are not responsible for any complications, including death, that may result from COUMADIN® use. Consultation with the health care professional or professionals responsible for prescribing the COUMADIN® and monitoring the patient's prothrombin time/INR is necessary and strongly recommended before a change in the patient's diet. The responsibility for the risks associated with COUMADIN® use remain with the patient and the health care professional or professionals described above. If the purchaser of this book does not wish to be bound by the above, the book may be returned to the publisher for a full refund.

The information set forth in the COUMADIN® Cookbook has been neither authorized nor approved by DuPont Pharmaceuticals Company ("DuPont Pharmaceuticals"). DuPont Pharmaceuticals is not responsible for the accuracy of such information and expressly disclaims any responsibility to correct such information. In no event will DuPont Pharmaceuticals be liable for damages, including special, incidental, consequential, or indirect damages arising from the use of the COUMADIN® Cookbook, however caused and/or under any theory of liability. This limitation will apply even if DuPont Pharmaceuticals has been advised of the possibility of any such damage.

The Authors

RENÉ DESMARAIS MD currently practices Cardiology with Peninsula Cardiology Associates on the Eastern Shore of Maryland and in Delaware. His practice includes the largest COUMADIN® Clinic on the Delmarva Peninsula. He received his BA from The Johns Hopkins University in 1983. He graduated from The University of Connecticut Medical School, where he was a Scholar in Medicine, in 1987. From 1987 to 1990, he trained in internal medicine at Francis Scott Key Medical Center, now know as Bayview Medical Center, a hospital affiliated with The Johns Hopkins Hospital, in Baltimore. MD. Subsequently, he completed a Fellowship in Cardiovascular Diseases at The University of Virginia Medical Center in 1993. After this training he began practicing on the Eastern Shore where he lives with his spouse, Cairy Packard, MD, and their three daughters. Dr. Desmarais' research has been published in *Circulation* and in the *Journal of The American College of Cardiology*.

GREGORY GOLDEN is a Registered Cardiac Sonographer currently working with Peninsula Cardiology Associates on the Eastern Shore of Maryland. Greg spent seven years in the U.S. Navy as an ordnance man training with some of the Navy's finest - HooYah! His spare time is taken kayaking, cycling and Martial Arts.

GAIL BEYNON is an enthusiastic gardener and cook who began cooking at the age of five. Gail continues to experiment with new recipes and ingredients growing the produce in her garden when she cannot find it locally. Despite 32 years as a full time computer specialist, Gail has developed a cooking data base with thousands of recipes. When she travels, Gail visits local grocery stores looking for unusual ingredients and new methods of preparation. While other folks may bring back artwork or jewelry, Gail brings home local foods and new recipe ideas to the enthusiastic reception of her family and friends.

TABLE OF CONTENTS

INTRODUCTION

by René Desmarais, MD

Welcome to the COUMADIN® Cookbook!

The goal of this cookbook is to allow the person on COUMADIN® to EASILY consume approximately the same amount of vitamin K each day in a heart-healthy way. This is essential for maintaining a PT/INR (prothrombin time/International Normalized Ratio) within the desired therapeutic range on a given COUMADIN® dose. The cookbook provides practical dietary guidelines for patients who take the anticoagulant COUMADIN®. Patients who take the generic form of COUMADIN®, warfarin sodium, can also use this cookbook. We intend to provide these guidelines in an enjoyable manner, primarily by furnishing the reader with recipes that are tasty, heart healthy, contain all food groups (including plenty of vegetables) and contain an accurate estimate of vitamin K content.

We want these guidelines to be easy to use and to understand. There are four major parts to this cookbook. The first part is this part, the introduction. The second part gives several useful tips on how to consume a more steady or consistent daily amount of vitamin K. The third part is a list of foods that contain very small amounts of vitamin K. The fourth part is the recipes themselves. Every food, drink and recipe included in this cookbook has a known amount of vitamin K per serving. So, by using all four parts of the cookbook, the patient on COUMADIN® can eat approximately the same amount of vitamin K every day AND have an enjoyable, healthy diet.

The amount of vitamin K that the patient on COUMADIN® consumes each day is crucial to keep the effect of COUMADIN® steady. COUMADIN® works to increase the time it takes for a patient's blood to clot by going against the action of vitamin K. By doing this, COUMADIN® PREVENTS harmful blood clots from forming. Likewise, vitamin K goes against the action of COUMADIN®. Vitamin K HELPS blood clot. Therefore, if patients do not consume a steady amount of vitamin K each day, while they are taking COUMADIN®, they are in danger of their blood forming unwanted clots too quickly or of prolonged bleeding from too much drug effect.

By using this cookbook, the person on COUMADIN® may have a more stable effect from his or her COUMADIN® dose. Also, a more stable COUMADIN® dose may lead to fewer prothrombin time/INR tests (the prothrombin time test is the blood test that your health care professional uses to monitor the effects of COUMADIN®).

Before we continue, it is necessary to make certain that all of our readers understand some basics about the use of the anticoagulant COUMADIN®. An anticoagulant is simply any drug that prevents blood from clotting as well as it should. Not all anticoagulants are COUMADIN®. The generic name for COUMADIN® is warfarin sodium. COUMADIN®, a trademark name belonging to The DuPont Merck Pharmaceutical Company, is the most commonly used warfarin sodium product in the U.S. today. Aspirin and heparin are drugs that also affect the blood's ability to form clots, but these products are not affected by vitamin K. COUMADIN® opposes the action of vitamin K in the body. One of the most important actions of vitamin K is to help the liver make proteins that circulate in our blood and cause blood to clot. These proteins are not the only things in our blood that make blood clot in the appropriate circumstances. Aspirin, for example, makes blood less likely to clot because it opposes blood cells called platelets. Platelets also help make blood clot, but platelets are not affected by COUMADIN®.

The typical patient on COUMADIN® receives contradictory advice regarding their diet. Often they are told to avoid foods with high vitamin K content so that vitamin K will not antagonize the effect of COUMADIN®. They are told this so their dose of COUMADIN® can be more easily managed. Further, they are told to "eat the same amount" of a given food each day, for example "You can eat spinach, but you have to have EXACTLY the same amount each day." This is very difficult to do in real life. Finally, the major food group they are told to avoid is vegetables. However, most, if not all, heart healthy dietary guidelines strongly emphasize the need to have a large amount of vegetables in the diet. So then, how does the average patient on COUMADIN® reconcile all of these inconsistent recommendations? The answer is simply that they often cannot. Thus, we hope to provide more practical guidelines to these patients, their loved ones, and their caregivers, if applicable.

If you have read this far, then you may be interested in this cookbook because you or a loved one has had a conversation like this with a physician or other health care professional:

DR: Hello Mr. or Ms. COUMADIN® Patient. Are you enjoying your supper? We have determined that you have blankety-blank (fill-in your particular diagnosis). This disorder requires that you begin COUMADIN® therapy.

Patient: Oh, can you tell me what that means?

DR: Yes, of course. First, you will take COUMADIN® so that your blood will not clot too much. It means you will have to have a lab test called a prothrombin time/INR on a regular basis. The prothrombin time/INR tells us how COUMADIN® is working and allows your health care professional to keep you within a desired therapeutic range. You may not be able to eat some of your favorite foods. In addition, you need to do this while staying on a heart healthy diet.

Patient: So, what exactly can I eat, since I am trying to stick to a heart healthy diet?

DR: Well, there are lots of things you can eat. However, there are also quite a few foods you really should try to stay away from.

Patient: Such as?

DR: Green leafy vegetables, such as spinach, lettuce and so forth. Also, you should avoid other green vegetables, like asparagus, peas, brussel sprouts, broccoli, seaweed, and so forth. There are other guidelines, outlined in that small pamphlet we gave you.

Patient: But aren't those foods good for me?

DR: Yes, of course they are!

Patient: I'm sorry doctor, but I'm a little confused about what I should eat. Can you help me with the foods I can and should eat?

Unfortunately, the answer to the patient's last question is not simple. However, one point is simple: If you are a patient on COUMADIN®, with or without atherosclerosis, (atherosclerosis = cholesterol plaques in arteries of the body), you may think your dietary choices are limited. You can try to eat the same, small amount of foods high in vitamin K each day, but this is extremely difficult. Or, you can try to eat foods that contain only a little vitamin K, but this is difficult, also. Thus, to help the patient on COUMADIN® consume a steady (or consistent) amount of vitamin K on a daily basis, every recipe and individual food item in this cookbook will have an accurate estimate of its vitamin K content. Because of small differences in the amount of vitamin K that are present even in the same quantity of any given food item, the best we can attain at this point is an accurate estimate of the amount of vitamin K in any recipe or food item. Nonetheless, we believe such an estimate is far superior to no estimate at all and, therefore, can only help in keeping the COUMADIN® effect steady.

Another important bit of knowledge the reader should have is the actual amount of vitamin K in a typical diet. The average amount of vitamin K a person in the U.S. consumes per day is approximately 60 to 80 micrograms (mcgs). One microgram (mcg) is one-millionth of a gram. Remember that twenty-nine (29) grams equal an ounce. Thus, you can see, we are talking about a tiny amount of vitamin K when we talk about the typical diet. Nonetheless, variations in small amounts of vitamin K can have a large effect on prothrombin time/INR in some patients.

As stated above, the patient on COUMADIN® is often instructed to limit the amount of vitamin K in his or her diet so as not to counteract the effect of the COUMADIN®. This advice has a few problems as regards the overall health of the patient. First, this leads to a decrease or entire lack in the consumption of many vegetables which provide many other essential nutrients and which are strongly recommended by most, if not all, heart healthy diets, including, for example, the DASH diet of the National Heart, Lung, and Blood Institute. Second, the importance and mechanism of action of vitamin K in tissues such as bone is not well known. The lack of vitamin K in these tissues could have unknown side effects for the individual on a low vitamin K diet. Third, the concept of a low vitamin K diet may not necessarily be the safest in terms of a relatively consistent "desired" or therapeutic effect of the COUMADIN® dose on a daily basis. More on this in the next paragraph.

We are ready to make firm recommendations regarding the daily intake of vitamin K in the diet of patients on COUMADIN®. As we have said, the patient on COUMADIN® is told to either take in a small amount of vitamin K daily, or to at least take in the same amount daily. But, if the patient tries to take in a small amount of vitamin K each day, then the patient can easily take in too much vitamin K by mistake. This would make the patient's blood more likely to develop unwanted clots, which could be dangerous. On the other hand, if the patient tries to take in the same amount of vitamin K each day, this is very difficult without accurate guidelines. This difficulty can cause the patient's blood to form unwanted clots or cause prolonged bleeding. It is important to understand that the typical patient on COUMADIN® does NOT need to STRICTLY limit his or her vitamin K intake, but rather to take in an amount consistent with the recommended daily allowance (RDA) in an ACCURATELY ESTIMATED manner. Therefore, we recommend that the patient on COUMADIN® uses the guidelines in this cookbook to try to take in approximately 100 micrograms of vitamin K each day. This may not be possible for every patient on COUMADIN®. Also, the intake of this amount of vitamin K daily may not be beneficial for every patient taking COUMADIN®. Each patient should, working with his or her doctor or other health care provider, find their own best daily vitamin K intake and use the guidelines in this book to keep their intake as steady as possible. Finally, since this approach must always be undertaken only with thorough understanding of the individual patient, we strongly recommend that the patient always consult his or her doctor prior to ANY change in his or her diet that may alter the COUMADIN® effect and laboratory test results.

By using the vitamin K content of the recipes and individual food items provided in this book, we hope that each reader can devise a diet on a daily basis that will provide a steady and consistent amount of vitamin K. This may be difficult, even if the vitamin K content of each individual recipe or food is known. Thus, we strongly encourage every reader to keep a diary. The diary should list the amount of vitamin K they have consumed that day. The diary must be carefully kept. For example, with each meal, the amount of vitamin K should be recorded in the diary, so that the patient on COUMADIN® can aim for a constant amount of vitamin K each day. Finally, the reader can continue to use some of his or her own heart healthy recipes, if all the ingredients contain very small amounts of vitamin K. We have provided a list of foods with very low vitamin K content that the patient can use in his or her own recipes. It should be noted, however, that not ALL foods have well-established levels of vitamin K.

USEFUL DIETARY TIPS FOR THE PATIENT ON COUMADIN®

In addition to the recipes provided in this cookbook, there are several important facts regarding the vitamin K content of foods that should be mentioned. By following the tips outlined in this section, the patient on COUMADIN® can improve the stability of the amount of vitamin K in their diet and, hopefully, the stability of the effect of COUMADIN®.

1. The vitamin K content of vegetables varies depending on the location where they are grown. Thus, the patient on COUMADIN® has to be careful when traveling since the vitamin K content of vegetables in one part of the country may be different from vegetables in another part of the country. Unfortunately, at this time, there is no easy solution to this problem. Currently, we recommend that the patients use the estimates provided in this cookbook.

2. The vitamin K content of recipes that contain fresh vegetables only apply when fresh vegetables are used. The effect of canning or drying on the vitamin K content of vegetables is unknown at this time. Thus, when using this cookbook, the patient must only use fresh veggies, unless stated otherwise.

3. Some multivitamins contain vitamin K. This does not mean you cannot take these vitamins, it just means that you have to take into account their vitamin K content in your daily diary when you take them.

4. Dried basil, thyme, and oregano contain a high amount of vitamin K. However, a teaspoon of fresh basil, thyme, or oregano would be expected to contain very small amounts of vitamin K. Notice that recipes in this book only use fresh basil, thyme and oregano and they are used only in small quantities.

5. Store-bought mayonnaise, and margarine are VERY BAD. The reason? They contain unknown quantities of various vegetable oils and therefore the amount of vitamin K in these foods is unpredictable. They should be avoided altogether. We have provided recipes for homemade mayonnaise that contain a known quantity of vitamin K. Only homemade mayonnaise should be used. Butter should be used instead of margarine. Butter contains almost no vitamin K. Some readers have worried about using butter instead of margarine for

heart-healthy reasons. Currently, it is not known for certain that margarine is more heart-healthy than butter. It is clear, however, that butter should be used only in moderation.

6. Store-bought salad dressings may contain unknown quantities of various vegetable oils. They may also contain unknown quantities of herbs that are high in vitamin K. Some store-bought salad dressings have a low amount of vitamin K and are safe to use. However, identifying the store-bought salad dressings that are low in vitamin K can be very difficult for the patient on COUMADIN®, Therefore we have provided several recipes for homemade salad dressings that contain a known quantity of vitamin K.

7. Watch out for foods that should be low in vitamin K, but are packed in vegetable oils. Certain types of vegetable oils can contain high amounts of vitamin K and when the quantity of oil and/or type of oil is unknown, this can lead to large variations in vitamin K in the diet. The best example of this is tuna fish. This is an excellent food choice for the patient on COUMADIN®, since it is both heart healthy and very low in vitamin K WHEN IT IS EATEN FRESH OR WHEN IT IS PACKED IN WATER. However, tuna is often packed in oil, and then the vitamin K content is much higher and UNKNOWN! Therefore, only consume tuna (and other canned items) that are packed in water, NOT OIL.

8. Factors other than vitamin K intake can affect COUMADIN®. Illness can affect your prothrombin time/INR. Also, MANY medications, both prescription and over-the-counter, can affect your prothrombin time/INR. Remember that the prothrombin time/INR is a laboratory test used to monitor the effects of COUMADIN®. Therefore, you should always tell your doctor when you are sick or when you are starting or stopping a new medicine or when the dose of one of your medicines is changed.

9. Vitamin K content of food is not altered by cooking or gamma irradiation.

10. Exposure of oils to sunlight or fluorescent light destroys approximately 85% of the vitamin K. Several recipes included in this cookbook use Canola oil or olive oil (we chose these oils because they are heart healthy). The vitamin K content of these oils can be quite high. Therefore, before using these oils, you must first expose them to sunlight or fluorescent light for at least 48 hours. This will destroy the majority of vitamin K in the oils and decrease the variability of vitamin K in the diet. When exposing the vegetable oils to sunlight, it is only

necessary to place the oil in a transparent container in the sun. The oil does not need to be open to the air. Interestingly, and distressingly, while researching this cookbook, we found wide variations in the amount of vitamin K levels reported to be present in various oils.

11. Beware of any food that contains vegetable oils in unknown quantities.

12. Fat in the diet is required for adequate vitamin K absorption. In fact, fat in the diet is required for the absorption of vitamins A, E and D as well. Thus, the use of VERY low fat diets is discouraged. Diets should contain approximately 25% fat.

13. The intake of large doses of vitamin E can affect the response of the body to vitamin K. Specifically, when taken in large doses, this vitamin may counteract the effect of vitamin K. Thus, intake of megadoses of vitamin E could further increase the patient's prothrombin time/INR and increase the effect of COUMADIN®. How vitamin E counteracts the effect of vitamin K is unknown. Thus, at this time, we can only recommend that a constant amount of this vitamin should be consumed on a daily basis. It would seem wise simply to take the RDA of this vitamin each day. However, the patient with coronary artery disease should consume 400 IU (international units) of vitamin E per day since this dose of vitamin E has been shown to have benefit in patients with coronary artery disease. There is no evidence that a constant intake of this amount of vitamin E per day would dangerously affect the prothrombin time/INR. However, we must again emphasize the importance of a constant amount of vitamin E.

14. NO GRAPEFRUIT or GRAPEFRUIT JUICE should be consumed by the patient on COUMADIN®!

Any drug taken by a patient is eventually removed by the body. The scientific name for this removal is metabolism. Grapefruit and grapefruit juice decrease the ability of the body to remove, or metabolize, COUMADIN®. This results in a higher level of COUMADIN in the patient's body. A higher level of COUMADIN in the body will lead to a greater anticoagulant effect.

COUMADIN® is not the only drug affected in this way by grapefruit and grapefruit juice. Many drugs are affected, including many of the medicines used to lower cholesterol and a few medicines used for high blood pressure. There are at least 75 different drugs whose metabolism is decreased by grapefruit and grapefruit juice.

15. BEWARE THE AVOCADO!! There are two reasons for this. First, the amount of vitamin K in avocado and avocado products such as guacamole can vary by as much as 40 times! Thus, the avocado represents a very unpredictable source of vitamin K. Second, there is some evidence that even small amounts of avocado can unpredictably alter the prothrombin time/INR.

16. Alcohol can alter the patient's response to COUMADIN® and thus increase or decrease the prothrombin time/INR. Alcohol should not be consumed by the patient on COUMADIN®. We have included some recipes for alcoholic beverages simply because we realize some patients will consume alcohol despite our recommendation to not consume alcohol.

17. The amount of vitamin K in leafy vegetables is highest in the outer, greener leaves when compared to the paler, inner leaves. The patient should take a balanced portion of the different leaves contained in the leafy vegetable. Also, the amount of vitamin K in iceberg lettuce is much lower than the amount of vitamin K in greener, more leafy types of lettuce.

How about eating SALADS? We suggest that the patient on COUMADIN® make salads out of iceberg lettuce only. Weigh the head of iceberg lettuce at the grocery store. At home, cut the lettuce into 8 to 10 equal portions (this is easy to do with a head of iceberg lettuce). Each portion of the head of lettuce will weigh about the same. Each ounce of iceberg lettuce contains about 9 micrograms of vitamin K. Simply multiply the number of ounces of lettuce you have in your salad by 9 (the number of micrograms of vitamin K per ounce of lettuce). The number you get is the number of micrograms of vitamin K in the portion of lettuce. For example, suppose your head of lettuce weighs 24 ounces. If you cut it into 8 equal portions, then each portion weighs 3 ounces. Each ounce contains 9 micrograms of vitamin K. Since 3 ounces times 9 micrograms per ounce equals 27 micrograms, there are 27 micrograms of vitamin K (approximately) in your portion of iceberg lettuce.

The effect of growing lettuce hydroponically is unknown and this type of lettuce should be avoided until more data is obtained in this regard. All data for lettuce available thus far is for lettuce grown the old-fashioned way.

18. Brewed black tea contains almost no vitamin K. Brewed green tea contains very little vitamin K. However, herbal teas should be avoided because they may contain herbs that may increase the effect of COUMADIN®.

19. A few words should be said about medicinal herbs. Garlic and ginger used in high doses as medicinals may increase the anticoagulant effect of COUMADIN®. However, garlic and ginger can be used in the amounts found in the recipes in this book. Gingko and Feverfew also increase the effect of COUMADIN®. Ginseng may decrease the effect of COUMADIN®.

20. Brussel sprouts should be avoided by patients taking COUMADIN. This is because brussel sprouts can lead to a lower level of COUMADIN in the body. This is the opposite effect that grapefruit and grapefruit juice have on COUMADIN,(see tip number 14 above).

LIST OF FOODS WITH VERY LOW VITAMIN K CONTENT

As stated previously, one of the purposes of this cookbook is to provide dietary guidelines so that the patient on COUMADIN® may consume approximately the same amount of vitamin K each day. To be successful, this cookbook must allow for a lot of different diets. Not everyone eats a big breakfast, for example. Towards this goal, this section contains a listing of foods with very little vitamin K content. With this list, patients on COUMADIN® can put into their diet any of the foods listed with little effect on their overall vitamin K intake. For example, if the patient prefers a small breakfast, he or she can enjoy a glass of cranberry juice, a cup of tea, and two pieces of toast without worrying about the vitamin K content. Similarly, of course, any other meal the patient wishes to make easily (from the standpoint of vitamin K calculation) could be made of a combination of the foods listed here. To take it one step further, this list also allows the easy addition of some food items to a meal that employs one or more of the recipes in the Recipe Section of the cookbook.

Please note that the criterion used to place a food on the following list was that it had to contain less than 2 micrograms (mcgs) of vitamin K per 100 grams (approximately 3 1/2 ounces) or milliliters.

- Apple juice
- Apple sauce
- Apple, skinless
- Bagel, plain
- Baking powder
- Banana
- Barley products (flour, bread)
- Beef
- Black olives
- Black pepper
- Bran flakes
- Bread (white, corn, or wheat)
- Cake (angel food)
- Chicken
- Coffee (caffeinated and decaffeinated)
- Cola
- Corn
- Corn flakes

- Corn oil
- Crackers (graham, wheat, or saltine, but watch out for additives, especially oils)
- Cranberry products (juice, sauce, etc.)
- Cream (Note: for every one per cent of fat in a milk product, there is only one-tenth of one microgram (mcg) of vitamin K per 100 grams or 100 milliliters)
- Cucumber, skinless
- Eel
- Egg white
- Egg yolk
- Eggplant
- Garlic and garlic powder
- Ginger ale
- Grapes, grape juice, grape jelly, etc.
- Honey
- Ice cream
- Jell-O
- Lemon juice, lemonade (the real stuff- not that artificial junk)
- Lemon peel
- Melon, cantaloupe
- Milk (see note above for "Cream")
- Millet
- Mushrooms
- Octopus
- Onions (but NOT spring onions)
- Oranges, orange juice
- Oysters
- Parsnips
- Peaches (canned)
- Peanuts (but NOT peanut butter)
- Pears (canned)
- Pineapple, pineapple juice
- Pork
- Pretzels
- Prunes, prune juice
- Radishes
- Raisins
- Rice, puffed rice, rice flour
- Sake
- Salmon
- Salt
- Sardine
- Shrimp
- Spaghetti

- Squid
- Sugar
- Tea, brewed (black and green, only)
- Tofu
- Turkey
- Turnips
- Vanilla
- Vinegar
- Wheat flour, wheat bread, puffed wheat, shredded wheat
- Wine
- Yellowtail (snapper)
- Yogurt, plain only

Some very common foods just missed making the list above. These include:
- Potato products which contain, when cooked, 10 micrograms of vitamin K per 100 grams,
- Tomato and tomato products (4 to 7 micrograms per 100 grams)
- Celery (12 micrograms per 100 grams)
- Cheddar cheese (3 micrograms per 100 grams)
- Oatmeal (3 micrograms per 100 grams)
- Peanut butter (10 micrograms per 100 grams)
- Squash (3 micrograms per 100 grams)

- *Remember to check the vitamin K content of the new ingredient when making substitutions in this book's recipes. If the food item is not listed in the vitamin "K" table (in the back of the book) you are using it at your own risk. We are constantly checking the USDA nutrition information to have the most up to date information on vitamin "K" for this book.*

USEFUL INFORMATION FOR THE COOK
by GAIL BEYNON

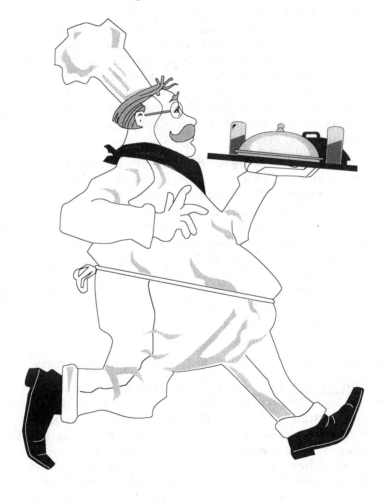

A few words from the cook

This book is not meant to be all things for all people. The recipes in the book are as wide a variety as possible to show the diversity in diet allowed while taking Coumadin®. If you are on a low fat diet some of these recipes will fit as they are, others will need adjustments and substitutions. If you are diabetic, use this book in conjunction with your diabetic rules and recipes. If you have high blood pressure, adjust the recipes accordingly. Substitute where necessary using the substitution list to help you.

Remember, when dealing with food and nutrition information there are many variables that determine the calories, fat content, carbohydrate content, etc. of each food item. The same food can have a different calorie count from state to state and brand to brand. The values on the Nutrition Facts Label are just an average. The exact numbers vary, depending on the season, weather and location. For instance avocados vary wildly from country to country, state to state and season to season. This is the reason we cannot include avocados in the Coumadin diet. You would have to do an analysis on every avocado to determine the amount of vitamin K and other nutritional values.

Considering the above facts, here comes the disclaimer.

Nutrition Analysis Disclaimer: The nutritional analysis of these recipes is calculated using the latest figures from the United States Department of Agriculture's nutrition data base and from Dr. Art Ulene's "The NutriBase Nutrition Facts Desk Reference." We cannot guarantee an exact nutrition duplication when you make the recipes because of the differences in food production around the world. It is important to note that all nutrient breakdowns for processed foods are subject to change by manufacturers without notice and may therefore vary.

ODDS AND ENDS

BREAD: When dealing with bread you need to make sure each slice you cut is approximately one ounce. (If you have a one pound loaf of bread and there are 16 slices then each slice is approximately one ounce.) When buying any uncut loaf of bread (Italian, French, etc.), note the weight of the loaf before cutting. That way you will be able to judge more accurately the weight of each slice and how much VITAMIN K you are getting.

CAULIFLOWER Adding a little milk to the water the Cauliflower is cooking in will help to keep it attractively white.

HIGH ALTITUDE BAKING (3500 to 6500 feet) takes longer than at lower altitudes. Increase your baking time by about 1/4 to 1/3.

ONIONS Do you have trouble digesting onions? Try using white onions rather than yellow onions. Some people are allergic to yellow onions but not white ones.

OVEN SPILLS If the juice from your fresh fruit pie runs over in the oven, shake some salt on the spill. This causes the juice to burn to a crisp for easy removal.

SLICING EGGS To keep egg yolks from crumbling, when slicing hard-cooked eggs, wet your knife between each cut.

TOO MUCH SALT? If your stew is over salted, try adding 1 teaspoon of vinegar and 1 teaspoon of sugar, and then reheat. Or add a few more potatoes.

WALNUT MEATS If you need to get walnut meats out whole, soak the nuts overnight in salt water before you crack them.

DON'T CHILL ALL YOUR PRODUCE! In our kitchens, the refrigerator is where we store most of our produce. But not every food item should be chilled. Anything that ripens <u>after</u> it's harvested should not be put into the refrigerator. This includes tomatoes, unripe pears and all melons except watermelon. Chilling at temperatures below 55 degrees Fahrenheit retards ripening. Some fruits and vegetables should not be chilled at all, while other types of produce can be refrigerated with a few easy precautions.

CITRUS FRUITS: For oranges, lemons and limes, refrigeration is a good way to preserve quality. Citrus fruits do not ripen further after harvest.

CUCUMBERS: While sensitive to cold, refrigerate cucumbers because they lose moisture rapidly even when they are lightly waxed. However, prolonged exposure to cold gives cucumbers pitted, mushy spots.

EGGPLANT: While sensitive to cold, refrigerate eggplant because they lose moisture rapidly. Store them in a paper bag in the refrigerator crisper drawer.

POTATOES AND SWEET POTATOES: When potatoes are refrigerated, their starch turns to sugar. While this condition can be reversed by removing the potatoes from the refrigerator, they will still retain some sugar, which causes them to brown when fried. Keep potatoes in a dark place slightly cooler than the normal temperature of the home, such as in a cool cupboard, in a basement storage area, or near the inside wall in a garage. In extremely cold conditions, covering the potatoes with a blanket or burlap will provide protection.

TOMATOES: Will lose their aroma and flavor after just 40 minutes in the refrigerator. Store tomatoes in a warm, dry area. You may store vine-ripened tomatoes this way for up to two weeks. Depending on how fast you want them to ripen, store tomatoes on a counter or on top of the refrigerator, out of sunlight. The warmer temperatures on top of a refrigerator will make a tomato ripen faster. You should store tomatoes so that none are touching, especially if the produce has cracks or lesions. The best place to store tomatoes is in an aerated basket that allows plenty of air flow.

TROPICAL FRUITS: Never refrigerate any tropical fruit (such as bananas, mangos, papayas and others.) Only chill bananas if you do not want them to ripen any further. The skins will turn nearly black but the inside flesh can still be a normal white. You can freeze bananas before cooking. Just thaw and use as if they were fresh in baked goods. Frozen bananas cannot be used in gelatin desserts, banana splits, trifles, banana cream pie, etc.

WINTER SQUASH OR MELONS: Refrigerate winter squash only after cooking, and refrigerate melons only after being cut open. These items maintain their best aroma and flavor at room temperature.

When storing produce, make liberal use of the crisper drawers. In most recently manufactured refrigerators, the crisper drawers can be adjusted for temperature and humidity. The crispers are usually marked 'fruits' or 'vegetables' or 'cool' and 'moist.' Store fruits and vegetables in paper or plastic bags with holes to slightly increase temperature and humidity.

Never store fruits and vegetables against the back wall of a refrigerator. The rear wall is the coldest area of any refrigerator and chilling injury or light freezing may occur.

If produce becomes frozen, handle the produce carefully. When a celery or cabbage freezes, the cells are very sensitive to touch. Damage and bruising will occur unless they are allowed to thaw slowly with very little handling.

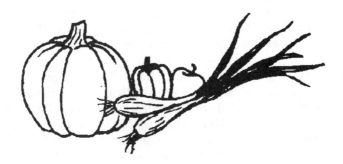

Meat Tips

Broiling

Score the edges of steaks, chops, and ham slices so they won't cup. Or, cook in a broiler basket to keep them flat.

Trim off the outer edge of fat from steaks, chops, and ham slices so drippings will not blaze up and become a problem.

When coals are completely hot, tap off the gray ash with fire tongs. Heat the grill top and grease it.

When small bubbles appear on the top surface of meat, it is ready to turn. Heat forces the juices to the uncooked surface. Flip steaks with tongs and turner, once, during cooking time.

Piercing with a fork wastes precious juices as does "mashing" the meat.

When you broil steaks or burgers in the oven, broil the second side a few minutes less than the first. The second side has a head start on heating. Turn meat only once.

For broiling steaks: Rub the steak well with oil before broiling. The heat will char the oil not the steak and seal in the juices.

Marinade: Marinate steak in 2 Tbsp wine vinegar, 2 Tbsp oil or melted butter, 1 clove crushed garlic and herbs of your choice for several hours, turning several times.

Broiling Basics: Place meat on the unheated rack of a broiler pan. For cuts less than 1 1/4 inches thick, broil 3 inches from the heat. For cuts 1 1/4 inches thick or thicker, broil 4 to 5 inches from the heat. Broil the meat for the time given below or until desired doneness, turning the meat over a little after half of the broiling time called for in the recipe.

Roasting

Place the meat, fat side up, on a rack in a shallow roasting pan. (Roasts with a bone do not need a rack.) For ham, if desired, score the top in a diamond pattern. Insert a meat thermometer. Do not add water or liquid, and do not cover. Follow the oven temperature and time directions in the individual recipe.

Pan-broiling And Pan-frying Basics

To pan-broil, preheat a heavy skillet over high heat until very hot. Do not add water or fat. (For beef steaks and veal, brush skillet lightly with cooking oil.) Add meat. Do not cover. Reduce heat to medium and cook for the time given or until done, turning meat over after half of the cooking time. If meat browns too quickly, reduce heat to medium low. Spoon off fat and juices as they accumulate during cooking.

To panfry, in a heavy skillet melt 1 to 2 tablespoons butter or margarine over medium-high heat. Add meat. Do not cover. Reduce heat to medium and cook for time given or until done, turning meat over after half of the cooking time.

Baking Temperature/Time Guide

Oven Temperatures

Slow	300 -- 325 F
Moderate	350 -- 375 F
Hot	400 -- 450 F
Very Hot	475 -- 500 F

Baking Times

Baked Items	Temperature	Time
Cakes		
Cupcakes	350 -- 375 F	20 -- 30 minutes
Foam or sponge type	350 -- 375 F	30 -- 60 minutes
Fruit Cakes	275 -- 300 F	2 hours or more
Jelly Roll	400 F	12 -- 15 minutes
Pound Cake	300 -- 325 F	1 -- 1 1/2 hours
Rectangular cakes	350 -- 375 F	35 -- 45 minutes
Round or square layers	350 -- 375 F	25 -- 40 minutes
Cookies		
Bar	350 -- 375 F	20 -- 35 minutes
Drop	350 -- 375 F	10 -- 15 minutes
Shaped or rolled	300 -- 425	5 -- 25 minutes
Pies		
Custard	400 -- 425 F	30 -- 45 minutes
Fruit	425 F	45 -- 60 minutes
Meringue	425 F	5 -- 8 minutes
Pie and Tart Shells	450 F	12 --15 minutes
Quick Breads		
Biscuits	450 F	10 -- 15 minutes
Coffee cakes, muffins	375 -- 425 F	5 -- 35 minutes
Fruit and nut loaves	350 F	55 --75 minutes
Yeast Breads		
Dinner rolls	375 -- 400 F	15 -- 20 minutes
Loaves	375 -- 400 F	45 -- 55 minutes
Sweet Rolls, coffee cakes	350 -- 400 F	20 -- 35 minutes

SUBSTITUTIONS

When you need an ingredient and you don't have it perhaps you can make a substitution

ALLSPICE - 1 teaspoon = 1/2 teaspoon cinnamon and 1/8 teaspoon ground cloves. (Unknown amount of vitamin K. Use sparingly.)

AMARETTO: - 3 ounces = 1 Tbsp light Karo plus 1 Tbsp almond extract plus 1/4 cup clear apple juice.

ARROWROOT - 2 teaspoon = 1 tablespoon cornstarch.

BAKING POWDER - 1 tsp. = 1/2 tsp. Cream of tartar plus 1/4 teaspoon baking soda. This will be a single-acting baking powder.

BRANDY: 1/4 cup apple juice plus 1 Tbsp brandy extract or flavoring.

BREAD CRUMBS - 1/4 cup dry bread crumbs = 1 slice bread, 1/2 cup soft bread crumbs = 1 slice.

BUTTER - 1 cup butter = 7/8 cup oil OR 1 cup mayonnaise.

BUTTERMILK - Add 1 tablespoon lemon juice or white vinegar to 1 cup of milk and let stand for about 10 minutes or use 1 cup plain lowfat yogurt. Some grocery, health food and specialty stores carry buttermilk powder. Use it as you would any other dried milk powder.

CATSUP - 1/2 cup = 1/2 cup tomato sauce, 2 tablespoons sugar, 1 tablespoon vinegar, 1/8 teaspoon ground cloves.

CHOCOLATE - For 1 ounce of unsweetened chocolate use 3 tablespoons cocoa plus 1 tablespoon unsalted butter or Canola oil, or 1-oz. Envelope pre-melted unsweetened chocolate product. For 1 2/3 ounces of sweetened chocolate use 1 ounce of unsweetened plus 4 teaspoon sugar.

COFFEE - 1/2 cup strong brewed coffee = 1 teaspoon instant coffee in 1/2 cup water.

CORNSTARCH - 1 tablespoon = 2 tablespoons of all-purpose flour

CRACKER CRUMBS - 3/4 cup = 1 cup bread crumbs.

CREAM, COFFEE - 1 cup coffee cream = 3 tablespoons butter, plus about 3/4 cup milk

CREAM, LIGHT - 1 cup light cream = 7/8 cup milk plus 1 tablespoon butter.

CREAM, HEAVY - 1 cup heavy cream = 1/3 cup butter, plus about 3/4 cup milk (it will not whip!) OR 2/3 cup well-chilled evaporated milk, whipped OR 1 cup nonfat dry milk powder whipped with 1 cup ice water.

CREAM, SOUR - 1 cup = 3 tablespoon butter plus 7/8 cup buttermilk or yogurt. For dips, 1 cup = 1 cup cottage cheese pureed with 1/4 cup yogurt or buttermilk, or 6 ounce cream cheese plus enough milk to make 1 cup.

EGG YOLKS (for thickening) - 2 egg yolks = 1 whole egg.

FLOUR, PASTRY - Use 2 parts bread flour to 3 parts cake flour OR 5 parts all-purpose flour to 1 part cake flour.

FLOUR, ALL PURPOSE - To substitute cake flour for all-purpose flour: add 2 additional tablespoons for every cup called for in the recipe.

FLOUR, CAKE - Use 3 parts all-purpose flour to 1 part cornstarch.

FLOUR, SELF-RISING - use 1 1/4 teaspoons baking powder plus a pinch of salt for every cup of all-purpose flour.

FLOUR, THICKENING - 1 tablespoon flour for thickening: use 1 tablespoon quick cooking tapioca OR 1 1/2 teaspoon cornstarch, potato starch or arrowroot.

GARLIC - 1 clove = 1/2 teaspoon powdered, OR 1 teaspoon garlic salt (reduce added salt by 1/2 teaspoon).

GELATIN - A 1/4 ounce envelope = a little less than one tablespoon.

GINGER - 1 tablespoon fresh = 1 teaspoon powdered or 1 tablespoon candied with sugar washed off.

HERBS - 1 tablespoon fresh = 1 teaspoon dried (Dried herbs are very high in VITAMIN K).

HONEY - For 1 cup: 1 cup molasses - or - use 1 1/4 cup sugar plus 1/3 cup liquid. For baking, also decrease the liquid in the recipe by 1/4 cup. If there is no liquid in the recipe, add an additional 1/4 cup flour. Unless sour cream or sour milk is used in the recipe, add a pinch of baking soda.

HOT PEPPER SAUCE - Few drops = dash of cayenne or red pepper.

LEMON JUICE - 1 teaspoon = 1/2 teaspoon vinegar. Juice of 1 lemon is about 2-3 tablespoons of lemon juice.

LIME JUICE - Use equivalent amount of lemon juice. Juice of 1 lime is about 2 tablespoons lime juice.

MILK, FRESH SWEET MILK: 1/2 cup evaporated milk plus 1/2 cup water OR 1/3 cup dried skim milk powder plus 1 cup water and 2 teaspoon melted butter or oil OR 1 cup skim milk plus 2 teaspoon melted butter or oil.

MILK, SOUR - 1 cup sour milk = 1 cup sweet milk plus 1 tablespoon vinegar or lemon juice

MILK, SKIM - 1/3 cup instant powdered milk plus 3/4 cup water. In baking: 1 cup whole milk = 1 cup fruit juice.

MILK, SWEETENED CONDENSED - 1 cup milk plus 2 tablespoons of nonfat powdered milk, 1/2 cup boiling water and 3/4 cup sugar. Beat for 10 minutes. Then chill. Use as a substitute for sweetened condensed milk.

MUSHROOMS - 6 ounces of canned drained mushrooms = 1/2 pound mushrooms.

MUSTARD - 1 tablespoon prepared = 1 teaspoon dry mustard plus 2 teaspoons vinegar.

OIL - In cakes you can usually replace 1/2 the oil with an equal amount of applesauce. Mayonnaise can be substituted for an equal amount of oil in most baked dishes.

OLIVE OIL - Use a good quality oil for the best flavor. If you do not use a lot of oil you should buy small quantities at a time. Oil will go rancid.

ONION - 1 small fresh chopped onion = 1 teaspoon onion powder, or 1 tablespoon dried minced or 1/4 cup frozen chopped onion.

ORANGE JUICE - Juice of 1 orange is about 1/3 to 1/2 cup orange juice.

RAISINS - 1/2 cup = 1/2 cup cut up pitted prunes or dates.

RUM: 1/4 cup apple juice plus 1 Tbsp rum extract.

SALT - When making a brine, do not use low sodium salt. Low sodium salt as a flavor enhancer is fine.

SOY SAUCE - 1/4 cup = 3 tablespoons of Worcestershire sauce plus 1 tablespoon water.

SUGAR, BROWN - Use 1 to 2 tablespoons molasses to 1 cup of granulated sugar OR substitute 1 cup granulated for 1 cup firmly packed brown sugar.

SUGAR, GRANULATED - To use honey, combine 3/4 cup honey, plus 1 tablespoon honey, plus a pinch of baking soda for every 1 cup of sugar. Reduce the liquid in the recipe by 3 tablespoons. Do not replace more than 1/3 of the sugar with honey. If using molasses, combine 1 cup molasses plus 1/2 teaspoon baking soda for every 1 cup sugar and reduce the liquid in the recipe by 4 teaspoons. Do not replace more than 1/2 of the sugar with the molasses. One cup sugar = 1 3/4 cups confectioner's sugar but do not substitute in baking.

SUGAR, TURBINADO - 1 cup = 1 cup granulated with a heavier molasses flavor.

TOMATO JUICE - Three cups = 1 1/2 cup tomato sauce plus 1 1/2 cup water OR one (6 ounce) can of tomato paste plus 3 cans of water and a dash of salt and pepper.

TOMATO PASTE - 1 tablespoon = 1 tablespoon catsup.

TOMATO PUREE - 1 cup puree = 1/2 cup paste plus 1/2 cup water.

TOMATO SAUCE - 1 cup tomato sauce = 1 can tomato paste plus 1 1/2 cans of water.

TOMATOES - 1 cup canned = 1 1/3 cup chopped fresh tomatoes simmered.

WINE FOR MARINADE - 1/2 cup wine = 1/4 cup vinegar plus 1 tablespoon sugar plus 1/4 cup water.

WINE, DRY RED: Use 1/2 cup (4 oz) carbonated cranberry drink plus 1 Tbsp lemon juice.

WINE, DRY WHITE: Welch's white grape juice plus 1 Tbsp white vinegar.

WINE, RED: (LAMBRUSCO OR SEMISWEET WINE): Carbonated cranberry drink.

SWEET WHITE WINE: Welch's white grape juice plus 1 Tbsp Karo corn syrup.

WORCESTERSHIRE SAUCE - 1 teaspoon Worcestershire sauce = 1 tablespoon soy sauce plus a dash of hot pepper sauce.

YEAST - 1 cake compressed yeast = 1 package dried, 1 package dried = 1 scant tablespoon.

YOGURT - 1 cup yogurt = 1 cup buttermilk.

ONE POUND (450 GRAMS) FOOD MEASURES

(16 ounces (dry) per pound, 4 ounces per 1/4 pound)

Brown sugar	2 1/4	cups
Butter	2	cups
Candied fruit	3	cups
Cheese, cheddar	4	cups grated
Cheese, cottage	2	cups
Chopped meats	2	cups
Coffee (ground)	5	cups or 80 tablespoons
Cornmeal	3	cups
Crumbs	4	cups
Diced potatoes	2	cups
Dried currants	2 2/3	cups
Dry beans	2 1/2	cups
Eggs, with shells	9-10	
Granulated sugar	2	cups
Liquid	2	cups
Long-grain rice	2 1/2	cups
Milk	2	cups
Oatmeal	2 2/3	cups
Pitted dates	2 1/2	cups
Powdered sugar	3 1/2	cups
Rye flour	3 3/4	cups
Seedless raisins	2 2/3	cups
Shelled almonds	2 1/2	cups
Shelled nuts (about)	4	cups
Shelled walnuts	3 2/3	cups
White flour	4	cups
Whole-wheat flour	3 3/4	cups
Whole potatoes	2	good-sized

ONE OUNCE (30 GRAMS) FOOD MEASURES

Bitter chocolate	1	square
Butter	2	tablespoons
Cocoa	1/3	cup
Dried hops	2 1/2	cups
Flour	4	tablespoons
Liquid	2	tablespoons
Salt	1	tablespoon
Soda	2	tablespoons
Sugar	2	tablespoons

MEASUREMENT ABBREVIATIONS

A short list of abbreviations used in this cookbook.

lb	=	pound
med	=	medium
oz	=	ounce
pkg	=	package
pn	=	pinch
tbsp	=	tablespoon
tsp	=	teaspoon

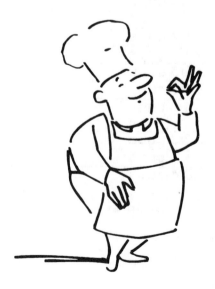

MEASUREMENT CHARTS

VOLUME MEASUREMENT EQUIVALENTS

Pinch or dash	= less than 1/8 teaspoon	
1 teaspoon	= 1/3 tablespoon	= 1/6 fluid ounce
1/2 tablespoon	= 1 1/2 teaspoons	= 1/4 fluid ounce
1/3 tablespoon	= 1 teaspoon	
3/4 tablespoon	= 2 1/4 teaspoons	
1 tablespoon	= 3 teaspoons	= 1/2 fluid ounce
2 tablespoons	= 1/8 cup	= 1 fluid ounce
4 tablespoons	= 1/4 cup	= 2 fluid ounces
8 tablespoons	= 1/2 cup	= 4 fluid ounces
12 tablespoons	= 3/4 cup	= 6 fluid ounces
16 tablespoons	= 1 cup	= 8 fluid ounces
1/8 cup	= 2 tablespoons	= 1 fluid ounce
1/4 cup	= 4 tablespoons	= 2 fluid ounces
1/3 cup	= 5 1/3 tablespoons	
1/2 cup	= 8 tablespoons	= 4 fluid ounces
3/4 cup	= 12 tablespoons	= 6 fluid ounces
1 cup	= 16 tablespoons	= 8 fluid ounces
2 cups	= 1 pint	= 16 fluid ounces
4 cups	= 2 pints	= 32 fluid ounces
8 cups	= 4 pints	= 64 fluid ounces
16 cups	= 8 pints	= 128 fluid ounces
1/2 pint	= 1 cup	= 8 fluid ounces
1 pint	= 2 cups	= 16 fluid ounces
2 pints	= 4 cups	= 32 fluid ounces
4 pints	= 8 cups	= 64 fluid ounces
8 pints	= 16 cups	= 128 fluid ounces
1/2 quart	= 2 cups	= 16 fluid ounces
1 quart	= 4 cups	= 32 fluid ounces
1 gallon	= 16 cups	= 128 fluid ounces

WEIGHT MEASUREMENT EQUIVALENTS

1 gram	= 0.035 ounce	
100 grams	= 3.527 ounces	
1 ounce		= 28.35 grams
1/4 pound	= 4 ounces	= 113.4 grams
1/3 pound	= 5 1/3 ounces	= 151.19 grams
1/2 pound	= 8 ounces	= 226.8 grams
2/3 pound	= 10 2/3 ounces	= 302.38 grams
3/4 pound	= 12 ounces	= 340.2 grams
1 pound	= 16 ounces	= 453.6 grams

Explanation of the Nutritional Analysis Tables
following each recipe:

Calories are calories
Fat is measured in grams
Cholesterol is measured in micrograms
Sodium is measured in micrograms
Protein is measured in grams
Carbohydrates are measured in grams
Fiber is measured in grams

APPETIZERS

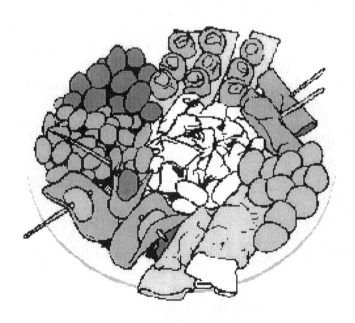

SHRIMP SPREAD
16 servings (less than 1 mcg of VITAMIN K per serving)

16	oz	Cream cheese, lowfat
1/2	lb	Shrimp
1	tbsp	Horseradish
1/4	tsp	Ground black pepper
1/4	cup	Lemon juice
1	tbsp	Green onions, chopped
1	tbsp	Worcestershire Sauce
1/8	tsp	Garlic powder

Bring the cream cheese to room temperature. (It needs to be soft.) Cook and chop the shrimp.

In a small mixing bowl, beat the cream cheese until fluffy. Gradually beat in lemon juice. Stir in remaining ingredients. Chill to blend flavors.

Garnish as desired. Serve with crackers or fresh vegetables.

Ingredient	Cal	Fat	Chol	Sod	Prot	Carb	Fiber
CREAM CHEESE	960	80	160	2560	48	32	0
SHRIMP	240	4	344	336	45.6	1.6	0
HORSERADISH	6	0.1	0	0	0.2	1.4	0.2
BLACK PEPPER	1	0	0	0	0.1	0.4	0.1
LEMON JUICE	12	0	0	0	2	4	0
GREEN ONIONS	4	0	0	2	0.5	1	0.5
WORCESTERSHIRE	10	0	0	200	0	2	0
GARLIC POWDER	1	0	0	0	0.1	0.3	0
Totals Per Serving:	**77**	**5.3**	**32**	**194**	**6**	**2.7**	**0**

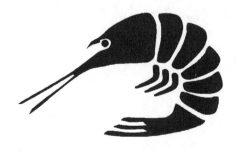

CHEDDAR-ALE CHEESE LOGS
16 servings (6 mcgs of VITAMIN K per serving)

1 1/2	lb	Cheddar cheese, shredded (about 6 cups)
4	oz	Cream cheese
4	tbsp	Butter
3/4	cup	Beer
1	tsp	Mustard, powdered
1/2	cup	Walnuts, chopped

Bring the cream cheese and butter to room temperature. Beat the cheddar, cream cheese and butter in a large bowl with an electric mixer until smooth. Gradually beat in the beer (or ale if you prefer) and mustard. If mixture is very soft, refrigerate until firm enough to hold shape.

Divide mixture in half and shape into two logs. Press a 3 inch round of wax paper onto the end of each log to keep the area free from walnuts. Put walnuts on a sheet of wax paper. Roll the cheese logs in the nuts to cover completely. Place on serving plates or boards, remove paper rounds. Decorate with pimiento.

To keep, cover with plastic wrap and refrigerate. Keeps well for several weeks. Do not roll in nuts or decorate until ready to use. Serve at room temperature.

Ingredient	Cal	Fat	Chol	Sod	Prot	Carb	Fiber
CHEDDAR	2640	216	720	4800	168	24	0
CREAM CHEESE	396	39.6	120	340	8	4	0
BUTTER	400	46	140	360	0	0	0
BEER	72	0	0	6	0.6	6	0
MUSTARD	19	0	0	0	0	0	0
WALNUTS	384	37.2	0	8	8.4	11.2	2.8
Totals Per Serving:	244	21.2	61	345	11.6	2.8	0.2

AMARETTO CHEESE SPREAD
24 servings (4 mcgs of VITAMIN K per serving)

16	oz	Cream cheese, lowfat
8	oz	Pineapple packed in juice, crushed, drained
1/2	cup	Bell pepper, chopped
3	tbsp	Green onions, chopped
3	tbsp	Amaretto liqueur
1	tsp	Seasoned salt (See Recipe Index)
4	oz	Almond slivers

Soften the cream cheese by letting it come to room temperature or use the microwave.

Lightly toast and chop the almonds.

Mix the first six ingredients and half of the almonds. Form the mixture into a ball. Roll in the remaining almonds.

Refrigerate several hours. Serve with crackers.

Ingredient	Cal	Fat	Chol	Sod	Prot	Carb	Fiber
CREAM CHEESE	960	80	160	2560	48	32	0
PINEAPPLE	144	0	0	16	0	36	1.6
BELL PEPPER	28	0	0	0	0.4	0.4	0.4
GREEN ONIONS	14	0	0	8	1.5	3	1.5
AMARETTO LIQUEUR	176	0.2	0	4	0	24	0
SEASONED SALT	4	0.1	0	1367	0.1	0.5	0
ALMOND SLIVERS	396	36.8	0	8	13.6	18	8
Totals Per Serving:	**72**	**4.9**	**7**	**204**	**2.8**	**4.7**	**0.5**

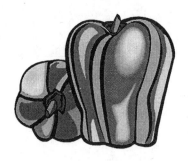

STUFFED MUSHROOMS
6 servings (3 mcgs of VITAMIN K per serving)

12	oz	White Mushrooms
1/4	lb	Butter
1	tbsp	Olive oil, treated (See Dietary Tip # 10)
1/4	tsp	Garlic powder
2	tbsp	White wine
1/4	tsp	Basil, fresh, minced
1/4	tsp	Oregano leaves, fresh, minced
1	cup	Bread crumbs, dry, plain
2	oz	Cheddar cheese (about 1/2 cup)

Wash the mushrooms and remove the stems. Put the caps on a baking sheet. Chop the stems and brown them in butter. Mix the stems and all the rest of the ingredients together. Stuff the caps.

Bake for 15 to 20 minutes until brown. (Shrimp added to this is good.)

Note: You can substitute Swiss cheese for the Cheddar cheese.

Ingredient	Cal	Fat	Chol	Sod	Prot	Carb	Fiber
WHITE MUSHROOMS	84	1.2	0	12	7.2	15.6	4.8
BUTTER	800	92	280	720	0	0	0
OIL	119	13.5	0	0	0	0	0
GARLIC POWDER	2	0	0	0	0.1	0.5	0
WHITE WINE	22	0	0	1	0	0.2	0
BASIL	0	0	0	0	0	0	0
OREGANO	0	0	0	0	0	0	0
BREAD CRUMBS	424	5.6	0	928	12	76.8	4
CHEDDAR	220	18	60	400	14	2	0
Totals Per Serving:	279	21.7	57	344	5.6	15.9	1.5

VERMONT CHEDDAR AND MAPLE CRACKERS
8 servings (4 mcgs of VITAMIN K per serving)

1/2	lb	Cheddar cheese, sharp, shredded (about 2 cups)
2/3	cup	Pecans, chopped
1/3	cup	BLENDER MAYONNAISE #2 (See Recipe Index)
1	tbsp	Maple syrup
1/2	tsp	Worcestershire Sauce
36	each	Whole-grain crackers

Mix the cheese, pecans, mayonnaise, maple syrup and Worcestershire Sauce together in a medium-sized bowl. Spread the mixture by rounded teaspoonfuls evenly on the crackers.

Place the crackers on a flat pan or cookie sheet and run it under the broiler until the cheese is melted and bubbling.

Transfer the crackers to a plate and serve at once. Makes 3 dozen puffs.

Ingredient	Cal	Fat	Chol	Sod	Prot	Carb	Fiber
CHEDDAR	880	72	240	1600	56	8	0
PECANS	528	53.3	0	0	6.4	14.9	5.3
MAYONNAISE	408	44.8	56	200	1.6	0.8	0
MAPLE SYRUP	37	0	0	2	0	9.5	0
WORCESTERSHIRE	2	0	0	33	0	0.3	0
CRACKERS	540	28.8	0	864	10.8	72	7.2
Totals Per Serving:	**299**	**24.9**	**37**	**337**	**9.4**	**13.2**	**1.6**

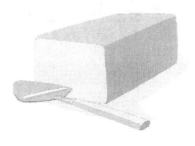

MIXED ANTIPASTO PLATTER
8 servings (11 mcgs of VITAMIN K per serving)

2	each	Cloves of garlic
1	lb	Bread, Italian, slice 1/2-inch thick, about 24 slices
8	oz	Ham or Prosciutto, sliced thin and cut in half
12	oz	Cheese, Provolone, sliced and cut in half
8	oz	Genoa salami, thinly sliced
1/2	lb	Mushrooms, marinated
1/2	lb	Artichoke, hearts, marinated
8	oz	Olives, pickled, Italian black olives, pitted
1/2	cup	Olive oil, extra-virgin, treated (See Dietary Tip # 10)
2	tbsp	Lemon Juice (1/2 lemon)
1	tsp	Oregano leaves, fresh, minced

Cut each clove of garlic in half and rub the cut sides over both sides of the bread. Arrange the bread in single layer on a serving platter.

Top each bread slice with the ham or prosciutto, cheese, salami, mushrooms, artichoke hearts and olives. Drizzle with oil. Squeeze lemon juice over top and sprinkle with oregano.

Ingredient	Cal	Fat	Chol	Sod	Prot	Carb	Fiber
GARLIC	4	0	0	2	0	0	0
BREAD	1232	16	0	2656	32	224	16
HAM	368	19.2	120	2896	41.6	5.6	0
PROVOLONE	1200	91.2	300	3000	84	12	0
GENOA SALAMI	880	80	72	3648	48	0	0
MUSHROOMS	80	0	0	360	6.4	16	0
ARTICHOKE HEARTS	104	0	0	216	8	24	16
OLIVES, BLACK	264	24	0	1976	1.6	16	8
OIL	960	108.8	0	0	0	0	0
LEMON JUICE	22	0.3	0	2	1.2	8.7	0
OREGANO	1	0	0	1	0	0	0
Totals Per Serving:	639	42.3	62	1845	27.9	38.3	5

CRACKERS DEL PASEO
10 servings (8 mcgs of VITAMIN K per serving)

1	cup	BLENDER MAYONNAISE #2 (See Recipe Index)
3	oz	Cheddar cheese, grated (about 3/4 cup)
1/2	tsp	Mustard, powdered
1/2	tsp	Caraway seeds
6	oz	Onion, thinly sliced (about 1 medium onion)
50	each	Butter crackers
1/2	cup	BLENDER MAYONNAISE #2 (See Recipe Index) for crackers

Mix the mayonnaise, cheese, mustard and caraway seeds.

Spread butter crackers with a thin layer of mayonnaise and top with a slice of onion. Add a teaspoonful of the mixture on top of the onion. Place under the broiler until hot. Serve immediately.

Ingredient	Cal	Fat	Chol	Sod	Prot	Carb	Fiber
MAYONNAISE	1224	134.4	168	600	4.8	2.4	0
CHEDDAR	330	27	90	600	21	3	0
MUSTARD	10	0	0	0	0	0	0
CARAWAY SEEDS	4	0.2	0	0	0.2	0.6	0.2
ONION	66	0	0	6	1.8	14.4	30
CRACKERS	900	50	0	1500	12.5	112.5	12.5
MAYONNAISE	612	67.2	84	300	2.4	1.2	0
Totals Per Serving:	315	27.9	34	301	4.5	13.7	4.5

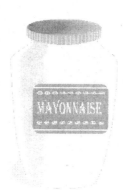

GARLICKY CLAM DIP
8 servings (Less than 1 mcg of VITAMIN K per serving)

8	oz	Cream cheese*
3	tsp	Garlic cloves
1/8	tsp	Black pepper, fresh ground
7	oz	Clams, drained and minced
1/4	cup	Clam broth (or juice)
1 1/2	tsp	Worcestershire Sauce
2	tsp	Lemon juice

*Or substitute lowfat or nonfat cream cheese.

Using a garlic press, squeeze the garlic pulp and juice into the softened cheese. Cream with a spoon until smooth.

Gradually add the remaining ingredients, blending until smooth. For thinner dip, add more clam broth.

Serve with crackers, chips or veggies.

Ingredient	Cal	Fat	Chol	Sod	Prot	Carb	Fiber
CREAM CHEESE	792	79.2	240	680	16	8	0
GARLIC	21	1.3	0	16	0.4	4	2.3
BLACK PEPPER	1	0	0	0	0	0.2	0
CLAMS	140	2.1	70	224	49	9.8	0
CLAM BROTH	2	0	2	122	0	0	0
WORCESTERSHIRE	5	0	0	100	0	1	0
LEMON JUICE	2	0	0	0	0.3	0.7	0
Totals Per Serving:	119	10.2	39	142	8.2	2.8	0.3

CRAB DIP
8 servings (12 mcgs of VITAMIN K per serving)

1	lb	Crab meat
1/2	cup	BLENDER MAYONNAISE #2 (See Recipe Index)
1/4	tsp	Garlic powder
2	tbsp	Onion, grated
2	tsp	Mustard (Dijon is best.)
2	tsp	Sugar, confectioners,
2/3	cup	White wine

Mix together all ingredients except the crab meat. Heat slowly on stove top or in Microwave oven.. Add the crab meat. Serve it warm with crackers.

Ingredient	Cal	Fat	Chol	Sod	Prot	Carb	Fiber
CRAB MEAT	400	4.8	352	1328	81.6	1.6	0
MAYONNAISE	612	67.2	84	300	2.4	1.2	0
GARLIC POWDER	2	0	0	0	0.1	0.5	0
ONION	11	0	0	1	0.3	2.4	0.5
MUSTARD	12	0.4	0	142	0.6	1	0
SUGAR	32	0	0	0	0	8.3	0
WHITE WINE	117	0	0	5	0	1.1	0
Totals Per Serving:	146	9.1	55	219	10.6	1.6	0.1

TANGY BLUE CHEESE DIP
8 servings (1.5 mcgs of VITAMIN K per serving)

2	oz	Blue cheese, crumbled
1 1/2	cups	Sour cream, lowfat
1	tsp	Garlic, peeled and minced
2	tbsp	Chives, fresh, finely chopped
1/8	tsp	Hot sauce

Blend the blue cheese and sour cream thoroughly. Add all the other ingredients, blending well. Cover and chill. Makes about 2 cups of dip.

SUGGESTED DIPPERS: Carrots, Cherry Tomatoes, Pineapple, Asian Pear, Cocktail Black Bread, Italian Or French Bread Chunks. (Remember to add the nutrition information of the dippers to the total nutrition count.)

Ingredient	Cal	Fat	Chol	Sod	Prot	Carb	Fiber
BLUE CHEESE	268	24.6	58	572	7.4	0.2	0
SOUR CREAM	480	24	60	420	24	48	0
GARLIC	4	0	0	2	0.2	1	0
CHIVES	9	0	0	1	1	1	1
HOT SAUCE	0	0	0	14	0	0	0
Totals Per Serving:	**95**	**6.1**	**15**	**126**	**4.1**	**6.3**	**0.1**

ARTICHOKE DIP

8 servings (less than 10 mcgs of VITAMIN K per serving)

4	oz	Parmesan cheese, grated (about 1 cup)
1	cup	BLENDER MAYONNAISE #2 (See Recipe Index)
6	oz	Artichoke hearts, cooked and chopped*
1/4	tsp	Garlic powder (or more)

*May use canned or frozen artichoke hearts.

Combine the Parmesan cheese and mayonnaise. Add garlic powder. Add the artichoke hearts and combine.

May be served cold or heated for 10 to 20 minutes in a 350 degree Fahrenheit oven until cheese melts. (Do not heat in microwave.) Serve with chips or as a spread on French bread.

Ingredient	Cal	Fat	Chol	Sod	Prot	Carb	Fiber
PARMESAN CHEESE	444	30	96	1816	40.4	3.6	0
MAYONNAISE	1224	134.4	168	600	4.8	2.4	0
ARTICHOKE HEARTS	78	0	0	162	6	18	12
GARLIC POWDER)	2	0	0	0	0.1	0.4	0
Totals Per Serving	**219**	**20.6**	**33**	**322**	**6.4**	**3**	**1.5**

DRIED TOMATO SMOKY SPREAD
12 servings (5 mcgs of VITAMIN K per serving)

16	oz	Cream cheese, lowfat
1	tsp	Liquid Smoke
1	oz	Sun-dried tomatoes, no oil
		Orange food coloring (optional)

Bring the cream cheese to room temperature. Mix all the ingredients in a food processor. Refrigerate for an hour.

Serve with crackers.

Ingredient	Cal	Fat	Chol	Sod	Prot	Carb	Fiber
CREAM CHEESE	960	80	160	2560	48	32	0
LIQUID SMOKE	0	0	0	0	0	0	0
SD TOMATOES	73	1	0	594	4	16	3
FOOD COLORING	0	0	0	0	0	0	0
Totals Per Serving:	86	6.8	13	263	4.3	4	0.3

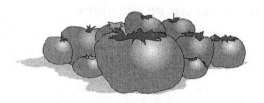

GOLDEN CITRUS-RAISIN DIP
12 servings (less than 3 mcgs of VITAMIN K per serving)

4	oz	Orange, peeled, seeded and quartered*
1	cup	Pecans, chopped
2	cups	Raisins, packed, golden
1/2	cup	BLENDER MAYONNAISE #2 (See Recipe Index)
8	oz	Yogurt, plain, nonfat

*About one medium orange.

Combine all the ingredients in a food processor or blender and process to a chunky consistency. Cover and chill. Makes about 4 1/2 cups of dip.

SUGGESTED DIPPERS: Ladyfingers, Plum Wafers, Pineapple, Ham, Chicken Drumettes, Celery.

You will need to add the nutrition counts of the dippers to the per serving totals.

Ingredient	Cal	Fat	Chol	Sod	Prot	Carb	Fiber
ORANGE, PEELED	248	0.8	0	0	4.8	61.6	12.4
PECANS	792	80	0	0	9.6	22.4	8
RAISINS	1008	1.6	0	64	8	264	22.4
MAYONNAISE	612	67.2	84	300	2.4	1.2	0
YOGURT, PLAIN	120	0	0	200	12	0	0
Totals Per Serving:	**232**	**12.5**	**7**	**47**	**3.1**	**29.1**	**3.6**

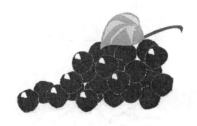

CAESAR MAYO DIP
12 servings (7.5 mcgs of VITAMIN K per serving)

2	each	Anchovy fillets
1 1/2	cups	BLENDER MAYONNAISE #2 (See Recipe Index)
1	tsp	Dijon mustard
1/2	oz	Parmesan cheese, grated (about 2 tablespoons)
1	tsp	Worcestershire Sauce
1	tbsp	Lemon juice
1/4	tsp	Ground black pepper

Chop and mash the anchovy fillets on a cutting board. Put in a bowl and blend in the mayonnaise. Add the remaining ingredients and blend well. Cover and chill. Makes about 1 3/4 cups of dip

SUGGESTED DIPPERS: Broccoli, Cauliflower, Carrot sticks, Green Bell pepper, Shrimp, Deli Roast Beef, Turkey or Radishes. You will need to add the nutrition counts of the dippers to the nutrition totals.

Ingredient	Cal	Fat	Chol	Sod	Prot	Carb	Fiber
ANCHOVY FILLETS	16	0.8	0	294	2.4	0	0
MAYONNAISE	1836	201.6	252	900	7.2	3.6	0
DIJON MUSTARD	5	0	0	120	0	0.2	0
PARMESAN CHEESE	56	3.8	12	227	5.1	0.5	0
WORCESTERSHIRE	3	0	0	67	0	0.7	0
LEMON JUICE	3	0	0	0	0.5	1	0
BLACK PEPPER	1	0	0	0	0.1	0.4	0.1
Totals Per Serving:	**160**	**17.2**	**22**	**134**	**1.3**	**0.5**	**0**

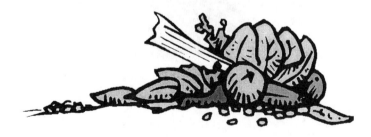

TIPSY TUNA DIP
12 servings (8 mcgs of VITAMIN K per serving)

1 1/2	tbsp	Brandy
8	oz	Cream cheese, lowfat, softened
1/4	cup	Sour cream, lowfat
1/4	cup	BLENDER MAYONNAISE #2 (See Recipe Index)
6	oz	Tuna, fresh, cooked, flaked*
2	tbsp	Onion, minced
1	tbsp	Lemon juice
1/8	tsp	Hot sauce

*Or you can substitute a 6 1/2,ounce can of tuna in water, well drained. This will add about 80 grams of sodium per serving.

Beat the brandy and cream cheese to a smooth and creamy consistency. Blend in the sour cream and mayonnaise. Mix in the tuna and onion, blending well. Add the remaining ingredients and blend until almost smooth. May be served at room temperature or chilled. Makes about 2 1/2 cups of dip.

SUGGESTED DIPPERS: French Bread Cubes, Cheese Crackers, Bread Sticks, Carrots & Radishes.

You will need to add the nutrition counts of the dippers to the per serving totals.

Ingredient	Cal	Fat	Chol	Sod	Prot	Carb	Fiber
BRANDY	49	0	0	0	0	0	0
CREAM CHEESE	480	40	80	1280	24	16	0
SOUR CREAM	80	4	10	70	4	8	0
MAYONNAISE	306	33.6	42	150	1.2	0.6	0
TUNA, FRESH,	174	0	78	60	36	0	0
ONION, MINCED	8	0	0	0	0.2	1.7	0.3
LEMON JUICE	3	0	0	0	0.5	1	0
HOT SAUCE	0	0	0	14	0	0	0
Totals Per Serving:	**92**	**6.5**	**18**	**131**	**5.5**	**2.3**	**0**

CAPONATA (EGGPLANT APPETIZER)
12 servings (less than 8 mcgs of VITAMIN K per serving)

1/4	cup	Olive oil, treated (See Dietary Tip # 10)
8	oz	Eggplant, peeled, cut in 1 inch cubes
1 1/2	cups	Celery, cut in 1/2-inch slices
1/2	cup	Olives, pitted black olives, chopped
6	oz	Onion, minced (about 1 cup)
1	tsp	Garlic, peeled and crushed
1/4	tsp	Dill weed, fresh
3/4	cup	Tomato puree
1/2	cup	Water
1/4	cup	Vinegar
1	tbsp	Sugar

Heat the oil in a large skillet and fry the eggplant cubes until lightly browned. Add the celery, olives, onion and garlic. Cook until vegetables are crisp tender.

Combine the tomato puree, water, vinegar and sugar. Pour over the vegetables in the skillet, stir lightly, add the dill and simmer for 1 minute. Remove from the heat. Cool and place in a covered container in the refrigerator until thoroughly chilled. Serve. Makes 3 to 4 cups.

Ingredient	Cal	Fat	Chol	Sod	Prot	Carb	Fiber
OIL	480	54.4	0	0	0	0	0
EGGPLANT	56	0	0	8	0.8	2.4	3.2
CELERY	24	0	0	156	1.2	7.2	1.2
OLIVES	132	12	0	988	0.8	8	4
ONION	66	0	0	6	1.8	14.4	30
GARLIC	4	0	0	2	0.2	1	0
DILL WEED, FRESH	0	0	0	0	0	0	0
TOMATO PUREE	66	0	0	60	0	18	6
VINEGAR	8	0	0	12	0	0	0
SUGAR	48	0	0	0	0	12.5	0
Totals Per Serving:	74	5.5	0	154	0.4	5.3	3.7

CRAB-MELT CANAPÉS

8 servings (3 mcgs of VITAMIN K per serving)

8	oz	Crab meat (about 1 cup)
1/4	lb	Cheese, Jarlsberg or Swiss cheese, shredded
1/4	cup	BLENDER MAYONNAISE #2 (See Recipe Index)
1/4	tsp	Mustard, powdered
30	each	Melba toast rounds
1/2	cup	Olives, sliced pitted black olives
3/4	tsp	Black pepper, coarsely ground

About 30 minutes before serving or early in the day, chop the crab meat. In a small bowl, with a fork, mix crab meat, cheese, mayonnaise, dry mustard, and 1/4 teaspoon coarsely ground black pepper.

Spread 1 heaping teaspoon of the crab meat mixture on each melba toast round. Place on cookie sheets, sprinkle with 1/2 teaspoon coarsely ground black pepper. If not serving right away, cover and refrigerate.

About 15 minutes before serving: preheat broiler. Broil canapés about 3 minutes or until cheese melts.

Top each canapé with a slice of ripe olive. Arrange canapés and garnish on platter. Serve immediately. Makes 2 1/2 dozen canapés.

Ingredient	Cal	Fat	Chol	Sod	Prot	Carb	Fiber
CRAB MEAT	200	2.4	176	664	40.8	0.8	0
CHEESE	400	28	64	520	28	4	0
MAYONNAISE	306	33.6	42	150	1.2	0.6	0
MUSTARD	5	0	0	0	0	0	0
MELBA TOAST	480	12	0	900	30	90	6
OLIVES	132	12	0	988	0.8	8	4
BLACK PEPPER	4	0.1	0	1	0.2	1.1	0.2
Totals Per Serving:	**191**	**11**	**35**	**403**	**12.6**	**13.1**	**1.3**

SALMON AND GOUDA PATE
15 servings (10 mcgs of VITAMIN K per serving)

7	oz	Cheese, Gouda, smoked, shredded
3	oz	Cream cheese, lowfat, cubed
3	tbsp	Milk, skim
1/4	cup	Butter
1/3	cup	BLENDER MAYONNAISE #2 (See Recipe Index)
1/4	cup	Green onion, finely chopped
2	tbsp	Lemon juice
1/8	tsp	Garlic powder
1/8	tsp	Hot sauce
1	lb	Salmon, cooked, skin and bones removed*
1/2	cup	Almond slivers, toasted
		Lemon slices
		Breads and crackers

*Or 14 ounce canned salmon, skin and bones removed.

Mix the gouda, cream cheese and milk. Set aside. Beat butter until fluffy. Beat in mayonnaise, green onion, lemon juice, garlic powder and hot pepper sauce. Add salmon, beat until combined. Line the bottom and sides of an 8 x 4 x 2 inch loaf pan with plastic wrap.

Sprinkle almonds in bottom of pan. Carefully spoon in half of the salmon mixture and spread evenly. Spread the cheese mixture on top of the salmon layer. Spread with the remaining salmon mixture. Cover and chill for 6 to 24 hours. Turn out onto a serving plate and carefully peel off the plastic wrap. Garnish with lemon slices. Serve with crackers and/or bread.

You will need to add the nutrition counts of the bread or crackers to the per serving totals.

Ingredient	Cal	Fat	Chol	Sod	Prot	Carb	Fiber
MILK, SKIM	16	0.2	2	24	1.5	2.3	0
BUTTER	400	46	140	360	0	0	0
MAYONNAISE #2	408	44.8	56	200	1.6	0.8	0
GREEN ONION	18	0	0	10	2	2	1
LEMON JUICE	6	0	0	0	1	2	0
GARLIC POWDER	1	0	0	0	0.1	0.3	0
HOT SAUCE	0	0	0	14	0	0	0
SALMON	656	27.2	176	208	121.6	0	0
ALMOND SLIVERS	396	36.8	0	8	13.6	18	8
CREAM CHEESE	180	15	30	480	9	6	0
CHEESE, GOUDA	700	56	0	1470	49	7	0
LEMON SLICES	0	0	0	0	0	0	0
Totals Per Serving:	**185**	**15.1**	**27**	**185**	**13.3**	**2.6**	**0.6**

If canned Salmon is used the per serving totals are as follows:

	Cal	Fat	Chol	Sod	Prot	Carb	Fiber
SALMON, CANNED	544	32	240	2064	80	3.2	0
Totals Per Serving:	**178**	**15.4**	**31**	**309**	**10.5**	**2.8**	**0.6**

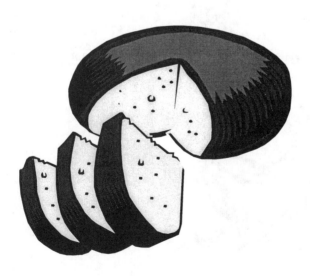

DEVILED EGGS
12 servings (Less than 1 mcg of VITAMIN K per serving)

6	each	Eggs, warm hard-cooked eggs
4	oz	Yogurt, plain, lowfat
1/2	tsp	Worcestershire Sauce
1/4	tsp	Mustard, powdered
1	tsp	Lemon juice
1/4	tsp	Salt
1/2	tsp	Paprika

Slice eggs in half lengthwise, remove the yolks and mash them. Add all remaining ingredients except the paprika. Mix until smooth. Fill egg whites with mixture, chill.

Dust with paprika and serve.

Ingredient	Cal	Fat	Chol	Sod	Prot	Carb	Fiber
EGGS	450	33.6	1278	378	37.8	3.6	0
YOGURT	64	2	8	100	8	8	0
WORCESTERSHIRE	2	0	0	33	0	0.3	0
MUSTARD	5	0	0	0	0	0	0
LEMON JUICE	1	0	0	0	0.2	0.3	0
SALT	0	0	0	575	0	0	0
PAPRIKA	3	0.2	0	1	0.2	0.6	0.2
Totals Per Serving:	44	3	107	91	3.8	1.1	0

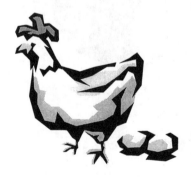

CANTALOUPE FRUIT SALAD
8 servings (less than 9 mcgs of VITAMIN K per serving)

2	med	Cantaloupes, peeled and seeded
2	cups	Pineapple chunks, fresh
1	cup	Raisins, packed
1	cup	Walnuts, chopped
1	med	Apple, peeled, cored and cut in small chunks
16	oz	Yogurt, vanilla lowfat

Cut the cantaloupes into small chunks and mix with all the other fruits and the walnuts in a large salad bowl.

Scoop yogurt into individual serving bowls. Pass the fruit salad so each can add the salad to the yogurt. Stir to coat and eat.

Ingredient	Cal	Fat	Chol	Sod	Prot	Carb	Fiber
CANTALOUPES	372	0.2	0	6	0.4	4.8	0.6
PINEAPPLE	224	1.6	0	0	1.6	56	4.8
RAISINS	504	0.8	0	32	4	132	11.2
WALNUTS	768	74.4	0	16	16.8	22.4	5.6
APPLE	73	0.4	0	1	0.3	19	1.1
YOGURT	256	0	16	352	32	32	0
Totals Per Serving	275	9.7	2	51	6.9	33.3	2.9

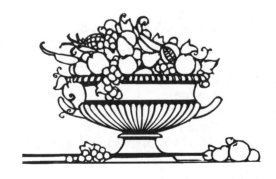

BLACK CHERRY YOGURT CREAM DIP
6 servings (1 mcg of VITAMIN K per serving)

8	oz	Yogurt, black cherry, lowfat
3	oz	Cream cheese, softened*
1	tbsp	Sugar, confectioners
1/4	tsp	Vanilla extract

*Or substitute nonfat.

In a blender, combine all the ingredients. Process 1-2 minutes or until smooth. Pour into a small serving bowl, refrigerate 2 hours or until slightly thickened.

Serve with fresh fruit dippers. (Change the dip flavor by changing the type of fruit yogurt.)

Ingredient	Cal	Fat	Chol	Sod	Prot	Carb	Fiber
YOGURT	40	0.8	0	0	0.8	8.8	4.8
CREAM CHEESE	297	29.7	90	255	6	3	0
SUGAR	29	0	0	0	0	7.5	0
VANILLA EXTRACT	3	0	0	0	0	0.1	0
Totals Per Serving:	62	5.1	15	43	1.1	3.2	0.8

SALMON MOUSSE
12 servings (2 mcgs of VITAMIN K per serving)

1	pack	Gelatin, unflavored
1/4	cup	Dry white wine*
1/2	cup	Boiling water
1/4	cup	Sour cream, lowfat
1/4	cup	BLENDER MAYONNAISE #2 (See Recipe Index)
1	tbsp	Lemon juice
1/8	tsp	Hot sauce
1	tbsp	Onion, minced
1/4	tsp	Paprika
5	oz	Salmon, canned (skin and bones removed, flaked)
1	cup	Heavy cream

*Water may be used instead.

In a large heat proof bowl, soften gelatin in cold wine or water. Slowly stir in boiling water until gelatin dissolves. Let cool to room temperature. Whisk in mayonnaise, sour cream, lemon juice, onion, paprika, and hot sauce until well blended. Refrigerate until mixture begins to thicken, about 20 minutes.

Mix in salmon.

In another large bowl, whip cream until soft peaks form. Fold whipped cream into salmon mixture, one-third at a time, until well blended. Pour mixture into an oiled 5 or 6 cup mold. Cover and refrigerate until firm, at least 4 hours or as long as 2 days. Unmold onto a serving plate and serve chilled.

COMMENTS: Serve this mild mousse with dark pumpernickel bread and peeled cucumber slices.

You will need to add the nutrition counts of the bread and cucumber to the per serving totals.

Ingredient	Cal	Fat	Chol	Sod	Prot	Carb	Fiber
GELATIN	25	0	0	10	0.5	5	0
DRY WHITE WINE*	44	0	0	2	0	1.4	0
BOILING WATER	0	0	0	0	0	0	0
SOUR CREAM	80	4	10	70	4	8	0
MAYONNAISE #2	306	33.6	42	150	1.2	0.6	0
LEMON JUICE	3	0	0	0	0.5	1	0
HOT SAUCE0	0	0	14	0	0	0	0
ONION	4	0	0	0	0.1	0.9	0.2
PAPRIKA	2	0.1	0	0	0.1	0.3	0.1
SALMON, CANNED	170	10	75	645	25	1	0
HEAVY CREAM	824	88	328	88	4.8	6.4	0
Totals Per Serving:	**122**	**11.3**	**38**	**82**	**3**	**2**	**0**

CARAMELIZED CARNITAS
10 servings (Less than 1 mcg of VITAMIN K per serving)

1 1/2	lb	Pork shoulder, lean boneless
2	tbsp	Brown sugar, packed
1	tbsp	Tequila
1	tbsp	Molasses
1/4	tsp	Ground black pepper
2	tsp	Garlic cloves, finely chopped
1/3	cup	Water
1	each	Green onion with top, sliced for garnish

Cut the pork into 1-inch cubes. Place the pork cubes in a single layer in a 10-inch skillet. Top with remaining ingredients except the green onion. Heat to boiling. Reduce heat. Simmer uncovered, stirring occasionally, until the water has evaporated and the pork is slightly caramelized, about 35 minutes.

Sprinkle with green onion and serve with wooden picks.

Ingredient	Cal	Fat	Chol	Sod	Prot	Carb	Fiber
PORK SHOULDER	960	48	432	552	144	0	0
SUGAR, BROWN	103	0	0	0	0	26.7	0
TEQUILA	35	0	0	0	0	0	0
MOLASSES, LIGHT	52	0	0	3	0	13.4	0
BLACK PEPPER	1	0	0	0	0.1	0.4	0.1
GARLIC CLOVE	8	0	0	4	0.3	2	0
GREEN ONION	9	0	0	5	1	1	0.5
Totals Per Serving:	**117**	**4.8**	**43**	**56**	**14.5**	**4.3**	**0.1**

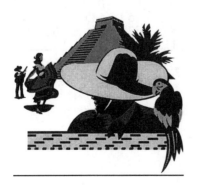

GRILLED BRUSCHETTA WITH FRESH MOZZARELLA AND TOMATOES
12 servings (5 mcgs of VITAMIN K per serving)

1	lb	Bread, Italian (cut 12 slices about 1 1/2 inch wide
1/2	cup	Olive oil, treated (See Dietary Tip # 10)
8	oz	Tomato, finely diced (about 1 cup)
2	tsp	Garlic cloves, crushed
12	slices	Cheese, mozzarella, nonfat (1 ounce per slice)
12	each	Basil, whole fresh leaves

Rub the bread slices with garlic and drizzle the olive oil over them. (An easier way, if you have a blender, is to puree the oil and garlic in the blender and then drizzle over the bread slices.)

Grill slices over an open flame, or under the broiler, turning once until crisp. Top with mozzarella and place in 375 degree Fahrenheit oven until cheese just begins to melt.

Remove to serving plates. Garnish with the diced tomato and basil leaves (one basil leaf per bruschetta).

Ingredient	Cal	Fat	Chol	Sod	Prot	Carb	Fiber
BREAD	1232	16	0	2656	32	224	16
OIL	952	108	0	0	0	0	0
TOMATO	40	0.8	0	16	1.6	8	2.4
GARLIC	8	0	0	4	0.3	2	0
MOZZARELLA	480	0	60	2400	108	12	0
BASIL	12	0	0	0	1.2	2.4	1.2
Totals Per Serving:	227	10.4	5	423	11.9	20.7	1.6

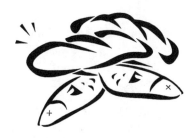

EGGPLANT CAVIAR
10 servings (6 mcgs of VITAMIN K per serving)

3	cups	Eggplant, peeled, raw (in 1/2 inch cubes)
1/3	cup	Bell pepper, chopped
3/4	cup	Onion, minced
1	tbsp	Garlic, peeled and minced
1/3	cup	Oil, olive or Canola, treated (See Dietary Tip # 10)
6	oz	Tomato paste
4	oz	Mushrooms, chopped
1/2	cup	Olives, pimiento stuffed olives
1/4	cup	Water
2	tbsp	Vinegar, red wine vinegar
1 1/2	tsp	Sugar
1	tsp	Seasoned salt (See Recipe Index)
1/2	tsp	Oregano leaves, fresh, minced
1/4	tsp	Ground black pepper

Put the eggplant, green pepper, onion, garlic and oil in skillet. Cover and cook gently for about 10 minutes, stirring occasionally. Add tomato paste, mushrooms and remaining ingredients. Cover and simmer 45 minutes to an hour to get a thick consistency. Turn into covered dish and refrigerate overnight to blend flavors.

Serve with crackers and chips. Makes about 1 quart and freezes well. To make this lower in fat, reduce the oil to 1 tablespoon. I have also left out the onion and it tastes great that way too.

Ingredient	Cal	Fat	Chol	Sod	Prot	Carb	Fiber
EGGPLANT	168	0	0	24	2.4	7.2	9.6
BELL PEPPER	19	0	0	0	0.3	0.3	0.3
ONION, MINCED	48	0	0	0	1.2	10.2	1.8
GARLIC	12	0.1	0	6	0.5	3	0
OIL	640	72.5	0	0	0	0	0
TOMATO PASTE	138	0	0	150	6	30	6
MUSHROOMS	28	0.4	0	4	2.4	5.2	1.6
OLIVES	132	12	0	988	0.8	8	4
VINEGAR	22	0	0	1	0	0.1	0
SUGAR	24	0	0	0	0	6.3	0
SEASONED SALT	0	0	0	2300	0	0	0
OREGANO	1	0	0	0	0	0	0
BLACK PEPPER	1	0	0	0	0.1	0.4	0.1
Totals Per Serving:	**123**	**8.4**	**0**	**467**	**1.6**	**7.1**	**2.3**

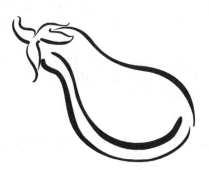

CROSTINI A LA PORCINI
8 servings (2 mcgs of VITAMIN K per serving)

1	oz	Mushrooms, dried Porcini mushrooms
3	tbsp	Olive oil, treated (See Dietary Tip # 10)
1	tbsp	Butter
1/2	lb	Mushrooms, fresh shiitake or chanterelle mushrooms, sliced (or white button, or a mixture)
1	tsp	Garlic, peeled and minced
1/4	cup	Heavy cream
3/4	oz	Parmesan cheese, fresh grated or Asiago cheese (about 3 tablespoons)
8	oz	Italian bread, 8 large or 16 small slices, lightly toasted

Soak the porcini in 1 cup of very hot water for 20 minutes. Drain and dice, removing any hard stem pieces. (Strain and save the liquid to use in soup.)

Heat the oil and butter in a large skillet until the butter foams. Add all the mushrooms and cook until lightly golden. Add garlic and cook and stir for one minute. Add cream and cook until slightly thickened, about 5 minutes. Season with a couple grinds of black pepper. Cool slightly (can be made ahead) and mound on toast.

Sprinkle with the Parmesan cheese and run under a preheated broiler until cheese is melted and all is bubbly and beginning to brown. Serve immediately.

Ingredient	Cal	Fat	Chol	Sod	Prot	Carb	Fiber
MUSHROOMS	7	0.1	0	1	0.6	1.3	0.4
GARLIC	4	0	0	2	0.2	1	0
OIL	357	40.5	0	0	0	0	0
BUTTER	100	11.5	35	90	0	0	0
MUSHROOMS	56	0.8	0	8	4.8	10.4	3.2
HEAVY CREAM	206	22	82	22	1.2	1.6	0
PARMESAN CHEESE	83	5.6	18	340	7.6	0.7	0
BREAD	616	8	0	1328	16	112	8
Totals Per Serving:	179	11.1	17	224	3.8	15.9	1.5

BREADS, SANDWICHES & SPREADS

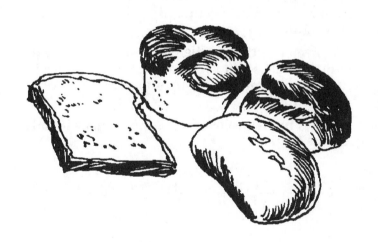

CHEDDAR BISCUITS
8 servings (VITAMIN K content = 6 mcg per serving)

2	cups	All purpose flour
1	tsp	Mustard, powdered
1	tsp	Paprika
1/4	tsp	Baking powder
1	cup	Butter, room temperature
10	oz	Cheddar cheese, sharp, grated (about 2 1/2 cups)
1	tsp	Worcestershire Sauce

Combine the flour, powdered mustard, paprika and baking powder in a medium bowl.

Beat the butter (either by hand or with an electric mixer at medium speed) until light and fluffy. Slowly beat in the cheddar cheese and Worcestershire Sauce. Gradually add the flour mixture, stirring with a fork, until well blended.

On a lightly floured surface, shape the dough into a long roll about 1 3/4- inches in diameter. Wrap in plastic wrap or foil. Place on a platter and refrigerate for at least 2 hours, or even better, overnight.

Preheat the oven to 325 degrees Fahrenheit. Slice the dough about 1/3 inch thick. With your hands, roll each slice into a ball. Flatten slightly and place on an ungreased baking sheet about 2 inches apart.

Bake 8 minutes in the preheated oven. Biscuits will only brown slightly on the bottom.

Ingredient	Cal	Fat	Chol	Sod	Prot	Carb	Fiber
FLOUR	800	3.2	0	0	22.4	176	0
MUSTARD	19	0	0	0	0	0	0
PAPRIKA	6	0.3	0	1	0.3	1.2	0.4
BAKING POWDER	1	0	0	51	0	0.1	0
BUTTER	1600	184	560	1440	0	0	0
CHEDDAR	1100	90	300	2000	70	10	0
WORCESTERSHIRE	3	0	0	67	0	0.7	0
Totals Per Serving:	441	34.7	108	445	11.6	23.5	0.1

GARDEN PIZZA
8 Servings (25 mcgs of VITAMIN K per serving)

1/2	each	PIZZA DOUGH (See Recipe Index)
1/2	lb	Mushrooms, sliced (about 2 cups)
1 1/2	cups	Carrot, peeled and shredded
1	cup	Zucchini, peeled and finely sliced
1/2	tsp	Garlic, peeled and minced
1/2	cup	Onion, chopped
1	tbsp	Olive oil, treated (See Dietary Tip # 10)
8	oz	Tomato sauce
1/2	tsp	Fennel seeds
1	tsp	Basil, fresh, minced
1	tsp	Oregano leaves, fresh, minced
1	tsp	Brown sugar
4	oz	Cheese, Mozzarella cheese (about 1 cup)
2	oz	Parmesan cheese, grated (about 1/2 cup)

Make and bake a 12 inch pizza crust according to the directions in the PIZZA DOUGH recipe.

Sauté mushrooms, carrots, zucchini, garlic and onion in oil over medium heat for 3 minutes.

When crust is prebaked, sprinkle with vegetables, tomato sauce, seasonings, sugar and cheeses.

Bake for 20 minutes. Remove from oven and cool for 3 minutes before serving.

Ingredient	Cal	Fat	Chol	Sod	Prot	Carb	Fiber
PIZZA DOUGH	820	22.8	0	920	19.5	140.7	0
MUSHROOMS	56	0.8	0	8	4.8	10.4	3.2
CARROT	72	1.2	0	60	1.2	18	1.2
ZUCCHINI	40	0	0	8	1.6	8	0.8
GARLIC	4	0	0	1	0.1	0.5	0
ONION	32	0	0	0	0.8	6.8	1.2
OIL	120	13.6	0	0	0	0	0
TOMATO SAUCE	88	0	0	1320	4	17.6	0
FENNEL SEEDS	4	0.2	0	1	0.2	0.6	0.2
BASIL	0	0	0	0	0	0	0
OREGANO	1	0	0	1	0	0	0
BROWN SUGAR	16	0	0	0	0	4.5	0
MOZZARELLA	360	28	100	720	24	4	0
PARMESAN	222	15	48	908	20.2	1.8	0
Totals Per Serving:	229	10.2	19	493	9.5	26.6	0.8

PIZZA DOUGH
8 servings (VITAMIN K content = 1 mcg per serving)

1	tbsp	Yeast, fresh or dry (1 scant tablespoon or 1 envelope)
1/4	cup	Warm water
1	tsp	Salt
1	tbsp	Honey
3	tbsp	Olive oil, treated (See Dietary Tip # 10)
3/4	cup	Cool water
3	cups	All purpose flour
1	tbsp	Olive oil, treated (See Dietary Tip # 10)

Dissolve yeast in the 1/4 cup warm water and let proof for 10 minutes. (It should get bubbly.)

Meanwhile, combine the salt, honey, olive oil and cool water in a small bowl and mix well.

Place the flour in a large bowl and make a well in the center. Pour the honey-water mixture and proofed yeast into the well.

Slowly incorporate the flour into the wet ingredients. When the dough ball forms, transfer it to a lightly floured surface and knead until smooth. (You can knead this in a mixer equipped with a dough hook.)

Use the 1 tablespoon of oil to oil a large bowl. Place the dough in the oiled bowl and let it rest, covered, for 30 minutes.

Divide the dough into 2 equal parts (or leave as one to make one very large pizza). Each part will make a 12 inch pizza crust.

Form each part into smooth, tight balls. Place on a flat dish, cover with a damp towel and refrigerate at least 2 hours. (If you only want to make one 12 inch crust at this time, wrap one of the balls of dough and put it in the freezer. When you are ready to use it, defrost to room temperature and proceed as follows.)

One hour before baking, remove the dough from the refrigerator.

Oil your pan (pizza pan or cookie sheet) well, flatten the dough and spread it in the pan making the outer edge thicker for the rim. At this point you can let the dough rise again for half an hour if you like a lighter dough. (Although you do not need to.)

Bake the dough at 350 degrees Fahrenheit for 10 to 12 minutes. Remove from oven. At this point you have a prebaked pizza dough crust to use for any type pizza. You can wrap and freeze for later use or use immediately.

Cover with sauce and your favorite toppings. Bake at 500 degrees Fahrenheit for 10 to 12 minutes.

If you have a baking stone, let the stone heat in a 500 degree Fahrenheit oven for at least 30 minutes to an hour before putting in the pizza.

(Do not forget to add the vitamin K content of the foods you use to top the pizza.)

Ingredient	Cal	Fat	Chol	Sod	Prot	Carb	Fiber
YEAST, ACTIVE DRY	42	0.5	0	7	5.5	5.5	3
HONEY	44	0	0	0	0.1	11.8	0
OIL	357	40.5	0	0	0	0	0
FLOUR	1200	4.8	0	0	33.6	264	0
SALT	0	0	0	2300	0	0	0
Totals Per Serving:	205	5.7	0	288	4.9	35.2	0.4

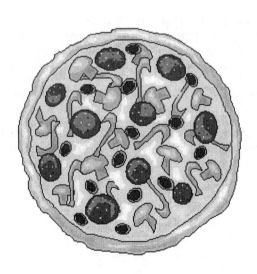

CHEDDAR FANS
12 fans (2 mcgs of VITAMIN K per serving)

5	oz	Cheddar cheese, sharp, grated (about 1 1/4 cups)
2	cups	All purpose flour, sifted
1	tbsp	Baking powder
1/2	tsp	Salt
1/2	cup	Butter
1/2	cup	Milk, skim
1/2	cup	Butter, softened
1/4	cup	Butter, melted

Grease the bottoms of a 12 cup muffin pan. Grate the cheese into a bowl, if not already grated, and set aside.

Sift the flour, baking powder and salt into a bowl. Cut in the butter with a pastry blender or two knives, until the mixture resembles coarse cornmeal.

Make a well in the center of the mixture and add the milk all at once. Stir with a fork until the dough forms a ball. Gently form the dough into a ball and put on a lightly floured surface. Knead it lightly with the fingertips 10 or 15 times.

Roll the dough into a 12 by 10-inch rectangle about 1/4-inch thick. Cut into 5 strips and spread with the softened butter. Sprinkle four strips with the grated cheddar cheese and stack the four on top of one another and top with the fifth strip.

Cut into 12 equal pieces and place on end in the muffin cups. Brush the tops of the rolls with the melted butter.

Bake at 450 degrees Fahrenheit for 10 to 15 minutes or until the biscuits are golden brown. Serve them hot with butter.

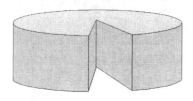

Ingredient	Cal	Fat	Chol	Sod	Prot	Carb	Fiber
CHEDDAR	550	45	150	1000	35	5	0
FLOUR	800	3.2	0	0	22.4	176	0
BAKING POWDER	6	0	0	612	0	1.4	0
SALT	0	0	0	1150	0	0	0
BUTTER	800	92	280	720	0	0	0
MILK, SKIM	44	0.4	4	64	4	6	0
BUTTER, SOFTENED	800	92	280	720	0	0	0
BUTTER, MELTED	400	46	140	360	0	0	0
Totals Per Serving:	**283**	**23.2**	**71**	**386**	**5.1**	**15.7**	**0**

QUICK AND EASY ROLLS
12 servings (1 mcg of VITAMIN K per serving)

2	cups	Self rising flour
1/4	cup	Buttermilk
6	tbsp	BLENDER MAYONNAISE #2 (See Recipe Index)
1	tbsp	Canola oil, treated (See Dietary Tip # 10)

Combine first 3 ingredients, stirring until moistened.

Spoon batter into oiled, (use the Canola oil) 12 cup muffin pan.

Bake at 375 degrees Fahrenheit for 12-15 minutes or until lightly browned.

Ingredient	Cal	Fat	Chol	Sod	Prot	Carb	Fiber
SELF RISING FLOUR	800	0	0	3040	20	164.8	0
BUTTERMILK	22	0.4	2	60	1.8	2.8	0
MAYONNAISE	459	50.4	63	225	1.8	0.9	0
OIL	120	13.6	0	0	0	0	0
Totals Per Serving:	**117**	**5.4**	**5**	**277**	**2**	**14**	**0**

MUFFINS, BASIC
12 servings (2 mcgs of VITAMIN K per serving)

2	cups	All purpose flour
1	tbsp	Baking powder
2	tbsp	Sugar, granulated
1	tsp	Salt
1	large	Egg
1	cup	Milk, skim
1/2	cup	Canola oil, treated (See Dietary Tip # 10)

Grease a 12 cup muffin pan. Heat the oven to 400 degrees Fahrenheit.

Sift the flour, baking powder, sugar and salt into a medium-sized bowl. Stir to mix well.

In a small bowl, beat the egg with a fork. Add the milk and oil. Add this all at once to the dry ingredients.

Stir the mixture until the dry ingredients are moistened. Batter will be lumpy. Drop the batter from a tablespoon into prepared muffin pans. Fill each cup half to two-thirds full.

Bake 15 to 20 minutes, or until golden brown. Remove from pan and serve hot.

Ingredient	Cal	Fat	Chol	Sod	Prot	Carb	Fiber
FLOUR	800	3.2	0	0	22.4	176	0
BAKING POWDER	6	0	0	612	0	1.4	0
SUGAR	97	0	0	0	0	25	0
SALT	0	0	0	2300	0	0	0
EGG	75	5	213	63	6.3	0.6	0
MILK, SKIM	88	0.8	8	128	8	12	0
OIL	964	112	0	0	0	0	0
Totals Per Serving:	**169**	**10.1**	**18**	**259**	**3.1**	**17.9**	**0**

GINGER MUFFINS:
12 servings (2 mcgs of VITAMIN K per muffin)

2	cups	All purpose flour
1	tbsp	Baking powder
2	tbsp	Sugar, granulated
1	tsp	Salt
1/2	cup	Ginger, candied, finely diced
1	large	Egg
1	cup	Milk, skim
1/2	cup	Canola oil, treated (See Dietary Tip # 10)

Grease a 12 cup muffin pan. Heat the oven to 400 degrees Fahrenheit.

Sift the flour, baking powder, sugar and salt into a medium-sized bowl. Stir to mix well. Stir in the candied ginger.

In a small bowl, beat the egg with a fork. Add the milk and oil. Add mixture all at once to the dry ingredients.

Stir the mixture only until the dry ingredients are moistened. Batter will be lumpy.

Drop the batter from a tablespoon into the prepared muffin pan, filling each cup half to two-thirds full.

Bake 15 to 20 minutes, or until golden brown. Remove from pan and serve hot.

Ingredient	Cal	Fat	Chol	Sod	Prot	Carb	Fiber
FLOUR	800	3.2	0	0	22.4	176	0
BAKING POWDER	6	0	0	612	0	1.4	0
SUGAR	97	0	0	0	0	25	0
SALT	0	0	0	2300	0	0	0
GINGER, CANDIED	384	0	0	68	0.4	98.8	0.8
EGG	75	5	213	63	6.3	0.6	0
MILK, SKIM	88	0.8	8	128	8	12	0
OIL	964	112	0	0	0	0	0
Totals Per Serving:	201	10.1	18	264	3.1	26.1	0.1

BANANA PECAN MUFFINS:
12 servings (VITAMIN K per muffin = 4 mcg)

2	tbsp	Canola oil, treated (See Dietary Tip # 10)
2	cups	All purpose flour
1	tbsp	Baking powder
2	tbsp	Sugar, granulated
1/4	tsp	Ground Nutmeg
1	tsp	Salt
1/2	cup	Pecans, chopped
1	large	Egg
1/2	cup	Milk, skim
1/2	cup	Canola oil, treated (See Dietary Tip # 10)
1	cup	Banana, peeled and mashed to make 1 cup

Grease a 12 cup muffin pan with the two tablespoons of Canola Oil.. Heat the oven to 400 degrees Fahrenheit.

Sift the flour, baking powder, sugar, nutmeg and salt into a medium-sized bowl. Stir to mix well. Add the chopped pecans.

In a small bowl, beat the egg with a fork. Add the milk, oil and banana. Mix well. Add mixture all at once to the dry ingredients. Stir the mixture only until the dry ingredients are moistened. Batter will be lumpy.

Drop the batter from a tablespoon into the prepared muffin pans, filling each cup half to two-thirds full.

Bake 15 to 20 minutes, or until golden brown. Remove from pan and serve hot.

Ingredient	Cal	Fat	Chol	Sod	Prot	Carb	Fiber
CANOLA OIL,	241	28	0	0	0	0	0
FLOUR	800	3.2	0	0	22.4	176	0
BAKING POWDER	6	0	0	612	0	1.4	0
SUGAR	97	0	0	0	0	25	0
GROUND NUTMEG	3	0.2	0	0	0	0.3	0.1
SALT	0	0	0	2300	0	0	0
PECANS	396	40	0	0	4.8	11.2	4
EGG	75	5	213	63	6.3	0.6	0
MILK, SKIM	44	0.4	4	64	4	6	0
CANOLA OIL,	964	112	0	0	0	0	0
BANANA	208	0.8	0	8	2.4	52.8	4
Totals Per Serving:	**236**	**15.8**	**18**	**254**	**3.3**	**22.8**	**0.7**

BLUEBERRY MUFFINS:
12 servings (VITAMIN K per muffin = 3 to 4 mcg)

2	cups	All purpose flour
1	tbsp	Baking powder
2	tbsp	Sugar, granulated
1	tsp	Salt
1	cup	Blueberries, washed and well drained
1	large	Egg
1	cup	Milk, skim
1/2	cup	Canola oil, treated (See Dietary Tip # 10)

Grease a 12 cup muffin pan. Heat the oven to 400 degrees Fahrenheit.

Sift the flour, baking powder, sugar and salt into a medium-sized bowl. Stir to mix well. Stir in the well-drained blueberries. (Fresh or frozen.)

In a small bowl, beat the egg with a fork. Add the milk and oil. Add the mixture all at once to the dry ingredients. Stir the mixture only until the dry ingredients are moistened. Batter will be lumpy.

Drop the batter from a tablespoon into the prepared muffin pan, filling each cup half to two-thirds full.

Bake 15 to 20 minutes, or until golden brown. Remove from the pan and serve hot.

Ingredient	Cal	Fat	Chol	Sod	Prot	Carb	Fiber
FLOUR	800	3.2	0	0	22.4	176	0
BAKING POWDER	6	0	0	612	0	1.4	0
SUGAR	97	0	0	0	0	25	0
SALT	0	0	0	2300	0	0	0
BLUEBERRIES	80	0.8	0	8	.8	20	3.2
EGG	75	5	213	63	6.3	0.6	0
MILK, SKIM	88	0.8	8	128	8	12	0
OIL	964	112	0	0	0	0	0
Totals Per Serving:	**176**	**10.2**	**18**	**259**	**3.1**	**19.6**	**0.3**

ORANGE MUFFINS:
12 servings (VITAMIN K per muffin = 2 mcg)

2	cups	All purpose flour
1	tbsp	Baking powder
2	tbsp	Sugar, granulated
1	tsp	Salt
2	each	Navel oranges, peeled
1	large	Egg
1	cup	Milk, skim
1/2	cup	Canola oil, treated (See Dietary Tip # 10)

Grease a 12 cup muffin pan. Heat the oven to 400 degrees Fahrenheit.

Sift the flour, baking powder, sugar and salt into a medium-sized bowl. Stir to mix well.

In a small bowl, beat the egg with a fork. Add the milk and oil. Add the mixture all at once to the dry ingredients. Stir the mixture only until the dry ingredients are moistened. Batter will be lumpy.

Drop the batter from a tablespoon into the prepared muffin pans, filling each cup half to two-thirds full.

When the batter is in the cup, place an orange section on top of each and sprinkle lightly with granulated sugar.

Bake 15 to 20 minutes, or until golden brown. Remove from the pan and serve hot.

Ingredient	Cal	Fat	Chol	Sod	Prot	Carb	Fiber
FLOUR	800	3.2	0	0	22.4	176	0
BAKING POWDER	6	0	0	612	0	1.4	0
SUGAR	97	0	0	0	0	25	0
SALT	0	0	0	2300	0	0	0
NAVEL ORANGES	124	0.4	0	0	2.4	30.8	6.2
EGG	75	5	213	63	6.3	0.6	0
MILK, SKIM	88	0.8	8	128	8	12	0
OIL	964	112	0	0	0	0	0
Totals Per Serving:	**180**	**10.1**	**18**	**259**	**3.3**	**20.5**	**0.5**

CHEESE MUFFINS:
12 servings (VITAMIN K per muffin = 3 mcg)

2	cups	All purpose flour
1	tbsp	Baking powder
2	tbsp	Sugar, granulated
1	tsp	Salt
1	large	Egg
1	cup	Milk, skim
1/2	cup	Canola oil, treated (See Dietary Tip # 10)
2	oz	Cheddar cheese, grated

Grease a 12 cup muffin pan. Heat the oven to 400 degrees Fahrenheit.

Sift the flour, baking powder, sugar and salt into a medium-sized bowl. Stir to mix well.

In a small bowl, beat the egg with a fork. Add the milk and oil. Add the mixture all at once to the dry ingredients. Fold 1/2 cup grated cheese into the muffin mix with the last few strokes. Stir mixture only until the dry ingredients are moistened. Batter will be lumpy.

Drop the batter from a tablespoon into the prepared muffin pans, filling each cup half to two-thirds full.

Bake 15 to 20 minutes, or until golden brown. Remove from pan and serve hot with scrambled eggs for a special breakfast.

Ingredient	Cal	Fat	Chol	Sod	Prot	Carb	Fiber
FLOUR	800	3.2	0	0	22.4	176	0
BAKING POWDER	6	0	0	612	0	1.4	0
SUGAR	97	0	0	0	0	25	0
SALT	0	0	0	2300	0	0	0
EGG	75	5	213	63	6.3	0.6	0
MILK, SKIM	88	0.8	8	128	8	12	0
OIL	964	112	0	0	0	0	0
CHEDDAR	220	18	60	400	14	2	0
Totals Per Serving	**188**	**11.6**	**23**	**292**	**4.2**	**18.1**	**0**

SURPRISE MUFFINS:
12 servings (VITAMIN K per muffin = 2 mcg)

2	cups	All purpose flour
1	tbsp	Baking powder
2	tbsp	Sugar, granulated
1	tsp	Salt
1	large	Egg
1	cup	Milk, skim
1/2	cup	Canola oil, treated (See Dietary Tip # 10)
6	tsp	Jelly, use your favorite

Grease a 12 cup muffin pan. Heat the oven to 400 degrees Fahrenheit.

Sift the flour, baking powder, sugar and salt into a medium-sized bowl. Stir to mix well.

In a small bowl, beat the egg with a fork. Add the milk and oil. Add the mixture all at once to the dry ingredients. Stir the mixture only until dry ingredients are moistened. Batter will be lumpy.

Fill the muffin cups 1/3 full of batter. Drop 1/2 teaspoon of your favorite jelly in the center of the batter. Add more batter to fill each cup 2/3 full.

Bake 15 to 20 minutes, or until golden brown. Remove from pan and serve hot. Kids just love these, as will you.

Ingredient	Cal	Fat	Chol	Sod	Prot	Carb	Fiber
FLOUR	800	3.2	0	0	22.4	176	0
BAKING POWDER	6	0	0	612	0	1.4	0
SUGAR	97	0	0	0	0	25	0
SALT	0	0	0	2300	0	0	0
EGG	75	5	213	63	6.3	0.6	0
MILK, SKIM	88	0.8	8	128	8	12	0
OIL	964	112	0	0	0	0	0
JELLY	77	0	0	10	0.1	20.1	0.3
Totals Per Serving:	176	10.1	18	259	3.1	19.6	0

BUTTERMILK BISCUITS
1 dozen (VITAMIN K content = 1 mcg per biscuit)

3	tbsp	Canola oil, treated (See Dietary Tip # 10)
2/3	cup	Buttermilk
2	cups	All purpose flour
2	tsp	Baking powder
1/4	tsp	Baking soda
1/4	tsp	Salt
2	tbsp	Sugar

Mix the dry ingredients together. Mix the buttermilk and oil and pour over the dry ingredients. Mix lightly.

Prepare a surface lightly covered with flour. Knead the dough on the flour-covered surface. Roll out the dough to 3/4 inch thickness. Cut in 2 to 3 inch squares.

Bake at 450 degrees Fahrenheit for 10 to 12 minutes until golden brown.

Ingredient	Cal	Fat	Chol	Sod	Prot	Carb	Fiber
OIL	362	42	0	0	0	0	0
BUTTERMILK	59	1.1	5	160	4.8	7.5	0
FLOUR	800	3.2	0	0	22.4	176	0
BAKING POWDER	4	0	0	408	0	0.9	0
BAKING SODA	0	0	0	205	0	0	0
SALT	0	0	0	575	0	0	0
SUGAR	97	0	0	0	0	25	0
Totals Per Serving:	**101**	**3.9**	**0**	**112**	**2.3**	**17.4**	**0**

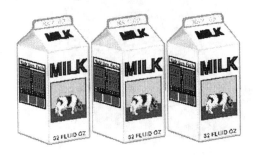

EGG PANCAKES
2 servings (3 mcgs of VITAMIN K per serving)

2	large	Eggs
1/2	cup	Milk, skim
1/2	cup	All purpose flour
1/4	cup	Butter

Mix the eggs, milk and flour until lumpy. Melt the butter in a pie plate. Pour the batter the into melted butter in the pie plate.

Bake in a 425 degree Fahrenheit oven for 20 minutes.

Serve with cooked apples, maple syrup, butter, powdered sugar, etc.

Ingredient	Cal	Fat	Chol	Sod	Prot	Carb	Fiber
EGGS	150	11.2	426	126	12.6	1.2	0
MILK, SKIM	44	0.4	4	64	4	6	0
FLOUR	200	0.8	0	0	5.6	44	0
BUTTER	400	46	140	360	0	0	0
Totals Per Serving:	**397**	**29.2**	**285**	**275**	**11.1**	**25.6**	**0**

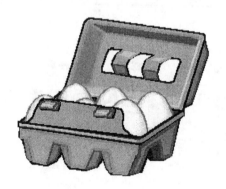

DATE OR RAISIN BRAN MUFFINS
12 servings (3.5 mcgs of VITAMIN K per serving)

1	cup	Oat Bran Flakes cereal (or any other bran cereal)
3/4	cup	Milk, skim
1	cup	All purpose flour
2 1/2	tsp	Baking powder
1/2	tsp	Salt
1/4	cup	Sugar, granulated
1/2	cup	Raisins, packed*
1/2	cup	Walnuts, chopped
1	each	Egg
1/4	cup	Canola oil, treated (See Dietary Tip # 10)

*For Date Muffins, substitute finely chopped pitted dates.

Mix the cereal and milk. Let stand a few minutes until most of the milk is absorbed.

Grease a 12 cup muffin pan. Heat the oven to 400 degrees Fahrenheit.

Sift the flour, baking powder, salt and sugar into a medium-sized bowl. Stir to mix well. Add the dates or raisins and nuts. Toss to mix.

Add the egg and oil to the soaked cereal and beat well with a fork. Pour the egg mixture into the flour mixture and stir only until the dry ingredients are moistened. Batter will be lumpy.

Drop the batter into prepared pans, filling each cup half to two-thirds full.

Bake about 30 minutes, or until browned. Remove from pan and serve hot with your favorite spread.

Ingredient	Cal	Fat	Chol	Sod	Prot	Carb	Fiber
OAT BRAN	480	9.6	0	16	36	144	20
MILK, SKIM	66	0.6	6	96	6	9	0
FLOUR	400	1.6	0	0	11.2	88	0
BAKING POWDER	5	0	0	510	0	1.1	0
SALT	0	0	0	1150	0	0	0
SUGAR	194	0	0	0	0	50	0
RAISINS	252	0.4	0	16	2	66	5.6
WALNUTS	384	37.2	0	8	8.4	11.2	2.8
EGG	75	5	213	63	6.3	0.6	0
OIL	482	56	0	0	0	0	0
Totals Per Serving:	195	9.2	18	155	5.8	30.8	2.4

CORN MEAL MUFFINS
12 servings (7 mcgs of VITAMIN K per muffin)

1	cup	All purpose flour
4	tsp	Baking powder
2	tbsp	Sugar, granulated
1	tsp	Salt
1	cup	cornmeal, yellow
2	large	Eggs
1	cup	Milk, skim
1/4	cup	Canola oil, treated (See Dietary Tip # 10)

Grease a 12 cup muffin pan.

Heat the oven to 425 degrees Fahrenheit.

Sift the flour, baking powder, sugar and salt into medium-sized bowl. Add cornmeal and stir to mix well.

In a small bowl, beat the eggs with fork. Add the milk and oil. Add the liquids all at once to the dry ingredients. Stir the mixture only until dry ingredients are moistened. Batter will be lumpy.

Drop batter from a tablespoon into the prepared muffin cups, filling each cup 1/2 to 2/3 full.

Bake 15 to 20 minutes, or until golden brown. Remove and serve hot.

Ingredient	Cal	Fat	Chol	Sod	Prot	Carb	Fiber
FLOUR	400	1.6	0	0	11.2	88	0
BAKING POWDER	8	0	0	816	0	1.8	0
SUGAR	97	0	0	0	0	25	0
SALT	0	0	0	2300	0	0	0
CORNMEAL	608	8	0	56	16	120	4
EGGS	150	11.2	426	126	12.6	1.2	0
MILK, SKIM	88	0.8	8	128	8	12	0
OIL	482	56	0	0	0	0	0
Totals Per Serving:	153	6.5	36	286	4	20.7	0.3

RICE PANCAKES

4 servings (Less than 2 mcgs of VITAMIN K per serving)

1/2	cup	All purpose flour
1	tsp	Baking powder
1/4	tsp	Salt
1	cup	Rice, white, cooked
2/3	cup	Milk, skim
2	each	Egg yolks
2	each	Egg whites, beaten stiff

Mix the dry ingredients together. Add the rice to the dry ingredients. Add the milk and egg yolks. Fold in the beaten egg whites last.

Bake on a greased griddle.

You can add chopped and drained fresh fruit to the batter if you like.

Ingredient	Cal	Fat	Chol	Sod	Prot	Carb	Fiber
FLOUR	200	0.8	0	0	5.6	44	0
BAKING POWDER	2	0	0	204	0	0.5	0
SALT	0	0	0	575	0	0	0
RICE	392	11.2	0	8	26.4	104	0.8
MILK, SKIM	59	0.5	5	85	5.3	8	0
EGG YOLKS	202	17.6	726	24	9.6	1	0
EGG WHITES	28	0	0	92	6	6	0
Totals Per Serving:	**221**	**7.5**	**183**	**247**	**13.2**	**40.9**	**0.2**

BACON AND ONION MUFFINS
12 servings (Less than 1 mcg of VITAMIN K per serving)

1/2	lb	Bacon, diced
1/4	cup	Onion, chopped
2 1/4	cup	All purpose flour, sifted
3	tsp	Baking powder
1/2	tsp	Baking soda
1/2	tsp	Salt
2	large	Eggs, beaten slightly
1/3	cup	Milk, skim
1	cup	Sour cream, nonfat

Fry the bacon in a skillet until crisp. Remove with a slotted spoon and drain on paper towels. Discard the bacon drippings except for 1 tablespoon.

Sauté the onion in the 1 tablespoon of bacon drippings until tender (do not brown). Set aside to cool.

Sift together the flour, baking powder, baking soda and salt in a large mixing bowl. Combine the eggs, milk and sour cream in a small bowl. Blend well. Add all the liquids at once to the dry ingredients, stirring just enough to moisten. Stir in the bacon and sautéed onion.

Spoon batter into a greased 12 cup muffin pan, fill each cup 2/3 full.

Bake in 375 degree Fahrenheit oven 18 to 20 minutes or until golden brown. Serve hot with jelly or jam.

Ingredient	Cal	Fat	Chol	Sod	Prot	Carb	Fiber
BACON	368	31.2	56	1016	18.4	0.8	0
ONION	16	0	0	0	0.4	3.4	0.6
BACON DRIPPINGS	126	12.8	12	104	0	0	0
FLOUR	900	3.6	0	0	25.2	198	0
BAKING POWDER	6	0	0	612	0	1.4	0
BAKING SODA	0	0	0	411	0	0	0
SALT	0	0	0	1150	0	0	0
EGGS	150	11.2	426	126	12.6	1.2	0
MILK, SKIM	29	0.3	3	43	2.7	4	0
SOUR CREAM	120	0	0	120	24	8	0
Totals Per Serving:	**143**	**4.9**	**41**	**299**	**6.9**	**18.1**	**0.1**

SAUSAGE, EGGPLANT, BASIL AND TOMATO PIZZA
8 servings (13 mcg of VITAMIN K per serving)

1/2	each	PIZZA DOUGH (See Recipe Index)
3/4	lb	Italian sausage, turkey, crumbled
1/2	cup	Onion, chopped
1 1/4	cups	Eggplant, in 1/2 inch slices (1 medium eggplant)
2	tbsp	Olive oil, treated ((See Dietary Tip # 10)
1/3	cup	Tomato sauce
1	oz	Parmesan cheese, grated
2	oz	Cheese, Mozzarella, shredded (about 1/2 cup)
6	oz	Tomato, diced (1 medium tomato)
2	tbsp	Basil, fresh, in thin strips

Make and bake a 12 inch pizza crust according to the directions in the PIZZA DOUGH recipe.

Cook the sausage for 6 to 8 minutes and set aside. Add the onion to the skillet and cook until the onion begins to brown, 5 to 8 minutes, cover and cook 5 minutes or until tender.

Meanwhile, (peel the eggplant if you wish) brush the eggplant with treated olive oil on both sides. Broil in the broiler until brown on both sides, turning once.

Spread the baked crust with sauce. Top with the sausage and onion mixture, eggplant, cheeses, tomatoes and basil.

Bake 10 minutes at 400 degrees Fahrenheit.

Ingredient	Cal	Fat	Chol	Sod	Prot	Carb	Fiber
PIZZA DOUGH	820	22.8	0	920	19.5	140.7	0
ITALIAN SAUSAGE	600	48	0	3000	48	10.8	0
ONION	32	0	0	0	0.8	6.8	1.2
EGGPLANT	70	0	0	10	1	3	4
OIL	238	27	0	0	0	0	0
TOMATO SAUCE	29	0	0	440	1.3	5.9	0
PARMESAN	111	7.5	24	454	10.1	0.9	0
MOZZARELLA	180	14	50	360	12	2	0
TOMATOES	30	0.6	0	12	1.2	6	1.8
BASIL	1	0	0	0	0.1	0.2	0.1
Totals Per Serving:	264	156	9	650	11.7	22	0.9

JUMBO POPOVERS
6 servings (Less than 1 mcg of VITAMIN K per serving)

2	large	Eggs
1	cup	Milk, skim
1	cup	All purpose flour, sifted
1/2	tsp	Salt

Butter 6 six-ounce custard cups with straight sides (popovers rise better in straight-sided containers).

Beat the eggs slightly with rotary beater. Add the other ingredients. Continue beating briskly 1 to 2 minutes. Mixture will be smooth and thin.

Pour it into the custard cups, about 1/2 full. Place cups on a cookie sheet, not touching each other.

Cook at 400 for 50 minutes or until puffed up and golden brown (do NOT peek until they are done - this may cause them to fall).

Ingredient	Cal	Fat	Chol	Sod	Prot	Carb	Fiber
EGGS	150	11.2	426	126	12.6	1.2	0
MILK, SKIM	88	0.8	8	128	8	12	0
FLOUR	400	1.6	0	0	11.2	88	0
SALT	0	0	0	1150	0	0	0
Totals Per Serving:	**106**	**2.3**	**72**	**234**	**5.3**	**16.9**	**0**

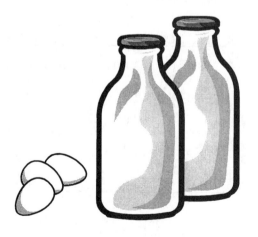

SMOKED SALMON-AND-CHIVE SANDWICHES
6 servings (15 mcgs of VITAMIN K per serving)

12	slices	Bread, Pumpernickel, thin slice
6	oz	Smoked salmon, thinly sliced
8	oz	Cream cheese, soft
4	oz	Butter, soft
1	tbsp	Grated lemon zest
1/4	tsp	Ground black pepper
3	tbsp	Chives, fresh, minced

Beat together the cream cheese and butter until smooth and light. Beat in the lemon zest and pepper to taste. Stir in the chives.

Lay out the bread. Carefully spread each slice with the cream cheese filling. Place the salmon, overlapping if necessary, in an even layer over the filling on 6 slices. Top with the remaining slices of bread, spread side down on the salmon.

Trim off the crusts and cut the sandwiches into quarters.

Ingredient	Cal	Fat	Chol	Sod	Prot	Carb	Fiber
BREAD	432	6	0	1140	12	78	12
SMOKED SALMON	198	7.2	42	1332	30	0	0
CREAM CHEESE	792	79.2	240	680	16	8	0
BUTTER	800	92	280	720	0	0	0
LEMON ZEST	0	0.1	0	0	0.2	3.6	0.1
BLACK PEPPER	1	0	0	0	0.1	0.4	0.1
CHIVES	14	0	0	2	1.5	1.5	1.5
Totals Per Serving:	373	30.7	94	646	10	15.2	2.3

TUNA BUNS
8 servings (6 mcgs of VITAMIN K per serving)

2	each	Eggs, hard cooked, chopped
6 1/2	oz	Tuna IN WATER, drained
4	oz	Cheddar cheese, shredded
1/4	cup	Bell pepper, green, chopped
2	tbsp	Onion, chopped
1/2	tsp	Mustard
1/2	cup	BLENDER MAYONNAISE #2 (See Recipe Index)
8	each	Hamburger buns, split

Mix the eggs, tuna, cheese, green pepper, onion, mustard and mayonnaise together. Fill the buns with the tuna mixture. Wrap each bun individually in aluminum foil. Place on a cookie sheet and heat them in the oven at 350 degrees Fahrenheit for about 20 minutes.

Ingredient	Cal	Fat	Chol	Sod	Prot	Carb	Fiber
EGGS	150	11.2	426	126	12.6	1.2	0
TUNA	214	0	58	624	45.5	0	0
CHEDDAR	440	36	120	800	28	4	0
BELL PEPPER	14	0	0	0	0.2	0.2	0.2
ONION	8	0	0	0	0.2	1.7	0.3
MUSTARD	2	0.1	0	30	0.2	0.2	0
MAYONNAISE	612	67.2	84	300	2.4	1.2	0
BUNS	640	13.6	0	1000	10.4	104	0
Totals Per Serving:	260	16	86	360	12.4	14.1	0.1

EARLY BIRD BUTTERMILK PANCAKES
4 servings (5 mcgs of VITAMIN K per serving)

1 1/2	cups	All purpose flour
1	tbsp	Sugar
1/2	tsp	Salt
2 1/4	tsp	Baking powder
1/2	cup	Buttermilk
2/3	cup	Milk, skim
1	large	Egg (beaten)
2	tbsp	Canola oil, treated (See Dietary Tip # 10)
1	tbsp	Canola oil, treated, for pan
1/2	cup	Milk, skim for thinning as needed

Sift together the flour, sugar, salt, and baking powder.

Beat together the buttermilk, milk, beaten egg and oil.

Pour the liquid into the dry ingredients and stir until well mixed. A few small lumps in the mixture will cook out.

The first pancake is a test pancake. (The batter should be thin for pancakes.) So thin the batter, if necessary, with milk (not buttermilk). The pan should be lightly oiled and hot enough to make a sprinkling of water dance, not just sit and sizzle.

Ladle about 1/8 cup of the batter into the hot pan. When the top of the pancake is full of bubbles and the bottom is golden, turn the pancake. Cook on the second side until done. Makes 15 (4 inch) pancakes.

Ingredient	Cal	Fat	Chol	Sod	Prot	Carb	Fiber
FLOUR	600	2.4	0	0	16.8	132	0
SUGAR	48	0	0	0	0	12.5	0
SALT	0	0	0	1150	0	0	0
BAKING POWDER	5	0	0	459	0	1	0
BUTTERMILK	44	0.8	4	120	3.6	5.6	0
MILK, SKIM	59	0.5	5	85	5.3	8	0
EGG, BEATEN	75	5.6	213	63	6.3	0.6	0
OIL	251	28	0	0	0	0	0
OIL	126	14	0	0	0	0	0
MILK, SKIM	44	0.4	4	64	4	6	0
Totals Per Serving:	**309**	**12.9**	**57**	**485**	**9**	**41.4**	**0**

BLUEBERRY BUTTERMILK PANCAKES
4 servings (5 mcgs of VITAMIN K per serving)

1	cup	All purpose flour
1/4	tsp	Salt
1	tsp	Baking soda
1	cup	Buttermilk
2	large	Eggs, beaten slightly
1	cup	Blueberries, washed and dried

Blend the flour, salt and baking soda.

In a separate bowl, combine the buttermilk, eggs and butter.

Stir the two mixtures together just long enough to blend them, but do not overbeat. Fold in the blueberries.

Heat 2-3 tablespoons of butter on a griddle or large skillet over medium heat. Spoon out 3-4 tablespoons of batter for each pancake. Cook until the bubbles that form on top begin to pop, then flip. Cook a minute or so more, then remove pancakes to heated dish. Serve with butter and syrup.

Ingredient	Cal	Fat	Chol	Sod	Prot	Carb	Fiber
FLOUR	400	1.6	0	0	11.2	88	0
SALT	0	0	0	575	0	0	0
BAKING SODA	0	0	0	821	0	0	0
BUTTERMILK	88	1.6	8	240	7.2	11.2	0
EGGS	150	11.2	426	126	12.6	1.2	0
BLUEBERRIES	80	0.8	0	8	0.8	20	3.2
Totals Per Serving:	**180**	**3.8**	**109**	**443**	**8**	**30.1**	**0.8**

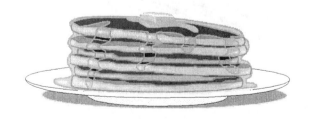

APPLE PANCAKE PUFF
4 servings (2 mcgs of VITAMIN K per serving)

4	tsp	Butter
3	med	Apples, peeled, cored and cut in 1/4 inch thick slices
2	tbsp	Raisins
3	tbsp	Sugar, granulated
2	tbsp	Orange juice
1	tsp	Cinnamon, ground
2	large	Eggs
1/2	cup	Milk, skim
6	tbsp	All purpose flour
1	tsp	Vanilla extract

In a heavy, medium sized, oven proof skillet, melt 2 teaspoons of the butter. Add the apples, raisins, 1 tablespoon of the sugar, orange juice and cinnamon. Cook, stirring frequently, 6 to 8 minutes, until apples are just tender. Remove the apples and raisins to a bowl. Preheat oven to 425 degrees Fahrenheit.

In a small bowl (with an electric mixer) beat the eggs until foamy. Gradually add the milk, flour, sugar and vanilla, beat 2 minutes longer, until the batter is smooth.

Add remaining 2 teaspoons of butter to the same skillet. Place in the oven to melt (about 1 minute.) Pour batter into skillet and bake 10 minutes. Remove from oven and spoon apple mixture into center of pancake. Return to oven and bake 12-15 minutes longer until puffed and golden. Cut into quarters.

Ingredient	Cal	Fat	Chol	Sod	Prot	Carb	Fiber
BUTTER	133	15.3	47	120	0	0	0
APPLES	219	1.2	0	3	0.9	57	3.3
RAISINS	63	0.1	0	4	0.5	16.5	1.4
SUGAR	146	0	0	0	0	37.5	0
ORANGE JUICE	17	0	0	0	0.2	3.2	0.1
CINNAMON	6	1	0	1	0.1	1.7	0.6
EGGS	150	11.2	426	126	12.6	1.2	0
MILK, SKIM	44	0.4	4	64	4	6	0
FLOUR	150	0.6	0	0	4.2	33	0
VANILLA EXTRACT	10	0	0	0	0	0.3	0
Totals Per Serving:	**235**	**7.5**	**119**	**80**	**5.6**	**39.1**	**1.4**

GARLIC BREAD
6 servings (6 mcgs of VITAMIN K per serving)

16	oz	Bread, Sourdough or Italian (1 loaf)
2	tbsp	Butter
3/4	cup	BLENDER MAYONNAISE #2 (See Recipe Index)
3	oz	Parmesan cheese, fresh grated
1	tbsp	Garlic, peeled and minced

Turn on the broiler

Cut the bread horizontally in half. Butter each half and brown them, butter side up, under the broiler.

Mix the remaining ingredients and spread each bread half evenly with the topping mixture.

Bake at 425 degrees Fahrenheit for about 15 to 20 minutes or until the crust is well browned.

Cut in wedges and serve hot or at room temperature.

Ingredient	Cal	Fat	Chol	Sod	Prot	Carb	Fiber
BREAD	1232	16	0	2656	32	224	16
BUTTER	200	23	70	180	0	0	0
MAYONNAISE	918	100.8	126	450	3.6	1.8	0
PARMESAN	333	22.5	72	1362	30.3	2.7	0
GARLIC	12	0.1	0	6	0.5	3	0
Totals Per Serving:	**449**	**27.1**	**45**	**776**	**11.1**	**38.6**	**2.7**

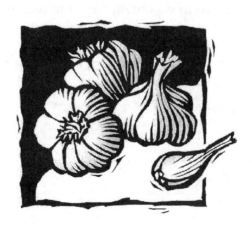

POTATO CRACKERS

20 servings (8 mcgs of VITAMIN K for the whole recipe)

3/4	cup	Oats, rolled
3/4	cup	All purpose flour
1/3	cup	Butter
2	cups	Potatoes, peeled, cooked and mashed
2	tbsp	Canola Oil, Treated (see Dietary Tip # 10.)

Combine the oats and flour in a bowl. Rub in the butter with your fingertips, then knead in the mashed potatoes to form a stiff dough.

Carefully roll out the dough onto a floured board and cut out thin rounds using a cookie cutter or an upside-down glass.

Cook the rounds on cookie sheets, greased with the Canola oil, at 350 degrees Fahrenheit for 20 minutes or until the crackers are crisp and lightly browned.

Ingredient	Cal	Fat	Chol	Sod	Prot	Carb	Fiber
OATS, ROLLED	420	12	0	6	29.4	112.8	27
FLOUR	300	1.2	0	0	8.4	66	0
BUTTER	533	61.3	187	480	0	0	0
POTATOES	272	0	0	16	6.4	64	0
CANOLA OIL	241	28	0	0	0	0	0
Totals Per Serving:	**88**	**5.1**	**9**	**25**	**2.2**	**12.1**	**1.4**

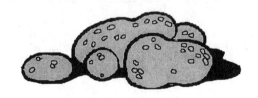

BASIC PANCAKES
4 servings (1.5 mcgs of VITAMIN K per serving)

3/4	cup	All purpose flour
1/2	tsp	Salt
1 1/2	tsp	Sugar
1	tsp	Baking powder
1	large	Egg
1 1/2	tsp	Canola oil, treated (See Dietary Tip # 10)
5	oz	Milk, skim
2	tbsp	Canola Oil, Treated (see Dietary Tip # 10.)

Sift the dry ingredients together into a bowl.

Combine the egg, oil and milk in another bowl.

Stir the wet ingredients into the dry ingredients until the batter is just smooth.

Lightly grease a large skillet or griddle with the Canola oil. When the griddle is hot, ladle the batter onto the griddle. Adjust the heat to medium-high.

When bubbles appear on the surface of the pancake, usually after 2 to 3 minutes, lift with a spatula to see that the underside is browned. Turn and cook the second side until browned (about 1 1/2 to 2 minutes.) Serve hot with butter and syrup.

Ingredient	Cal	Fat	Chol	Sod	Prot	Carb	Fiber
FLOUR	300	1.2	0	0	8.4	66	0
SALT	0	0	0	1150	0	0	0
SUGAR	24	0	0	0	0	6.3	0
BAKING POWDER	2	0	0	204	0	0.5	0
EGG	75	5	213	63	6.3	0.6	0
OIL	60	7	0	0	0	0	0
MILK, SKIM	55	0.5	5	80	5	7.5	0
CANOLA OIL	120	14	0	0	0	0	0
Totals Per Serving:	**159**	**6.9**	**55**	**374**	**4.9**	**20.2**	**0**

SCOTTISH SCONES
8 servings (1 mcg of VITAMIN K per serving)

2	cups	All purpose flour
1	tsp	Salt
1	tsp	Baking soda
2	tsp	Cream of tartar
3	tbsp	Butter, room temperature
1	large	Egg, room temperature, lightly beaten
1/2	cup	Buttermilk, room temperature
1	tbsp	Canola Oil, Treated (see Dietary Tip # 10.)

In a bowl, mix the flour, salt, baking soda and cream of tartar. Stir thoroughly.

With your fingers, rub the butter into the dry ingredients.

Gradually stir the beaten egg and buttermilk into the flour mix. If it is a bit too moist and sticks to your hands, add a bit of flour.

Turn the dough onto a lightly floured work surface and knead as little as possible to achieve a soft, pliable dough ball.

Divide the dough into 2 equal parts. Flatten each with the knuckles into a round disc (about 6 inches in diameter and 1/2 inch thick). Prick about a dozen times with fork. Then cut in four sections each.

Use the Canola oil to grease a baking sheet. Place the scones on the baking sheet and bake at 375 degrees Fahrenheit for about 15 minutes, or until the scones are a light tan in color. (You can add 1/2 cup raisins or currants if you wish.)

Ingredient	Cal	Fat	Chol	Sod	Prot	Carb	Fiber
FLOUR	800	3.2	0	0	22.4	176	0
SALT	0	0	0	2300	0	0	0
BAKING SODA	0	0	0	821	0	0	0
CREAM OF TARTAR	16	0	0	1	0	0.6	0
BUTTER	300	34.5	105	270	0	0	0
EGG, BEATEN	75	5.6	213	63	6.3	0.6	0
BUTTERMILK	44	0.8	4	120	3.6	5.6	0
CANOLA OIL	120	14	0	0	0	0	0
Totals Per Serving:	169	7.2	40	447	4	22.9	0

APPLESAUCE BANANA BREAD
12 servings (Less than 1 mcg of VITAMIN K per serving)

2 1/2	cup	All purpose flour
2	tsp	Baking powder
1	tsp	Baking soda
1	tsp	Cinnamon, ground
1/2	cup	Applesauce, unsweetened
1	cup	Sugar, granulated
3	each	Egg whites
4	large	Bananas, whole, very ripe
1	tsp	Vanilla extract
1	tbsp	Butter

Preheat the oven to 350 degrees Fahrenheit.

Coat an 8 by 4 by 3 inch loaf pan with butter.

Combine the flour, baking powder, baking soda, and cinnamon. Set aside.

Peel and mash the bananas. There should be about 2 cups.

In a large mixing bowl, whisk together the apple sauce, sugar, egg whites, banana and vanilla. Add the flour mixture all at once and stir gently to blend.

Pour the batter into a prepared loaf pan and bake for 50-60 minutes or until a knife, inserted into the center, comes out clean. Cool the bread completely before slicing.

NOTE: The loaf can be wrapped tightly and stored for up to one week or frozen for up to 2 months.

Ingredient	Cal	Fat	Chol	Sod	Prot	Carb	Fiber
FLOUR	1000	4	0	0	28	220	0
BAKING POWDER	4	0	0	408	0	0.9	0
BAKING SODA	0	0	0	821	0	0	0
CINNAMON	6	1	0	1	0.1	1.7	0.6
APPLESAUCE	48	0	0	4	0.8	0	0
SUGAR	776	0	0	0	0	200	0
EGG WHITES	42	0	0	138	9	9	0
BANANAS	480	4	0	0	4	112	12
VANILLA EXTRACT	10	0	0	0	0	0.3	0
BUTTER	100	11.5	35	90	0	0	0
Totals Per Serving:	**206**	**1.7**	**3**	**122**	**3.5**	**45.3**	**1.1**

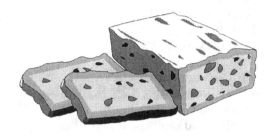

ORANGE SPREAD
4 servings (2 mcgs of VITAMIN K per serving)

1	med	Orange (about 2 5/8 inches in diameter)
8	oz	Cream cheese
1	tbsp	Honey
2	tbsp	Pecans, chopped
4	each	Bagels, 5 ounce size

Grate the orange rind. Peel, seed and chop the orange. Soften the cream cheese. Add the pecans. Mix all the ingredients together and serve on bagels.

Ingredient	Cal	Fat	Chol	Sod	Prot	Carb	Fiber
ORANGE	62	0.2	0	0	1.2	15.4	3.1
CREAM CHEESE	792	79.2	240	680	16	8	0
HONEY	44	0	0	0	0.1	11.8	0
PECANS	99	10	0	0	1.2	2.8	1
BAGELS	772	0	0	1500	32	160	10
Totals Per Serving:	**442**	**22.4**	**60**	**545**	**12.6**	**49.5**	**3.5**

IRISH SODA BREAD
8 servings (1 mcg of VITAMIN K per serving)

3	tbsp	Butter, soft
2 1/2	cup	All purpose flour
2	tbsp	Sugar
1	tsp	Baking soda
1	tsp	Baking powder
1/2	tsp	Salt
1/3	cup	Raisins, packed
3/4	cup	Buttermilk
2	tsp	Canola Oil, Treated (see Dietary Tip # 10.)

Heat the oven to 375 degrees Fahrenheit. . Mix together the dry ingredients except the raisins. Cut the butter into the flour mixture until it resembles fine crumbs. Stir in the raisins and enough buttermilk to make a soft dough.

Turn the dough onto a lightly floured surface. Knead it until smooth, about 1 to 2 minutes. Shape into a round loaf about 6 1/2 inches in diameter. Oil the baking sheet with the Canola oil. Place the loaf on the greased baking sheet.

Cut an X about 1/4-inch through the center of the loaf using a floured knife. Bake until golden brown, 35 to 45 minutes. Brush with butter if desired. Delicious warm, or cool to slice more easily.

Ingredient	Cal	Fat	Chol	Sod	Prot	Carb	Fiber
BUTTER	300	34.5	105	270	0	0	0
FLOUR	1000	4	0	0	28	220	0
SUGAR	97	0	0	0	0	25	0
BAKING SODA	0	0	0	821	0	0	0
BAKING POWDER	2	0	0	204	0	0.5	0
SALT	0	0	0	1150	0	0	0
RAISINS	168	0.3	0	11	1.3	44	3.7
BUTTERMILK	66	1.2	6	180	5.4	8.4	0
CANOLA OIL	80	9.3	0	0	0	0	0
Totals Per Serving:	214	6.2	14	330	4.3	37.2	0.5

BEEF

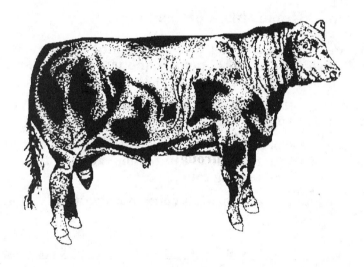

BEEF STIR FRY

6 Servings (VITAMIN K content of beef stir fry (without rice or tortilla) = 4 mcg per cup)

3	cups	Beef sirloin steak, lean, cut into small pieces, either thin strips or small cubes, with fat trimmed
1	tsp	Garlic cloves, minced
12	oz	Onion, sliced (about 2 medium onions)
1 1/2	cups	Tomatoes, sliced
2	tsp	Olive oil, treated (See Dietary Tip # 10)
1	tsp	Vinegar
1/4	tsp	Ground black pepper

Sauté the garlic in a skillet with the oil until the garlic is golden brown, then add the steak, pepper and vinegar. Cook until the steak is brown, approximately 5 to 10 minutes.

Add the vegetables and cook until the onions and tomatoes are at the desired tenderness.

This recipe is especially good served with white rice or on a tortilla. (Remember to add the nutrition values of the rice or tortillas to the per serving total.)

Neither white rice nor tortillas contain a significant amount of VITAMIN K.

Ingredient	Cal	Fat	Chol	Sod	Prot	Carb	Fiber
SIRLOIN STEAK	1296	40.8	600	432	196.8	0	0
GARLIC	4	0	0	2	0.2	1	0
ONION	132	0	0	12	3.6	28.8	60
TOMATOES	60	1.2	0	24	2.4	12	3.6
OIL	80	9.3	0	0	0	0	0
VINEGAR	1	0	0	1	0	0	0
BLACK PEPPER	1	0	0	0	0.1	0.4	0.1
Totals Per Serving:	**262**	**8.6**	**100**	**79**	**33.8**	**7**	**10.6**

SAUCY MEATLOAF
8 servings (3 mcgs of VITAMIN K per serving)

1	cup	Catsup
2	tbsp	Dijon mustard
1 1/2	tbsp	Brown sugar
2	lb	Beef, lean, ground coarse
4	oz	Onion, diced (about 1/2 cup)
1/2	tsp	Garlic, peeled and minced
1/4	cup	Bell pepper, green, diced
3/4	cup	Bread crumbs, dry, plain
2	large	Eggs*
1/2	tsp	Ground black pepper

*Or 1/2 cup egg substitute. (This will change the nutrition values.)

Combine the ketchup, mustard and sugar for a sauce.

Mix the meat with all the remaining ingredients. Pat into a loaf shape and turn out into a baking pan with sides.

Put 2/3 cup of sauce on top of the loaf. Bake in a preheated 350 degree Fahrenheit oven about 45 minutes to an hour or until a quick-read thermometer says 130.

Serve with remaining sauce.

Ingredient	Cal	Fat	Chol	Sod	Prot	Carb	Fiber
CATSUP	232	0.8	0	2688	3.2	64.6	3.2
DIJON MUSTARD	30	0	0	720	0	1	0
BROWN SUGAR	72	0	0	0	0	20.3	0
BEEF	2112	160	640	608	160	0	0
ONION, DICED	44	0	0	4	1.2	9.6	20
GARLIC	2	0	0	1	0.1	0.5	0
BELL PEPPER	14	0	0	0	0.2	0.2	0.2
BREAD CRUMBS	318	4.2	0	696	9	57.6	3
EGGS	150	11.2	426	126	12.6	1.2	0
BLACK PEPPER	3	0.1	0	1	0.1	0.7	0.2
Totals Per Serving:	**373**	**22**	**133**	**606**	**23.3**	**19.1**	**3.3**

BEEF STROGANOFF
8 servings (1 mcg of VITAMIN K per serving)

1 1/2	lb	Beef, sirloin
1/4	tsp	Ground black pepper
3	tbsp	Butter
1 1/2	cups	MUSHROOM CREAM SAUCE (See Recipe Index.)*
1	cup	Beef broth, hot
1	tsp	Dijon mustard
2	tbsp	Catsup
1/2	cup	Onion, sliced or chopped
2	tsp	Worcestershire Sauce
1/2	cup	Sour cream, lowfat**
3	tbsp	Brandy
1	tbsp	Paprika

*OR 1 can Cream of mushroom soup, low fat.

**OR 1/2 cup yogurt, plain, lowfat (Adjust the nutrition values accordingly.)

Remove all the fat and gristle from the meat. Cut it into narrow strips about 2 inches long and 1/2 inch thick. Season the strips with pepper and paprika.

In a saucepan, melt 1 1/2 tablespoons of butter. Add the meat strips and brown. Remove the beef from the pan and keep it warm.

Add the other 1 1/2 tablespoons of butter, add the onion and sauté until golden.

Put the beef back into the pan. Add the brandy and cook for two minutes on medium heat.

Add the hot beef stock and the Mushroom Cream Sauce or the Cream of Mushroom Soup. Stir until well blended. Stir in mustard and Worcestershire Sauce. Add the sour cream and heat over a brisk flame for 3 minutes.

Serve sauce and meat over buttered noodles.

Ingredient	Cal	Fat	Chol	Sod	Prot	Carb	Fiber
SIRLOIN	1296	40.8	600	432	196.8	0	0
BLACK PEPPER	1	0	0	0	0.1	0.4	0.1
BUTTER	300	34.5	105	270	0	0	0
MUSHROOM SAUCE	420	24	84	804	16.8	37.2	3.6
BEEF BROTH	40	0	0	1744	8	0	0
DIJON MUSTARD	5	0	0	120	0	0.2	0
CATSUP	29	0.1	0	336	0.4	8	0
ONION	44	0	0	4	1.2	9.6	20
WORCESTERSHIRE	7	0	0	133	0	1.3	0
SOUR CREAM	160	8	20	140	8	16	0
BRANDY	98	0	0	0	0	0	0
PAPRIKA	18	0.9	0	3	0.9	3.6	1.2
Totals Per Serving:	**302**	**13.5**	**101**	**498**	**29**	**9.5**	**3.1**

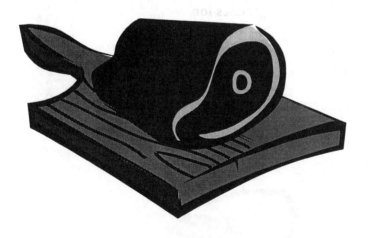

MEATLOAF

4 servings (VITAMIN K for entire loaf = 154 mcgs or almost 40 mcgs per serving)

1	lb	Beef, lean, ground
1/4	cup	Bread crumbs, dry, plain
1/2	cup	Tomato paste
1/4	cup	Onion, chopped
1/4	cup	Bell pepper, green
1	cup	Tomato, chopped
1/2	tsp	Mustard
1/2	tsp	Ground black pepper
2	tsp	Garlic cloves, minced
1/4	cup	Scallions, chopped

Mix all the ingredients together and bake at 325 degrees Fahrenheit for 1 hour.

Ingredient	Cal	Fat	Chol	Sod	Prot	Carb	Fiber
BEEF GROUND	1056	80	320	304	80	0	0
BREAD CRUMBS	106	1.4	0	232	3	19.2	1
TOMATO PASTE	92	0	0	100	4	20	4
ONION	16	0	0	0	0.4	3.4	0.6
BELL PEPPER	14	0	0	0	0.2	0.2	0.2
TOMATO	40	0.8	0	16	1.6	8	2.4
MUSTARD	2	0.1	0	30	0.2	0.2	0
BLACK PEPPER	3	0.1	0	1	0.1	0.7	0.2
GARLIC	8	0	0	4	0.3	2	0
SCALLIONS	8	0.2	0	4	0.4	1.6	0.4
Totals Per Serving:	**336**	**20.6**	**80**	**173**	**22.5**	**13.8**	**2.2**

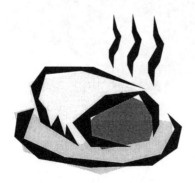

BREADED VEAL CUTLET (WEINERSCHNITZEL)
6 servings (Less than 1 mcg of VITAMIN K per serving)

2	lb	Veal steak, 1/2 inch thick
1/4	tsp	Ground black pepper
1	cup	Bread crumbs, dry, plain
1	large	Egg, beaten
1	tbsp	Olive oil, treated (See Dietary Tip # 10)
2	tsp	Lemon juice
6	each	Eggs, fried in Canola or olive oil
1	tbsp	Canola Oil, Treated (see Dietary Tip # 10.)

Cut the veal steak in pieces for serving. Sprinkle with the pepper, dip it in the cracker or bread crumbs, then in the beaten egg, then again in crumbs. Let stand a few minutes then fry the veal steaks in olive oil on both sides.

Sprinkle with lemon juice and garnish with a fried egg per portion.

Ingredient	Cal	Fat	Chol	Sod	Prot	Carb	Fiber
VEAL STEAK	992	22.4	704	704	182.4	0	0
BLACK PEPPER	1	0	0	0	0.1	0.4	0.1
BREAD CRUMBS	424	5.6	0	928	12	76.8	4
EGG, BEATEN	75	5.6	213	63	6.3	0.6	0
OIL	238	27	0	0	0	0	0
LEMON JUICE	2	0	0	0	0.3	0.7	0
EGGS, FRIED	450	33.6	1278	378	37.8	3.6	0
CANOLA OIL	120	14	0	0	0	0	0
Totals Per Serving:	384	18	366	346	39.8	13.7	0.7

BEEF TACOS

6 servings (34 mcgs of VITAMIN K per serving or 17 mcgs per taco)

1	lb	Beef, lean, ground
3/4	cup	Onion, chopped (about 1 medium onion)
1/2	cup	Bell pepper, green, chopped
1 1/2	cups	Potatoes, peeled, cooked and diced
1	cup	Tomato, chopped
1/2	tsp	Sugar
1	tbsp	Chili powder
1	tsp	Coriander, ground
1/4	tsp	Ground black pepper
1/2	cup	Olives, black chopped
12	each	Tortilla shells, pre-made, corn
1	cup	Tomato, chopped
2	tbsp	ITALIAN HERB DRESSING (See Recipe Index)
4	oz	Cheddar cheese, grated (about 1 cup)
1	cup	Sour cream, lowfat

Sauté the beef, green pepper and onion until the meat is brown and the veggies are translucent.

Add the potato, tomatoes, sugar, chili powder, coriander and pepper and stir to blend, cooking a few minutes more.

Mix in the olives. Cook for about 10 minutes more, stirring constantly.

Put the pre-shaped taco shells in the oven and heat, to crisp them.

Place a heaping tablespoon of meat mixture in each shell and stuff with tomato and cheese that have been tossed with the ITALIAN HERB DRESSING. Top with sour cream.

Ingredient	Cal	Fat	Chol	Sod	Prot	Carb	Fiber
BEEF GROUND	1056	80	320	304	80	0	0
ONION	66	0	0	6	1.8	14.4	30
BELL PEPPER	28	0	0	0	0.4	0.4	0.4
POTATOES	180	0	0	12	4.8	42	3.6
TOMATO	40	0.8	0	16	1.6	8	2.4
SUGAR	8	0	0	0	0	2.1	0
CHILI POWDER	16	0	0	0	0	0	0
CORIANDER	14	0.8	0	2	0.6	2.6	1.4
BLACK PEPPER	1	0	0	0	0.1	0.4	0.1
OLIVES	132	12	0	988	0.8	8	4
TORTILLA SHELLS	600	27.6	0	540	7.2	78	8.4
TOMATO	40	0.8	0	16	1.6	8	2.4
ITALIAN DRESSING	162	18.1	0	173	0	0.1	0
CHEDDAR	440	36	120	800	28	4	0
SOUR CREAM	320	16	40	280	16	32	0
Totals Per Serving:	**517**	**32**	**80**	**523**	**23.8**	**33.3**	**8.8**

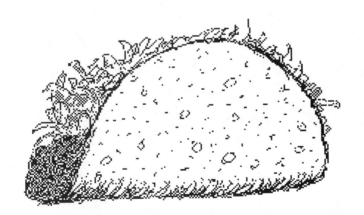

CROCK POT CHILI CON CARNE
6 servings (12 mcgs of VITAMIN K per serving)

1	lb	Beef, lean, ground
4	oz	Onion, chopped (about 1 small onion)
1	each	Bay leaf
1	tsp	Chili powder
1	tsp	Worcestershire Sauce
16	oz	Tomato sauce
32	oz	Kidney beans, canned, drained

In a skillet (or crock pot with a browning unit) break up the beef with a fork and cook until lightly browned. Pour off any excess fat.

In a crock pot, combine the meat with the onion, chili powder, bay leaf, Worcestershire Sauce, tomato sauce, and kidney beans.

Cover and cook on high for 2 to 3 hours. Remove the bay leaf. Serve hot.

Ingredient	Cal	Fat	Chol	Sod	Prot	Carb	Fiber
BEEF GROUND	1056	80	320	304	80	0	0
ONION	44	0	0	4	1.2	9.6	20
BAY LEAF	0	0	0	0	0	0	0
CHILI POWDER	6	0	0	0	0	0	0
WORCESTERSHIRE	3	0	0	67	0	0.7	0
TOMATO SAUCE	176	0	0	2640	8	35.2	0
KIDNEY BEANS	1056	16	0	2624	64	192	38.4
Totals Per Serving:	**390**	**16**	**53**	**940**	**25.5**	**39.6**	**9.7**

HAMBURG CASSEROLE
5 Servings (VITAMIN K content = 18 mcg per cup)

1	lb	Beef, lean, ground
1	cup	Bell pepper, green, diced
1/2	tsp	Ground black pepper
1	cup	Carrots, peeled and diced
6	oz	Onion, diced, (about 1 cup)
1	cup	Celery, diced
3 1/2	cup	Tomatoes, diced
1	cup	Peas, green, fresh or frozen
1	cup	Rice, white uncooked
1 1/2	cups	Water

Brown the beef in a skillet, then drain any fat.

Add the remainder of the ingredients, mix and cook over medium heat until boiling.

Cover skillet and cook on low heat for 35 minutes. Serve hot.

Ingredient	Cal	Fat	Chol	Sod	Prot	Carb	Fiber
BEEF GROUND	1056	80	320	304	80	0	0
BELL PEPPER	56	0	0	0	0.8	0.8	0.8
BLACK PEPPER	3	0.1	0	1	0.1	0.7	0.2
CARROTS	48	0.8	0	40	0.8	12	0.8
ONION, DICED	66	0	0	6	1.8	14.4	30
CELERY, DICED	16	0	0	104	0.8	4.8	0.8
TOMATOES, DICED	140	2.8	0	56	5.6	28	8.4
PEAS	184	0.8	0	8	12	32.8	8
RICE	824	1.6	0	8	16	181.6	2.4
Totals Per Serving:	**479**	**17.2**	**64**	**105**	**23.6**	**55**	**10.3**

TEXAS CHILI

8 servings (12 mcgs of VITAMIN K per serving. Add a 16 ounce can of Navy beans and increase the VITAMIN K count to 13 mcgs per serving)

2	tbsp	Olive oil, treated (See Dietary Tip # 10)
2	lb	Beef, lean, ground
12	oz	Onion, chopped (about 2 cups)
2	tsp	Garlic cloves, chopped
28	oz	Tomatoes, canned, peeled and chopped
12	oz	Beer
5	tbsp	Chili powder
2	each	Jalapeno pepper, seeded and chopped (Optional)
1	tbsp	Cumin
2	tsp	Paprika
1	tsp	Sugar
1/2	tsp	Black pepper, ground
1/4	tsp	Cayenne pepper
4	oz	Cheddar cheese, shredded (about 1 cup)
4	oz	Onion, chopped (about 1 small to medium onion)
1	cup	Sour cream, lowfat

Heat the oil in 6-quart saucepan.

Add the ground beef, onions and garlic and sauté until the meat is browned. Stir in the next 7 ingredients and bring to boil over medium-high heat.

Reduce heat to medium-low and simmer, uncovered, about 45-55 minutes. Taste and season with pepper and cayenne pepper, if desired.

Ladle into bowls. Garnish with cheese, chopped raw onion and sour cream.

If you like your chili with beans, you can add 1 to 3 cups of canned navy beans to the pot during the last 20 minutes of cooking time. Remember to add the beans to the nutrition totals. The beans will have a negligible effect on the vitamin K content per serving.

Ingredient	Cal	Fat	Chol	Sod	Prot	Carb	Fiber
OIL	241	28	0	0	0	0	0
BEEF GROUND	2112	160	640	608	160	0	0
ONION	132	0	0	12	3.6	28.8	60
GARLIC	8	0	0	4	0.3	2	0
TOMATOES	224	0	0	1540	8.4	33.6	0
BEER	144	0	0	12	1.2	12	0
CHILI POWDER	82	0.1	0	0	0	0	0
JALAPENO PEPPER	18	0	0	0	0	4	2
CUMIN	21	0	0	12	1.2	1.8	0.6
PAPRIKA	12	0.6	0	2	0.6	2.4	0.8
SUGAR	16	0	0	0	0	4.2	0
BLACK PEPPER	3	0.1	0	1	0.1	0.7	0.2
CAYENNE PEPPER	1	0.1	0	0	0.1	0.3	0.1
CHEDDAR	440	36	120	800	28	4	0
ONION	44	0	0	4	1.2	9.6	20
SOUR CREAM	320	16	40	280	16	32	0
Totals Per Serving:	**477**	**30.1**	**100**	**409**	**27.6**	**16.9**	**10.5**

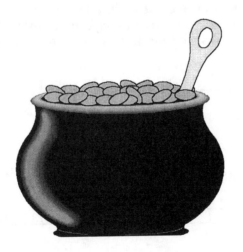

ENCHILADA PIE
8 servings (1 mcg of VITAMIN K per serving)

1	lb	Beef, lean, ground
4	oz	Onion, chopped (about 1/2 to 2/3 cup)
4	oz	Tomato sauce
1	tsp	Chili powder
1/2	tsp	Cumin
1/4	tsp	Ground black pepper
8		Corn tortillas
3	oz	Cheddar cheese shredded (about 3/4 cup)
1/2	cup	Water
1	tbsp	Canola oil, treated (See Dietary Tip # 10)

Cook the beef and onion until browned. Stir in the tomato sauce and seasonings and cook until heated.

Layer the tortillas, meat sauce and cheese in a 2 quart casserole coated with the Canola oil. Pour the water over top.

Cover and bake in the oven at 400 degrees Fahrenheit for 20 minutes. (If you fry the tortillas in Canola oil before adding to this dish they will stay together more. It does add the extra fat.)

Ingredient	Cal	Fat	Chol	Sod	Prot	Carb	Fiber
BEEF GROUND	1056	80	320	304	80	0	0
ONION	44	0	0	4	1.2	9.6	20
TOMATO SAUCE	44	0	0	660	2	8.8	0
CHILI POWDER	6	0	0	0	0	0	0
CUMIN	4	0	0	2	0.2	0.3	0.1
BLACK PEPPER	1	0	0	0	0.1	0.4	0.1
CORN TORTILLAS	360	0	0	80	8	72	0
CHEDDAR	330	27	90	600	21	3	0
OIL	120	13.5	0	0	0	0	0
Totals Per Serving:	328	20.1	68	275	18.7	15.7	3.4

VEAL PARMIGIANA
6 servings (3 mcgs of VITAMIN K per serving)

1	large	Egg, beaten
1/4	tsp	Ground black pepper
1/4	cup	Bread crumbs, soft
1/4	oz	Parmesan cheese, grated (about 1 tablespoon)
1	lb	Veal cutlet, thin, cut into 6 serving size pieces
8	oz	Tomato sauce
2	oz	Cheese, Mozzarella cheese
2	tbsp	Olive oil, treated (See Dietary Tip # 10)

Combine the egg and pepper and beat with a wire whisk until blended.

Combine the bread crumbs and Parmesan cheese, stirring well.

Dip the veal into the egg mixture, and dredge in the bread crumbs mixture.

Put the oil into a large skillet. Sauté the veal until golden brown. Transfer the veal to a shallow baking dish. Pour the tomato sauce over the veal, and top with cheese slices.

Bake at 350 degrees Fahrenheit for 15-20 minutes. Serve immediately.

Ingredient	Cal	Fat	Chol	Sod	Prot	Carb	Fiber
EGG, BEATEN	75	5.6	213	63	6.3	0.6	0
BLACK PEPPER	1	0	0	0	0.1	0.4	0.1
BREAD CRUMBS	106	1.4	0	232	3	2	0
PARMESAN CHEESE	28	1.9	6	114	2.5	0.2	0
VEAL CUTLET	480	8	352	288	96	0	0
TOMATO SAUCE	88	0	0	1320	4	17.6	0
MOZZARELLA	180	14	50	360	12	2	0
OIL	251	28	0	0	0	0	0
Totals Per Serving:	200	9.8	104	396	20.6	3.8	0

VEAL MARSALA
6 servings (20 mcgs of VITAMIN K per serving)

1	lb	veal, leg, lean, thin, cut in medallion sized pieces (cutlet)
1/3	cup	Parmesan Cheese
10	tbsp	Butter
1	tsp	Garlic, chopped
1/4	cup	Green onions, sliced
1/4	cup	Chicken broth
3	cups	Mushrooms, sliced
1/4	cup	Marsala wine
1/4	tsp	Ground black pepper
		Lemon slices

Pound the veal thin and coat it with Parmesan.

In a pan, melt the butter over medium to high heat, add garlic and sauté the veal until golden brown. Remove the veal to a platter and keep it warm. Discard garlic.

In the same pan, add the stock to deglaze the pan. Add the onions, mushrooms, and wine.

Simmer to reduce the sauce to one half. Pour the sauce over veal and garnish with lemons.

Ingredient	Cal	Fat	Chol	Sod	Prot	Carb	Fiber
VEAL	480	0	352	288	96	0	0
PARMESAN CHEESE	109	7.5	21	453	10.1	1.1	0
BUTTER	1000	115	350	900	0	0	0
GARLIC	0	0	0	0	0	0	0
GREEN ONIONS	18	0	0	10	2	2	1
CHICKEN BROTH	8	0	0	330	0.4	1.4	0
MUSHROOMS	168	0	0	24	14.4	31.2	9.6
MARSALA WINE	20	0	0	2	0	2	0
BLACK PEPPER	1	0	0	0	0.1	0.4	0.1
LEMON SLICES	0	0	0	0	0	0	0
Totals Per Serving:	301	20.4	121	335	20.5	6.3	1.8

VEAL NORMANDE
4 servings (1 mcg of VITAMIN K per serving)

1 1/2	tbsp	Butter
1 1/2	tbsp	Olive oil, treated (See Dietary Tip # 10)
1	lb	Veal cutlets, thinly sliced or pieces of boneless chicken breasts
1/2	cup	Shallots, chopped
5	tbsp	Brandy
1 1/2	cups	MUSHROOM CREAM SAUCE (See Recipe Index.)
1	med	Granny Smith apple, peeled, cored and sliced
2	cups	Wild rice, cooked

Melt the butter with the oil in a large skillet over medium-high heat. Add the veal and brown, turning once. Transfer to a platter.

Add the brandy and shallots to the skillet and stir, scraping up any browned bits clinging to the bottom of the pan. Blend in the MUSHROOM CREAM SAUCE.

Return the veal to the pan with the peeled apple. Reduce the heat and simmer, stirring once or twice, until heated through. Serve over rice.

Ingredient	Cal	Fat	Chol	Sod	Prot	Carb	Fiber
BUTTER	150	17.3	52	135	0	0	0
OIL	180	20.4	0	0	0	0	0
VEAL CUTLETS	480	8	352	288	96	0	0
SHALLOTS	56	0.4	0	8	2.8	13.6	0.8
BRANDY	162	0	0	0	0	0	0
MUSHROOM SAUCE	84	1.2	0	12	7.2	15.6	4.8
APPLE	73	0.4	0	1	0.3	19	1.1
WILD RICE	464	0	0	16	16	96	16
Totals Per Serving:	**412**	**11.9**	**101**	**115**	**30.6**	**36.1**	**5.7**

VEAL CHILI
2 servings (30 mcgs of VITAMIN K per serving)

1	tbsp	Canola oil, treated (See Dietary Tip # 10)
1/2	cup	Onion, diced
1/2	each	Jalapeno pepper, minced
1/2	lb	Veal, lean, ground
1 1/2	cups	Tomatoes canned with liquid, chopped
1/2	cup	Tomato sauce
1	tbsp	Chili powder
1	tsp	Mustard, powdered
1/4	tsp	Ground black pepper
1/4	tsp	Basil, fresh, minced
1/4	tsp	Oregano leaves, fresh, minced
4	oz	Kidney beans, canned, low-salt, drained
2	tbsp	Dry white wine
1	tsp	Lemon juice

Sauté the onion and jalapeno pepper, in the Canola oil, over medium heat for about 2 minutes.

Add the veal and cook for 5-7 minutes until the pink color is gone.

Add the tomatoes with their liquid, tomato sauce and seasonings. Stir to combine. Reduce the heat to low and let simmer until flavors blend, about 5 minutes.

Add the remaining ingredients and stir to combine. Cook 15 minutes longer. Serve.

Ingredient	Cal	Fat	Chol	Sod	Prot	Carb	Fiber
OIL	126	14	0	0	0	0	0
ONION, DICED	32	0	0	0	0.8	6.8	1.2
JALAPENO PEPPER	4	0	0	0	0	1	0.5
VEAL	256	8	192	192	48	0	0
TOMATOES	60	0	0	504	0	12	0
TOMATO SAUCE	44	0	0	660	2	8.8	0
CHILI POWDER	16	0	0	0	0	0	0
MUSTARD	19	0	0	0	0	0	0
BLACK PEPPER	1	0	0	0	0.1	0.4	0.1
BASIL	0	0	0	0	0	0	0
OREGANO	0	0	0	0	0	0	0
KIDNEY BEANS	132	2	0	328	8	24	4.8
DRY WHITE WINE	22	0	0	1	0	0.7	0
LEMON JUICE	1	0	0	0	0.2	0.3	0
Totals Per Serving:	354	12	96	843	29.5	27	3.3

VEAL PICCATA
4 servings (Less than 1 mcg of VITAMIN K per serving)

1/4	cup	All purpose flour
1	lb	Veal, leg, lean, sliced very thin and cut into 3x4 inch pieces (cutlet)
1/4	cup	Olive oil, treated (See Dietary Tip # 10)
2	tbsp	Butter
2	tbsp	Lemon juice
1/4	cup	Dry white wine
		Lemon slices
1/4	tsp	Ground black pepper

Lightly flour the veal on both sides. Shake off the excess.

In a large heavy skillet, heat the oil and butter. When bubbling, add the veal and sauté about 2 minutes on each side. When the veal is nearly cooked, sprinkle with lemon juice.

Remove the veal from the pan and keep it warm.

Add wine to the pan and deglaze over high heat, stirring constantly. Reduce the liquid to about 3 tablespoons. Pour the sauce over the veal.

Lemon slices - Slice the lemon to paper thinness and put a slice on each veal scallop. Sprinkle with pepper and serve.

Ingredient	Cal	Fat	Chol	Sod	Prot	Carb	Fiber
FLOUR	100	0.4	0	0	2.8	22	0
VEAL	480	0	352	288	96	0	0
OIL	502	56	0	0	0	0	0
BUTTER	200	23	70	180	0	0	0
LEMON JUICE	6	0	0	0	1	2	0
DRY WHITE WINE	44	0	0	2	0	1.4	0
LEMON SLICES	0	0	0	0	0	0	0
BLACK PEPPER	1	0	0	0	0.1	0.4	0.1
Totals Per Serving:	**328**	**19.9**	**106**	**118**	**25**	**6.4**	**0**

VEAL SCALOPPINI
6 servings (1 mcg of VITAMIN K per serving)

1 1/2	lb	Veal steak, 1/2 inch thick, fat removed
1/4	cup	All purpose flour
1/4	cup	Olive oil, treated (See Dietary Tip # 10)
1/2	cup	Onion, sliced thin
1	each	Bell pepper, green, cut in strips
1 1/2	cups	Chicken broth
1/4	lb	Mushrooms
1	tbsp	Butter

MARINADE/SAUCE

1	tsp	Paprika
1/2	cup	Olive oil, treated (See Dietary Tip # 10)
1/4	cup	Lemon juice
1	tsp	Garlic cloves, split
1	tsp	Mustard
1/4	tsp	Nutmeg, ground
1/2	tsp	Sugar

In a sauce pan, combine all the sauce ingredients and bring to a boil.

Pound the veal with a meat hammer to 1/4 inch thick and lay flat in a baking dish. Pour the sauce over the veal and turn to coat thoroughly. Let stand 15 minutes. Discard garlic.

Remove the veal from the sauce and dredge in the flour.

Brown the veal in hot oil in a heavy skillet. Add the onion and green pepper.

Combine the chicken broth with the sauce and pour over the veal.

Cover the baking dish and cook slowly in the oven, preheated to 350 degrees Fahrenheit, until veal is very tender, about 40 minutes.

Clean and slice the mushrooms. Brown lightly in butter.

Place the mushrooms on the veal and ladle the sauce over the top. Cook 5 minutes more. May be served over noodles.

Ingredient	Cal	Fat	Chol	Sod	Prot	Carb	Fiber
VEAL STEAK	744	16.8	528	528	136.8	0	0
FLOUR	100	0.4	0	0	2.8	22	0
OIL	480	54.4	0	0	0	0	0
ONION	44	0	0	4	1.2	9.6	20
BELL PEPPER	7	0	0	0	0.1	0.1	0.1
CHICKEN BROTH	48	0	0	1980	2.4	8.4	0
MUSHROOMS	28	0.4	0	4	2.4	5.2	1.6
BUTTER	100	11.5	35	90	0	0	0
MARINADE/SAUCE							
PAPRIKA	6	0.3	0	1	0.3	1.2	0.4
OIL	960	108.8	0	0	0	0	0
LEMON JUICE	12	0	0	0	2	4	0
GARLIC	0	0	0	0	0	0	0
MUSTARD	3	0.2	0	60	0.3	0.3	0
NUTMEG	3	0.2	0	0	0	0.3	0.1
SUGAR	8	0	0	0	0	2.1	0
Totals Per Serving:	**424**	**32**	**94**	**445**	**24.7**	**8.9**	**3.7**

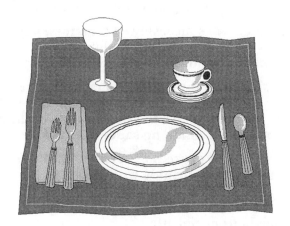

STEAK PARMIGIANA
6 servings (8 mcgs of VITAMIN K per serving)

1 1/2	lb	Steak, top round,1/2 inch thick, fat removed
1/3	cup	Bread crumbs, dry, plain,
1 1/2	oz	Parmesan cheese, grated
1	each	Egg, beaten
1/3	cup	Canola oil, treated (See Dietary Tip # 10)
1	cup	Onion, chopped
8	oz	Tomato sauce
16	oz	Tomatoes, stewed, 'No Salt Added'
1/4	tsp	Ground black pepper
1	tsp	Basil, fresh, minced
1/2	tsp	Oregano leaves, fresh, minced
6	oz	Mozzarella cheese, grated (about 1 1/2 cups)

Trim the excess fat from the steak and cut it into 6 pieces. Pound each piece with a heavy mallet to 1/4-inch thickness.

Combine the bread crumbs and Parmesan cheese. Dip each piece of meat into the beaten egg and then in the crumb mixture.

Heat the oil in a large skillet, brown the steak well on both sides. Remove the steak to paper towels to drain.

Add the onion, tomato sauce, stewed tomatoes, pepper, basil and oregano to the skillet, stir to combine. Bring the mixture to a boil, lower the heat and simmer, uncovered, for 30 minutes.

Spoon 5 tablespoons of the cooked tomato mixture into the bottom of a 13x9x2 inch baking dish (enough to lightly cover the bottom of the dish). Place the steak on top of the sauce in a single layer, pour the remaining sauce over the steak.

Bake in preheated 350 degrees Fahrenheit oven for 1 hour. Remove from oven and sprinkle with cheese.

Bake 15 minutes longer, or until cheese is melted.

Serve with spaghetti or polenta.

Remember to add the spaghetti or polenta to the nutrition totals. The spaghetti will have a negligible effect on the vitamin K content per serving. The polenta will add less than 7 mcgs of vitamin K per serving.

Ingredient	Cal	Fat	Chol	Sod	Prot	Carb	Fiber
STEAK, TOP ROUND	1344	33.6	624	288	240	0	0
BREAD CRUMBS	141	1.9	0	309	4	25.6	1.3
PARMESAN CHEESE	166	11.3	36	681	15.2	1.4	0
EGG, BEATEN	75	5.6	213	63	6.3	0.6	0
OIL	669	74.7	0	0	0	0	0
ONION	64	0	0	0	1.6	13.6	2.4
TOMATO SAUCE	88	0	0	1320	4	17.6	0
TOMATOES	128	0	0	1008	0	32	0
BLACK PEPPER	1	0	0	0	0.1	0.4	0.1
BASIL	0	0	0	0	0	0	0
OREGANO	1	0	0	0	0	0	0
MOZZARELLA	540	42	120	1140	36	6	0
Totals Per Serving:	**532**	**28.2**	**166**	**802**	**51.2**	**16.2**	**0.6**

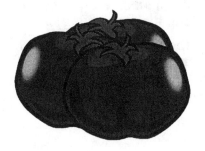

VEAL SALTIMBOCCA A LA ROMANA
6 servings (Less than 1 mcg of VITAMIN K per serving)

3 1/2	lb	Veal steak, cut 1/2 inch thick
1/2	tsp	Sage, fresh, chopped
1/2	tsp	Black pepper, freshly ground
1/4	lb	Prosciutto ham, sliced paper-thin*
4	tbsp	Butter
2	tbsp	Olive oil, treated (See Dietary Tip # 10)
3	tbsp	All purpose flour
3/4	cup	Marsala wine

*Smoked or boiled ham may be used if prosciutto is unavailable.

Preheat the oven to 325 degrees Fahrenheit.

Bone and trim the fat from the meat. Pound with a meat mallet to 1/8 inch thickness. Rub the meat on one side with the sage and pepper. Cut it into 4 to 5 inch squares. Lay the ham over the seasoned side of the veal pieces. Carefully roll up each piece and secure with wooden toothpicks.

Heat the butter and oil together in a large skillet over high heat.

Brown the veal rolls on all sides. Remove to a 13 1/2 inch by 9 inch by 2 inch baking dish, reserving the pan drippings.

Stir the flour into the drippings. Stir in 1-1/2 cups water and the Marsala and bring to a boil. Pour over the veal rolls. Cover the baking dish with aluminum foil and bake in preheated oven for 35 minutes or until tender.

Serve.

Ingredient	Cal	Fat	Chol	Sod	Prot	Carb	Fiber
VEAL STEAK	1736	39.2	1232	1232	319.2	0	0
SAGE, FRESH	1	0	0	0	0	0	0
BLACK PEPPER	3	0.1	0	1	0.1	0.7	0.2
PROSCIUTTO HAM	184	9.6	60	1448	20.8	2.8	0
BUTTER	400	46	140	360	0	0	0
OIL	251	28	0	0	0	0	0
FLOUR	75	0.3	0	0	2.1	16.5	0
MARSALA WINE	60	0	0	6	0	6	0
Totals Per Serving:	450	20.5	239	508	57	4.3	0

ITALIAN MEAT LOAF
4 servings (5 mcg of VITAMIN K per serving)

1 1/4	lb	Beef, lean, ground
1	each	Egg, beaten
1/4	cup	Tomato sauce or tomato puree
6	tbsp	Bread crumbs, soft
1/2	tsp	Oregano leaves, fresh, minced
1	tsp	Garlic cloves, crushed
1/4	tsp	Ground black pepper
2 1/2	oz	Salami, chopped
3	oz	Mozzarella cheese, nonfat, chopped

Preheat the oven to 350 degrees Fahrenheit.

In a bowl, combine the egg, tomato sauce, bread crumbs, oregano, garlic and pepper.

Add the ground beef. Mix well.

Place the meat on a sheet of aluminum foil. Shape it into a 7x9 inch rectangle. Evenly sprinkle the salami over the top. Sprinkle the cheese over the salami, leaving a narrow margin around the edges. Beginning from the 7 inch end, roll the meat, jelly roll fashion, using the foil to help you roll. Press to seal the edges. Discard the foil.

Place the loaf seam side down in a greased baking pan. Bake at 350 degree Fahrenheit for 1 hour or until done. Drain fat. Slice. Serve immediately.

Ingredient	Cal	Fat	Chol	Sod	Prot	Carb	Fiber
BEEF GROUND	1320	100	400	380	100	0	0
EGG, BEATEN	75	5.6	213	63	6.3	0.6	0
TOMATO SAUCE	22	0	0	330	1	4.4	0
BREAD CRUMBS	159	2.1	0	348	4.5	3	0
OREGANO	1	0	0	0	0	0	0
GARLIC	4	0	0	2	0.2	1	0
BLACK PEPPER	1	0	0	0	0.1	0.4	0.1
SALAMI	175	15	0	950	10	2.5	0
MOZZARELLA	120	0	15	600	24	3	0
Totals Per Serving:	469	30.7	157	668	36.5	3.7	0

UPSIDE DOWN PIZZA
8 servings (5 mcgs of VITAMIN K per serving)

FILLING
1 1/2	lb	Beef, lean, ground
1	cup	Onion, chopped
1	cup	Bell pepper, green, chopped
1	tsp	Garlic cloves, minced
1/2	tsp	Oregano leaves, fresh, minced
1/2	cup	Water
1/8	tsp	Hot pepper sauce
1	pkg	Spaghetti sauce mix (1.5 oz.)

BATTER
1	cup	Milk, skim
1	cup	All purpose flour
1/2	tsp	Salt
1	tbsp	Olive or Canola oil, treated (See Dietary Tip # 10)
2	each	Eggs

MISCELLANEOUS
7	oz	Cheese, Mozzarella or Monterey Jack, slices
1/2	cup	Parmesan cheese, grated

Pre- the heat oven to 400 degrees Fahrenheit

FILLING

In a large skillet, brown the beef and drain. Stir in the onion, green pepper, garlic, oregano, water, hot pepper sauce, tomato sauce and sauce mix. Simmer about 10 minutes stirring occasionally.

BATTER

In a bowl, combine the milk, oil and eggs, beat 1 minute on medium speed. Add the flour and salt, beat 2 minutes or until smooth.

ASSEMBLY

Pour the hot meat mixture into a 13x9 inch pan and top with the cheese slices. Pour the batter over the cheese, covering the filling completely. Sprinkle with Parmesan cheese. Bake at 400 degrees Fahrenheit for 25-30 minutes or until puffed and brown. To serve, cut in squares and lift out with a spatula.

Ingredient	Cal	Fat	Chol	Sod	Prot	Carb	Fiber
FILLING							
BEEF GROUND	1584	120	480	456	120	0	0
ONION	64	0	0	0	1.6	13.6	2.4
BELL PEPPER	56	0	0	0	0.8	0.8	0.8
GARLIC	7	0.4	0	5	0.1	1.3	0.8
OREGANO	1	0	0	0	0	0	0
HOT PEPPER SAUCE	1	0	0	0	0	0.2	0
SPAG SAUCE MIX	22	0.1	0	0	0.6	4	0.1
BATTER							
MILK, SKIM	88	0.8	8	128	8	12	0
FLOUR	400	1.6	0	0	11.2	88	0
OIL	126	14	0	0	0	0	0
EGGS	150	11.2	426	126	12.6	1.2	0
SALT	0	0	0	1150	0	0	0
MISCELLANEOUS							
MOZZARELLA	630	49	175	1260	42	7	0
PARMESAN	164	11.2	32	680	15.2	1.6	0
Totals Per Serving:	**411**	**26**	**140**	**475**	**26.5**	**16.2**	**0.5**

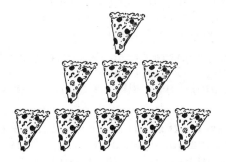

GARLIC MEATBALLS
4 servings (6 mcgs of VITAMIN K per serving)

1 1/2	cups	Onion
2	tbsp	Butter
1	lb	Beef, lean, ground
3	tsp	Garlic cloves, minced
1	cup	Bread crumbs, dry, plain
1/4	tsp	Ground black pepper
1	tbsp	Olive oil, treated (See Dietary Tip # 10)
2	cups	Tomato juice, canned, with out salt
2	tsp	Lemon juice
2	tsp	Sugar
1	tbsp	Cornstarch
2	tbsp	Cold water

Mince 1/2 cup of onion and reserve. Slice the remaining onion.

In a large skillet, melt the butter. Add the sliced onion and cook over medium heat, stirring often, until golden brown, about 8 minutes. Transfer to a plate and set the skillet aside.

In a medium bowl, combine the beef, minced onion, garlic, bread crumbs and pepper. Using about 2 tablespoons for each, form into 12 large meatballs.

In the same skillet the onions were cooked in, heat the oil. Add the meatballs and cook over medium high heat, turning often, until browned all over, about 8 minutes.

Return the cooked onions to the skillet. Stir in the tomato juice, lemon juice, and sugar. Bring to a boil, reduce the heat to low, cover and simmer until meatballs are cooked through, about 10 minutes.

In a small bowl dissolve the cornstarch in 2 tablespoons cold water. Stir into the tomato sauce and cook, stirring, until thickened, about 1 minute. (If your tomato juice is very thick, you may not need to do this last step.)

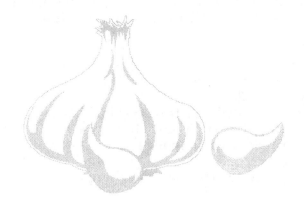

Ingredient	Cal	Fat	Chol	Sod	Prot	Carb	Fiber
ONION	132	0	0	12	3.6	28.8	60
BUTTER	200	23	70	180	0	0	0
BEEF	1056	80	320	304	80	0	0
GARLIC CLOVE	12	0.1	0	6	0.5	3	0
BREAD CRUMBS	424	5.6	0	928	12	76.8	4
BLACK PEPPER	1	0	0	0	0.1	0.4	0.1
OLIVE OIL	119	13.5	0	0	0	0	0
TOMATO JUICE	80	0	0	48	0	16	0
LEMON JUICE	2	0	0	0	0.3	0.7	0
SUGAR	32	0	0	0	0	8.3	0
CORNSTARCH	54	0	0	2	0.1	13	0.2
Totals Per Serving:	**528**	**30.5**	**98**	**370**	**24**	**36.7**	**16.1**

VEAL OSCAR WITH SHRIMP

1 serving (20 mcgs of VITAMIN K per serving with asparagus. Less than 1 mcg of VITAMIN K per serving without asparagus)

3	oz	Veal cutlet
1/4	tsp	Ground black pepper
1	tsp	All purpose flour
1	tsp	Olive oil, treated (See Dietary Tip # 10)
1/4	cup	BEARNAISE SAUCE OR HOLLANDAISE SAUCE, (See Recipe Index.)
2	each	asparagus spears
1/2	cup	Shrimp, peeled, deveined and chopped
1/4	cup	Mushrooms, sliced
1/4	cup	Onion, chopped

Season the veal with the pepper, dust with the flour and sauté 2-3 minutes on both sides. Place the veal on a plate and cover with the Béarnaise or Hollandaise sauce.

Place 2 asparagus spears on top of the veal one inch apart and fill the space with shrimp mixture.

SHRIMP MIXTURE: Sauté the onions and mushrooms in butter until tender, add the shrimp, sauté 5 more minutes, season to taste.

You can also use crab instead of shrimp

Ingredient	Cal	Fat	Chol	Sod	Prot	Carb	Fiber
VEAL CUTLET	90	1.5	66	54	18	0	0
BLACK PEPPER	1	0	0	0	0.1	0.4	0.1
FLOUR	8	0	0	0	0.2	1.8	0
OIL	40	4.5	0	0	0	0	0
BEARNAISE SAUCE	316	186	32	260	7.2	5.8	0.4
ASPARAGUS SPEARS	14	0	0	2	2	2	2
SHRIMP	76	1.2	112	108	14.4	0.8	0
MUSHROOMS	14	0	0	2	1.2	2.6	0.8
ONION	16	0	0	0	0.4	3.4	0.6
Totals Per Serving:	**575**	**193.3**	**210**	**426**	**43.5**	**16.8**	**3.9**

OVEN-BAKED BOURGUIGNONNE
8 servings (5 mcg of VITAMIN K per serving)

2	lb	Beef chuck, boneless, fat removed, cut into 1 inch cubes
1/4	cup	All purpose flour
1 1/3	cups	Carrots, peeled and sliced
14 1/2 oz		Tomatoes, canned, peeled tomatoes, undrained and chopped or use crushed tomatoes
1	each	Bay leaf
1	pkg	Onion Soup Mix
1/2	cup	Red wine
8	oz	Mushrooms, whole
1	cup	Rice, white uncooked*

*OR 8 ounces of medium or broad egg noodles.

In a 2-quart casserole, toss the beef with the flour. Add the carrots, tomatoes, bay leaf, and mushrooms then add the onion soup mix blended with the wine.

Cook at 250 degrees Fahrenheit for 7 hours or until the beef is tender. Remove the bay leaf.

Meanwhile, cook the rice or noodles according to the package directions. To serve, arrange the Bourguignonne over the rice or noodles.

Ingredient	Cal	Fat	Chol	Sod	Prot	Carb	Fiber
BEEF CHUCK	2112	96	896	576	284.8	0	0
FLOUR	100	0.4	0	0	2.8	22	0
CARROTS	64	1.1	0	53	1.1	16	1.1
TOMATOES	72	0	0	609	0	14.5	0
BAY LEAF	0	0	0	0	0	0	0
ONION SOUP MIX	75	1	0	2469	2	17	2
RED WINE	88	0	0	4	0	0.4	0
MUSHROOMS	56	0.8	0	8	4.8	10.4	3.2
RICE	824	1.6	0	8	16	181.6	2.4
Totals Per Serving:	**424**	**12.6**	**112**	**466**	**38.9**	**32.7**	**1.1**

POULTRY

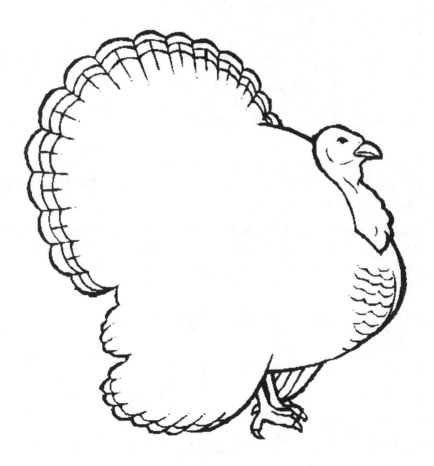

CHICKEN RAGOUT
6 servings (VITAMIN K content = 5 mcg per cup)

2 1/2	lb	Chicken, skinless pieces, fat removed
1	tsp	Garlic cloves, minced
1/2	cup	Onion, diced
2	cups	Tomato, chopped
1	tsp	Parsley, fresh, chopped
1/4	cup	Celery, diced
2	cups	Potato, peeled and diced
1	cup	Carrots, peeled and diced
1/2	tsp	Ground black pepper
1	cup	Water

Combine the chicken, tomatoes, parsley, water, onion, garlic and pepper in a large pan and cook on low heat for 30 minutes.

Remove the chicken.

Add the potatoes, celery, and carrots and cook until vegetables are at desired tenderness (approximately 10 to 15 minutes).

Add the chicken back to the pan. Heat and serve.

Ingredient	Cal	Fat	Chol	Sod	Prot	Carb	Fiber
CHICKEN	1360	40	800	880	240	0	0
GARLIC	4	0	0	2	1	1	0
ONION, DICED	32	0	0	0	0.8	6.8	1.2
TOMATO	80	1.6	0	32	3.2	16	4.8
PARSLEY, FRESH	1	0	0	1	0	0.1	0
CELERY, DICED	4	0	0	26	0.2	1.2	0.2
POTATO	240	0	0	16	6.4	54.4	4.8
CARROTS	48	0.8	0	40	0.8	12	0.8
BLACK PEPPER	3	0.1	0	1	0.1	0.7	0.2
Totals Per Serving:	295	7.1	133	166	41.9	15.4	2

CHICKEN-FILLED TORTILLAS

5 servings (VITAMIN K content = 9 mcg per cup of chicken mixture with cheese. Tortillas contain negligible amounts of VITAMIN K)

1	tbsp	Canola oil or olive oil, treated (See Dietary Tip # 10)
1 1/2	lb	Chicken, lean, ground
1/2	cup	Onion, chopped
4	oz	Cheese, Mozzarella or Cheddar, grated
1/2	cup	Tomato, finely chopped
1	tsp	Garlic cloves, minced
1	cup	Bell pepper, green, chopped

Sauté the chicken in the Canola oil on low heat until the chicken is white.

Add the vegetables and garlic to the skillet and cook until vegetables are tender. Allow to cool a little, then mix in the cheese.

Serve on flour tortillas (can be corn or white flour tortillas.)

Remember to add the nutrition values of the tortillas to your per serving total.

Ingredient	Cal	Fat	Chol	Sod	Prot	Carb	Fiber
OIL	120	14	0	0	0	0	0
CHICKEN	1008	48	432	528	144	0	0
ONION	32	0	0	0	0.8	6.8	1.2
CHEESE,	360	28	100	720	24	4	0
TOMATO	20	0.4	0	8	0.8	4	1.2
GARLIC CLOVE	4	0	0	2	0.2	1	0
BELL PEPPER	56	0	0	0	0.8	0.8	0.8
Totals Per Serving:	320	18.1	106	252	34.1	3.3	0.6

CROCKPOT BAKED CHICKEN BREASTS
4 servings (4 mcgs of VITAMIN K per serving)

1 1/2	lb	Chicken breast, skinless (at least 4 pieces)
2	tsp	Butter
1	can	Cream of Chicken soup, lowfat
1/2	cup	Dry sherry
1	tsp	Rosemary, fresh, minced
1	tsp	Worcestershire Sauce
1/4	tsp	Garlic powder
4	oz	Mushrooms, sliced

Put the chicken breasts in the bottom of a crock pot.

In a bowl, mix the other ingredients and then pour over the chicken.

Cover and cook on low 5-7 hours. Serve over rice or baked potatoes.

Ingredient	Cal	Fat	Chol	Sod	Prot	Carb	Fiber
CHICKEN BREAST	744	0	384	432	168	0	0
BUTTER	67	7.7	23	60	0	0	0
CHICKEN SOUP	20	0.8	3	208	0.9	2.5	0.9
DRY SHERRY	120	0	0	0	0	2	0
ROSEMARY	1	0	0	0	0	0	0
WORCESTERSHIRE	3	0	0	67	0	0.7	0
GARLIC POWDER	2	0	0	0	0.1	0.5	0
MUSHROOMS	28	0.4	0	4	2.4	5.2	1.6
Totals Per Serving:	**246**	**2.2**	**103**	**193**	**42.9**	**2.7**	**0.6**

JAMAICAN JERK CHICKEN
8 servings (VITAMIN K content = 10 mcg per cup)

3	lb	Chicken pieces, skinless, boneless
3/4	tsp	Cinnamon, ground
2	tsp	Ground black pepper
1	tbsp	Jalapeno pepper
1	tsp	Oregano leaves, fresh, minced
1	tsp	Thyme leaves, fresh, minced
6	tsp	Garlic cloves, minced
1	cup	Onion, chopped
1/4	cup	Vinegar
4	tbsp	Brown sugar

Place all the ingredients in a large bowl and mix. Marinate in the refrigerator for at least 6 hours.

Place all the ingredients in a baking pan and bake covered for 20 minutes and then 20 to 40 minutes uncovered until the chicken is cooked and tender.

Ingredient	Cal	Fat	Chol	Sod	Prot	Carb	Fiber
CHICKEN	1632	48	960	1056	288	0	0
CINNAMON	5	0.8	0	1	0.1	1.3	0.5
BLACK PEPPER	10	0.2	0	2	0.4	2.8	0.8
JALAPENO PEPPER	4	0	0	0	0	1	0.5
OREGANO LEAVES	1	0	0	1	0	0	0
THYME LEAVES	1	0	0	0	0	0	0
GARLIC CLOVE	24	0.1	0	12	0.9	6	0
ONION	64	0	0	0	1.6	13.6	2.4
VINEGAR	8	0	0	12	0	0	0
SUGAR	206	0	0	0	0	53.4	0
Totals Per Serving:	244	6.1	120	136	36.4	9.8	0.5

QUICK CHICKEN CREOLE

3 to 4 servings (VITAMIN K content of recipe without rice =
16 mcg per cup. The rice contains an insignificant amount of
VITAMIN K when cooked.)

1	lb	Chicken breast, skinless, boneless, cut into small chunks
14	oz	Tomatoes, canned 'no salt added' plus juice
1	cup	Bell pepper, green, chopped
1/2	cup	Celery, chopped
1/2	cup	Onion, chopped
2	tsp	Garlic cloves, minced
1	tsp	Basil, fresh, minced
1	tsp	Crushed dried red pepper
1/2	tsp	Chili powder
1	tsp	Canola oil, treated (See Dietary Tip # 10)

Cook the chicken using the teaspoon of oil in a hot skillet,
turning often so that the chicken is not burned. Cook the
chicken in this way until it is fully cooked.

Remove the chicken from the pan and keep it warm. Add the
remaining ingredients, bring to a boil, then cook on low heat
for 20 to 30 minutes.

Add the chicken back to the pan. Heat.

Best served on white rice.

Ingredient	Cal	Fat	Chol	Sod	Prot	Carb	Fiber
CHICKEN BREAST	496	0	256	288	112	0	0
TOMATOES	126	0	0	70	4.2	28	0
BELL PEPPER	56	0	0	0	0.8	0.8	0.8
CELERY	8	0	0	52	0.4	2.4	0.4
ONION	32	0	0	0	0.8	6.8	1.2
GARLIC CLOVE	8	0	0	4	0.3	2	0
BASIL	0	0	0	0	0	0	0
DRIED RED PEPPER	6	0.3	0	1	0	0.1	0
CHILI POWDER	3	0	0	0	0	0	0
OIL	40	4.5	0	0	0	0	0
Totals Per Serving:	**194**	**1.2**	**64**	**104**	**31.4**	**10.6**	**0.6**

CHICKEN GUMBO
4 to 6 servings (VITAMIN K content = 29 mcg per cup)

1 1/2	lb	Chicken, skinless, boneless pieces
3	cups	Water
1	tsp	Canola oil, treated (See Dietary Tip # 10)
1/4	cup	All purpose flour
1	cup	Potatoes, peeled and chopped
1	cup	Onion, chopped
2	cups	Carrots, peeled and chopped
1	cup	Celery, chopped
4	tsp	Garlic cloves, minced
1/2	cup	Green onions, chopped
1/2	tsp	Thyme leaves, fresh
1	tsp	Ground black pepper
1	cup	Okra, sliced, fresh or frozen

Place the oil and flour in a large pot and heat the mixture until the flour is golden brown.

Stir in the water. Add the remaining ingredients except the okra and bring to a boil. Cook on low heat for 30 minutes.

Add the okra and cook on low heat for 15 more minutes or until okra is the desired tenderness.

Ingredient	Cal	Fat	Chol	Sod	Prot	Carb	Fiber
CHICKEN	816	24	480	528	144	0	0
OIL	40	4.7	0	0	0	0	0
FLOUR	100	0.4	0	0	2.8	22	0
POTATOES	120	0	0	8	3.2	32	2.4
ONION	64	0	0	0	1.6	13.6	2.4
CARROTS	96	1.6	0	80	1.6	24	1.6
CELERY	16	0	0	104	0.8	4.8	0.8
GARLIC	16	.1	0	8	0.6	4	0
GREEN ONIONS	36	0	0	20	4	8	4
THYME LEAVES	0	0	0	0	0	0	0
BLACK PEPPER	5	0.1	0	1	0.2	1.4	0.4
OKRA	96	0.8	0	16	4.8	17.6	2.4
Totals Per Serving:	**351**	**7.9**	**120**	**191**	**40.9**	**31.9**	**3.5**

SAUCY HAM AND CHICKEN
8 servings (15 mcgs of VITAMIN K per serving)

8	lb	Broiler chickens, cut up (2 or 3 chickens)
2	tsp	Canola oil, treated (See Dietary Tip # 10)
1	cup	Ham, fully cooked, in strips
1 1/2	cups	Onion, quartered (about 1 1/2 medium onions)
10	oz	Tomato (about 1 1/4 cups or 2 medium tomatoes)
2	cups	CHEDDAR CHEESE SAUCE (See Recipe Index)
1	tsp	Basil, fresh, minced
1/8	tsp	Ground black pepper

Remove the chicken skin and any visible fat.

Brown the chicken on all sides in hot oil, drain. Transfer to a crock pot.

Layer the ham on top of the chicken.

Chop one tomato, combine with the cheddar cheese sauce and basil, pour the sauce over the meat.

Cover and cook on low 6-8 hours (or high 3-4 hours).

Garnish with tomato wedges (from the remaining tomato) and serve.

Ingredient	Cal	Fat	Chol	Sod	Prot	Carb	Fiber
CHICKEN	4352	128	2560	2816	768	0	0
OIL	80	9	0	0	0	0	0
HAM	296	11.2	104	2896	44	2.4	0
ONION	132	0	0	12	3.6	28.8	60
TOMATO	60	0	0	30	0	10	0
CHEESE SAUCE	768	56	192	1600	33.6	38.4	0
BASIL	0	0	0	0	0	0	0
PEPPER, BLACK	1	0	0	0	0	0.2	0
Totals Per Serving:	356	12.8	179	460	53.1	5	3.8

RASPBERRY CHICKEN BREASTS
4 servings (2 mcgs of VITAMIN K per serving)

1 1/2	lb	Chicken breast, skinless, boneless (4 pieces)
2	tbsp	Butter
1/4	cup	Raspberry preserves, seedless
2	tbsp	Balsamic vinegar

Sauté the chicken breast in butter until just barely done. Slide the chicken to the side of the skillet.

Add the jam and vinegar, stir until the jam is melted and mixed with the vinegar, toss the chicken in the mixture to coat.

Serve chicken with the sauce poured over the top.

Ingredient	Cal	Fat	Chol	Sod	Prot	Carb	Fiber
CHICKEN	744	0	384	432	168	0	0
BUTTER	200	23	70	180	0	0	0
PRESERVES	216	0	0	30	0	48	0
BALSAMIC VINEGAR	4	0	0	6	0	0	0
Totals Per Serving:	291	5.8	114	162	42	12	0

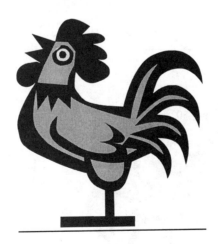

LEMON ONION CHICKEN
4 servings (VITAMIN K content = less than 1 mcg per cup)

1 1/2	lb	Boneless, skinless chicken
1/2	cup	Lemon juice
2	tbsp	Vinegar
1/2	cup	Lemon peel, fresh minced
1	tsp	Oregano leaves, fresh, minced
3/4	cup	Onion, chopped

Put all the ingredients into a baking dish and marinate for a few hours.

Bake at 400 degrees Fahrenheit until the chicken is cooked. About 20 to 30 minutes depending on the thickness of the chicken pieces.

Ingredient	Cal	Fat	Chol	Sod	Prot	Carb	Fiber
CHICKEN	816	24	480	528	144	0	0
LEMON JUICE	24	0	0	0	4	8	0
VINEGAR	4	0	0	6	0	0	0
LEMON PEEL	88	1.2	0	8	4.8	34.8	0
OREGANO	1	0	0	1	0	0	0
ONION	48	0	0	0	1.2	10.2	1.8
Totals Per Serving:	**245**	**6.3**	**120**	**136**	**38.5**	**13.3**	**0.5**

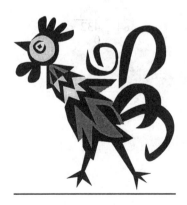

CHICKEN BREASTS DIANE
4 servings (24 mcgs of VITAMIN K per serving)

1 1/2	lb	Chicken breast, skinless, boneless
2	tbsp	Olive oil, treated (See Dietary Tip # 10)
1/2	tsp	Ground black pepper
2	tbsp	Butter
3	tbsp	Chives or green onions, fresh
1 1/2	tbsp	Lime or lemon juice
2	tbsp	Brandy or cognac
2	tsp	Dijon mustard
1/4	cup	Chicken broth

Place the chicken breast halves between sheets of waxed paper or plastic wrap. Pound slightly with a mallet to even out the thickness of each piece. Sprinkle with pepper.

Heat 1 tablespoon each of oil and butter in a large skillet. Cook the chicken over high heat for 2 minutes on each side. Do not cook longer or they will be overcooked and dry. Transfer the chicken to a warm serving platter and keep it warm.

Add the chives or green onions, lime juice, brandy and mustard to the pan. Cook 15 seconds, whisking constantly. Whisk in the broth. Stir until the sauce is smooth. Whisk in the remaining butter and oil.

Pour the sauce over the chicken. Serve immediately.

Ingredient	Cal	Fat	Chol	Sod	Prot	Carb	Fiber
CHICKEN BREAST	744	0	384	432	168	0	0
OIL	238	27	0	0	0	0	0
BLACK PEPPER	3	0.1	0	1	0.1	0.7	0.2
BUTTER	200	23	70	180	0	0	0
CHIVES	14	0	0	2	1.5	1.5	1.5
LIME JUICE	16	0.2	0	2	0.9	6.5	0
BRANDY	60	1.2	0	2	4.5	18	2.5
DIJON MUSTARD	10	0	0	240	0	0.3	0
CHICKEN BROTH	8	0	0	330	0.4	1.4	0
Totals Per Serving:	323	12.9	114	297	43.9	7.1	1.1

CHICKEN PICCATA
2 servings (1 mcgs of VITAMIN K per serving)

1	lb	Chicken breast, skinless, boneless and flattened
1/4	tsp	Ground black pepper
1 1/2	tbsp	All purpose flour
1/2	tbsp	Butter
1/2	tbsp	Olive oil, treated (See Dietary Tip # 10)
1	tsp	Garlic cloves, minced
1/4	lb	Mushrooms, sliced
1	tsp	Lemon juice
1/4	cup	Dry white wine

Dredge the chicken in the pepper and flour.

In a sauté pan, over medium heat, melt the butter with the olive oil. Add the garlic and sauté briefly.

Add the chicken breast and sauté for 1 to 2 minutes on each side and set aside.

Add the mushrooms and sauté for 1 minute.

Return the chicken to the pan and stir in the lemon juice and wine. Simmer, covered, for 5 to 10 minutes or until cooked through.

Put the chicken on a platter, spoon any remaining sauce over the chicken.

A nice touch would be to garnish with lemon slices.

Ingredient	Cal	Fat	Chol	Sod	Prot	Carb	Fiber
CHICKEN BREAST	544	16	320	352	96	0	0
BLACK PEPPER	1	0	0	0	0.1	0.4	0.1
FLOUR	38	0.2	0	0	1.1	8.3	0
BUTTER	50	5.8	18	45	0	0	0
OLIVE OIL	60	6.8	0	0	0	0	0
GARLIC CLOVE	4	0	0	2	0.2	1	0
MUSHROOMS	28	0.4	0	4	2.4	5.2	1.6
LEMON JUICE	1	0	0	0	0.2	0.3	0
DRY WHITE WINE	44	0	0	2	0	1.4	0
Totals Per Serving:	385	14.5	169	203	49.9	8.3	0.9

TURKEY SPAGHETTI SAUCE
6 servings (20 mcgs of VITAMIN K per serving)

1/4	cup	Onion, chopped
1	tsp	Garlic cloves, minced
1	tsp	Olive oil, treated (See Dietary Tip # 10)
28	oz	Tomatoes, canned, 'no salt added', cut up
6	oz	Tomato paste
1	tsp	Basil, fresh, chopped
1	tsp	Thyme leaves, fresh chopped
3	cups	Turkey, cooked, chopped
1	lb	Noodles, uncooked

Sauté the onion and garlic in the oil until lightly browned. Add the tomatoes, tomato paste, basil, thyme and turkey.

Simmer for 20 to 25 minutes while cooking the noodles.

Serve sauce over noodles.

Ingredient	Cal	Fat	Chol	Sod	Prot	Carb	Fiber
ONION	16	0	0	0	0.4	3.4	0.6
GARLIC CLOVE	4	0	0	2	0.2	1	0
OIL	40	4.5	0	0	0	0	0
TOMATOES	252	0	0	140	8.4	56	0
TOMATO PASTE	138	0	0	150	6	30	6
BASIL	0	0	0	0	0	0	0
THYME LEAVES	1	0	0	0	0	0	0
TURKEY, COOKED	624	21.6	720	600	201.6	0	0
NOODLES	1728	16	432	96	64	320	16
Totals Per Serving:	**467**	**7**	**192**	**165**	**46.8**	**68.4**	**3.8**

CHICKEN BREASTS WITH DRIED BEEF
8 servings (1 mcg of VITAMIN K per serving)

2	lb	Chicken breasts, skinless, boneless and flattened
4	oz	Dried beef slices (not cured)
8	oz	Bacon, 8 slices
1	tbsp	Canola oil, treated (See Dietary Tip # 10)
1 1/2	cups	MUSHROOM CREAM SAUCE (See Recipe Index)
1/2	cup	White wine
1	cup	Sour cream, lowfat
2	oz	Almonds, slivered (about 1/2 cup)

Place the beef slices in the flattened chicken breast and roll them into rolls. Wrap bacon slices around the chicken rolls.

Grease an an 8x12x2 inch pan with the Canola oil. Place the remaining slices of beef into the greased pan. Put the chicken rolls on top of the beef.

Mix the sour cream, white wine and mushroom sauce. Pour over chicken.

Bake at 350 degrees Fahrenheit for 1 hour uncovered. After the first 30 minutes, sprinkle the almonds on top. Finish baking.

Serve with rice, noodles or mashed potatoes.

Ingredient	Cal	Fat	Chol	Sod	Prot	Carb	Fiber
CHICKEN	992	0	512	576	224	0	0
DRIED BEEF SLICES	320	40	96	76	33.6	0	0
BACON, 8 SLICES	1264	128	152	1656	16	0	0
CANOLA OIL	120	14	0	0	0	0	0
MUSHROOM SAUCE	84	1.2	0	12	7.2	15.6	4.8
WHITE WINE	88	0	0	4	0	0.8	0
SOUR CREAM	320	16	40	280	16	32	0
ALMONDS	122	3.2	260	88	16.6	2.2	0
Totals Per Serving:	414	25.3	133	337	39.2	6.3	0.6

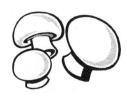

MARSALA CHICKEN BREASTS
8 servings (Less than 1 mcg of VITAMIN K per serving)

2	lb	Chicken breasts, skinless, boneless
1/4	tsp	Ground black pepper
2	tbsp	Butter
1	tbsp	Canola oil or Olive oil, treated (See Dietary Tip # 10)
1	lb	Mushrooms, halved
2	tbsp	All purpose flour
3/4	cup	Marsala wine
1/2	cup	Chicken broth
1	tsp	Garlic cloves, minced
		Lemon slices for garnish

Pepper the chicken breasts. Melt the butter in a skillet and add the oil. Sauté the chicken breasts on both sides, until browned. Remove to a platter.

Add the mushrooms to the skillet and sauté for 2 minutes. Sprinkle with the flour, blending well. Add the wine to the skillet. Stir up any browned bits in the pan into the wine. Add the garlic and chicken broth. Heat until thickened.

Cut the chicken into bite size pieces, return to the skillet and toss with the ingredients. Turn onto a serving platter and garnish with lemon slices. This is also excellent made with veal.

Ingredient	Cal	Fat	Chol	Sod	Prot	Carb	Fiber
CHICKEN	992	0	512	576	224	0	0
BLACK PEPPER	1	0	0	0	0.1	0.4	0.1
BUTTER	200	23	70	180	0	0	0
OIL	126	14	0	0	0	0	0
MUSHROOMS	112	1.6	0	16	9.6	20.8	6.4
FLOUR	50	0.2	0	0	1.4	11	0
MARSALA WINE	60	0	0	6	0	6	0
CHICKEN BROTH	16	0	0	660	0.8	2.8	0
GARLIC	4	0	0	2	0.2	1	0
LEMON SLICES	0	0	0	0	0	0	0
Totals Per Serving:	194	4.9	73	180	29.5	5.2	0.8

CHICKEN SAUTÉ BOURGUIGNONNE
6 servings (2 mcgs of VITAMIN K per serving)

3	lb	Chicken breasts, skinless, boneless, split in half
1/4	tsp	Ground black pepper
4	tbsp	Butter
1/2	lb	Mushrooms, trimmed and sliced
1/2	cup	Onion, chopped
1	each	Bay leaf
1	tsp	Garlic cloves, chopped
1/2	tsp	Thyme leaves, fresh
1	tbsp	All purpose flour
1/2	cup	Chicken broth
1	cup	Red wine, dry

Flatten the chicken breasts between waxed paper to 1/4 inch thickness. Season with pepper. Cut each cutlet into quarters.

Heat 2 tablespoons of the butter in a large heavy skillet. Cook the chicken 5 minutes or until no longer pink in center, turning over halfway through cooking.

Transfer the chicken to a platter. Add the mushrooms to the skillet, cook 2 minutes. Add the onion, shallot, bay leaf, garlic and thyme, cook and stir for 1 minute.

Sprinkle with flour, stirring to blend. Stir in the broth and wine. Simmer 2 minutes.

Whisk in the remaining butter to thicken slightly. Add the chicken to the skillet and heat through. Season with pepper.

Remove the bay leaf. Serve the chicken with the sauce poured over top.

Ingredient	Cal	Fat	Chol	Sod	Prot	Carb	Fiber
CHICKEN	1488	0	768	864	336	0	0
BLACK PEPPER	1	0	0	0	0.1	0.4	0.1
BUTTER	400	46	140	360	0	0	0
MUSHROOMS	56	0.8	0	8	4.8	10.4	3.2
ONION	32	0	0	0	0.8	6.8	1.2
BAY LEAF	0	0	0	0	0	0	0
GARLIC	4	0	0	2	.2	1	0
THYME	0	0	0	0	0	0	0
FLOUR	25	0.1	0	0	0.7	5.5	0
CHICKEN BROTH	16	0	0	660	0.8	2.8	0
RED WINE, DRY	176	0	0	8	0	0.8	0
Totals Per Serving:	**366**	**7.8**	**151**	**317**	**57.2**	**4.6**	**0.8**

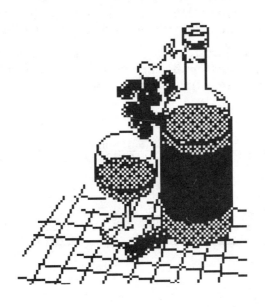

ROAST TURKEY
14 servings (2 mcgs of VITAMIN K per serving)

12	lb	Turkey*
1	tbsp	Canola oil, treated (See Dietary Tip # 10)
1/2	tsp	Ground black pepper
6	oz	Onion, peeled (about 1 medium onion)
1	each	Bay leaf
1	tsp	Thyme leaves, fresh

*Nutrition values are calculated on meat only. No skin or fat.

Preheat the oven to 350 degrees Fahrenheit. Sprinkle the turkey, inside and out, with pepper. Put the bay leaf and thyme inside the cavity. Rub the turkey all over with oil.

Put the turkey, breast side up, on a rack, in a roasting pan and arrange the onion, neck and gizzard around it. Bake for 1 hour and then cover loosely with a sheet of aluminum foil. (If there is no liquid in the pan add water or wine to make a liquid.)

Continue baking and baste at 10-minute intervals, for about 1 1/2 hours longer. Transfer the turkey to a platter and pour off the pan drippings into a strainer and remove fat. Serve with the natural juices.

Ingredient	Cal	Fat	Chol	Sod	Prot	Carb	Fiber
TURKEY	6528	192	3456	3840	1152	0	0
CANOLA OIL	120	14	0	0	0	0	0
BLACK PEPPER	3	0.1	0	1	0.1	0.7	0.2
ONION, PEELED	66	0	0	6	1.8	14.4	30
BAY LEAF	0	0	0	0	0	0	0
THYME	1	0	0	0	0	0	0
Totals Per Serving:	480	14.7	247	275	82.4	1.1	2.2

SAUTEED CHICKEN BREAST WITH MUSHROOMS
2 servings (2 mcgs of VITAMIN K per serving)

8	oz	Chicken breasts (2), boneless, skinless
1	cup	Mushrooms, quartered
4	tbsp	Butter
1/4	cup	All purpose flour for dredging
1/4	tsp	Ground black pepper
1	cup	Water
1 1/2	tbsp	Lemon juice

Pound the chicken breasts until they are thin. Dredge in the flour and shake off excess.

In a large skillet, melt the butter and add the chicken breasts. Brown lightly on both sides.

Add the mushrooms, lemon juice and pepper and toss. Add the water, reduce over high heat until sauce thickens slightly.

Remove the breasts and place on a warmed serving plate. Spoon the sauce and mushrooms over the chicken. Garnish with a twist of lemon.

Ingredient	Cal	Fat	Chol	Sod	Prot	Carb	Fiber
CHICKEN	248	0	128	144	56	0	0
MUSHROOMS	56	0.8	0	8	4.8	10.4	3.2
BUTTER	400	46	140	360	0	0	0
FLOUR	100	0.4	0	0	2.8	22	0
BLACK PEPPER	1	0	0	0	0.1	0.4	0.1
LEMON JUICE	4	0	0	0	0.8	1.5	0
Totals Per Serving:	**405**	**23.6**	**134**	**256**	**32.2**	**17.1**	**1.7**

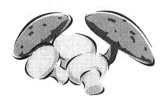

LAMB

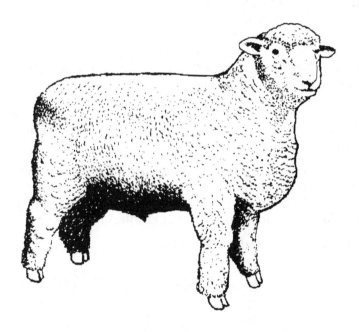

OVEN-COOKED LAMB STEW
6 servings (5 mcg of VITAMIN K per serving)

3	lb	Lamb stew meat,1 1/2 inch cubes
3	tbsp	All purpose flour
1 1/2	cups	Water
1 1/4	cups	Red wine
1/8	tsp	Pepper
1	each	Bay leaf
1	tsp	Garlic cloves, minced
3/4	cup	Onion, chopped
1/2	cup	Celery, coarse, diced
1/2	cup	Carrot, peeled and diced
1	tbsp	Canola OIL, treated (See Dietary Tip # 10)
1	cup	Tomatoes, canned

Brown the lamb in a skillet. Add the flour, water, wine and bay leaf. Bring to a boil, pour into a large casserole with a tight-fitting cover.

Sauté the garlic and vegetables in oil until limp, add them with the tomatoes to the lamb and gravy mixture. Cover the casserole and bake in a preheated 350 Fahrenheit oven for 1 1/2 hours, or until the lamb and vegetables are tender.

Remove the bay leaf before serving.

Ingredient	Cal	Fat	Chol	Sod	Prot	Carb	Fiber
LAMB	1632	43.2	912	1056	283.2	0	0
FLOUR	75	0.3	0	0	2.1	16.5	0
RED WINE	220	0	0	10	0	1	0
PEPPER	1	0	0	0	0	0.2	0
BAY LEAF	0	0	0	0	0	0	0
GARLIC	4	0	0	2	0.2	1	0
ONION	48	0	0	0	1.2	10.2	1.8
CELERY	8	0	0	52	0.4	2.4	0.4
CARROT	24	0.4	0	20	0.4	6	0.4
OIL	120	13.6	0	0	0	0	0
TOMATOES	40	0	0	336	0	8	0
Totals Per Serving:	**362**	**9.6**	**152**	**246**	**47.9**	**7.5**	**0.4**

GREEK-ROAST LEG OF LAMB
5 servings (Less than 2 mcg of VITAMIN K per serving)

6	lb	Leg of Lamb
1/2	cup	Olive oil, treated (See Dietary Tip # 10)
3	tsp	Garlic cloves, crushed
1	tsp	Oregano leaves, fresh, minced
1/8	tsp	Black pepper, freshly ground

For rare lamb, allow the lamb to come to room temperature before cooking.

Heat your oven to 400 degrees Fahrenheit.

Mix the oil, garlic and oregano together and rub the leg completely with the mixture. Season with black pepper and place on a baking rack in a pan. Insert a meat thermometer into the thickest part of the leg, being careful not to touch the bone.

Bake at 400 degrees Fahrenheit for 40 minutes so the meat can brown. Turn the oven down to 325 degrees Fahrenheit and bake for an additional 40 to 50 minutes, or until the thermometer registers 140 degrees Fahrenheit.

Remove the meat from the oven and allow it to sit 1/2 hour before slicing. It will continue to cook during this time. For medium lamb: Follow the above instructions but cook a bit longer so that the thermometer registers 145 to 150 degrees Fahrenheit.

Slice thinly and serve with some of the pan juices.

The nutrition values are calculated after all visible fat has been removed and discarded.

Ingredient	Cal	Fat	Chol	Sod	Prot	Carb	Fiber
LAMB	1824	48	864	912	288	0	0
OLIVE OIL	476	54	0	0	0	0	0
GARLIC CLOVE	12	0.1	0	6	0.5	3	0
OREGANO LEAVES	1	0	0	1	0	0	0
BLACK PEPPER	1	0	0	0	0	0.2	0
Totals Per Serving:	386	17	144	153	48.1	0.5	0

LEG OF LAMB
8 servings (2 mcgs of VITAMIN K per serving)

8	lb	Leg of lamb
2	tsp	Garlic cloves, slivered
1/4	cup	Butter
1/2	tsp	Rosemary, fresh, minced
1 1/2	tbsp	Lemon juice
12	each	Pearl onions (optional)
1/4	tsp	Ground black pepper

Peel the onions. Wash and dry the lamb. Make incisions in the roast and stuff them with slivers of garlic. Place in a roasting pan along with the pearl onions.

Melt the butter, add rosemary and the lemon juice and spread the mixture over the lamb in the roasting pan.

Bake at 325 degrees Fahrenheit for 2-1/2 to 3 hours. Serve with rice and vegetables.

Ingredient	Cal	Fat	Chol	Sod	Prot	Carb	Fiber
LAMB	2432	64	1152	1216	384	0	0
GARLIC CLOVE	8	0	0	4	0.3	2	0
BUTTER	400	46	140	360	0	0	0
ROSEMARY	0	0	0	0	0	0	0
LEMON JUICE	4	0	0	0	0.8	1.5	0
PEARL ONIONS	132	0	0	12	3.6	28.8	60
BLACK PEPPER	1	0	0	0	0.1	0.4	0.1
Totals Per Serving:	**372**	**13.8**	**162**	**199**	**48.6**	**4.1**	**7.**

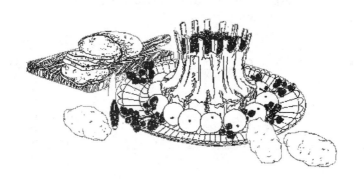

CROWN ROAST OF LAMB

6 to 8 servings (Less than 1 mcg of VITAMIN K per serving)

4	lb	Crown roast of lamb, trimmed (2 or more ribs per person, depending on size)
3	tsp	Garlic cloves peeled and cut in slivers
1/4	cup	Olive oil, treated (See Dietary Tip # 10)
2	tsp	Ground black pepper
2	lb	New potatoes, peeled (allow 2-to-3 for each diner)

Preheat the oven to 450 degrees Fahrenheit.

Make small incisions in the meaty part of the lamb every few inches and insert slivers of garlic. Paint the meat well with olive oil. Sprinkle all over with pepper.

Crumple a ball of aluminum foil and stuff in the center. Place on a small rack and surround with the potatoes in a low roasting pan just large enough to hold everything.

Place the pan in the oven and immediately turn the heat down to 400 degrees Fahrenheit. Roast until done, depending upon weight and size, about 30 minutes or until internal temperature reaches 140 degrees Fahrenheit.

Remove the foil ball. Remove the lamb to a warmed platter, and let rest 5-to-10 minutes before serving. If waiting longer, cover with foil to retain heat.

To serve, place paper frills on the rib bones and fill the center with vegetables or stuffing, surround with potatoes and garnish with watercress or curly endive. (Do not eat the watercress or endive. The VITAMIN K content is too high. Garnish only.)

Any sauce would be served on the side.

Ingredient	Cal	Fat	Chol	Sod	Prot	Carb	Fiber
CROWN ROAST	2560	108.8	1344	960	364.8	0	0
GARLIC CLOVE	12	0.1	0	6	0.5	3	0
OLIVE OIL	476	54	0	0	0	0	0
BLACK PEPPER	10	0.2	0	2	0.4	2.8	0.8
POTATOES*, PEELED	704	0	0	64	19.2	163.2	16
Totals Per Serving:	470	20.4	168	129	48.1	21.1	2.1

MUSTARD & WINE MARINATED LAMB CHOPS
4 servings (1 mcg of VITAMIN K per serving)

2	lb	Sirloin lamb chops, 4 chops, 1 inch thick
3	tbsp	Mustard, stone ground
1/4	tsp	Ground black pepper
1	cup	Red wine

Trim all visible fat from the lamb chops.

Rub both sides of the chops with mustard. Sprinkle with pepper. Cover with wine and marinate overnight in the refrigerator.

Rub again with mustard just before broiling or pan-frying to desired doneness.

Ingredient	Cal	Fat	Chol	Sod	Prot	Carb	Fiber
LAMB CHOPS	1216	44.8	576	576	185.6	0	0
MUSTARD	30	1.8	0	540	2.7	3	0
BLACK PEPPER	1	0	0	0	0.1	0.4	0.1
RED WINE	176	0	0	8	0	0.8	0
Totals Per Serving:	**356**	**11.7**	**144**	**281**	**47.1**	**1**	**0**

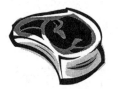 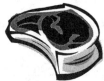

ARTILLERY RACK OF LAMB
8 servings (1 mcg of VITAMIN K per serving)

4	lb	Lamb, 2 racks with 8 to 9 chops each
3	tsp	Garlic cloves, split
1/8	tsp	Ground black pepper
1/2	tsp	Rosemary, fresh, minced

Have butcher "French" bone ends of racks.

Rub each rack generously with garlic. Lightly season with pepper and rosemary. Cover the exposed bone tips with small pieces of foil.

Place the lamb on racks in shallow baking pans and roast at 375 degrees Fahrenheit. Roast until the thermometer placed in the thickest part of the chops registers 140 degrees Fahrenheit for medium rare, 160 degrees Fahrenheit for medium or 170 degrees Fahrenheit for well done.

Remove the roasts from the oven and place the bone sides together, intertwining the ends of the rib bones to resemble stacked rifles.

Discard the foil and cover the bone tips with paper frills, if desired. Allow to stand 10 minutes before carving.

Ingredient	Cal	Fat	Chol	Sod	Prot	Carb	Fiber
LAMB	2560	108.8	1344	960	364.8	0	0
GARLIC	12	0.1	0	6	0.5	3	0
BLACK PEPPER	1	0	0	0	0	0.2	0.1
ROSEMARY	0	0	0	0	0	0	0
Totals Per Serving:	**323**	**13.6**	**168**	**121**	**45.7**	**0.4**	**0**

ATHENIAN LAMB STEW
8 servings (16 mcgs of VITAMIN K per serving)

3/4	cup	Onion, minced
1	tsp	Garlic cloves, crushed
1	tbsp	Basil, fresh, chopped
2	lb	Lamb, lean shoulder or leg, cubed
3	tbsp	Olive oil, treated (See Dietary Tip # 10)
1/8	tsp	Ground black pepper
28	oz	Tomatoes, crushed, canned
1/2	cup	Rose wine
1	cup	Carrots, peeled, cut in 1/2 inch slices
1	lb	Potatoes, peeled and quartered
1	each	Cinnamon, 2 inch stick

Sauté the onion, garlic and basil with the lamb in oil until the onion is tender. Season with pepper.

Continue cooking until lamb is lightly browned. Add crushed tomatoes and wine. Cook 10 minutes.

Add carrots, potatoes and cinnamon stick. Cover and cook over low heat 1 to 1 1/2 hours, or until lamb is very tender. Remove the cinnamon stick.

Serve with rice or noodles.

Ingredient	Cal	Fat	Chol	Sod	Prot	Carb	Fiber
ONION	48	0	0	0	1.2	10.2	1.8
GARLIC CLOVE	4	0	0	2	0.2	1	0
BASIL	0	0	0	0	0.1	0.1	0.1
LAMB	1184	48	576	608	179.2	0	0
OIL	357	40.5	0	0	0	0	0
BLACK PEPPER	1	0	0	0	0	0.2	0.1
TOMATOES	252	0	0	1036	0	56	28
ROSE WINE	88	0	0	0	0	11.2	0
CARROTS	48	0.8	0	40	0.8	12	0.8
POTATOES	352	0	0	32	9.6	81.6	8
CINNAMON	0	0	0	0	0	0	0
Totals Per Serving:	389	14.9	96	286	31.8	28.7	6.4

GRILLED LAMB AND SAUSAGE KEBABS
6 servings (4 mcg of VITAMIN K per serving)

1	lb	Lamb shoulder, boneless, cut into 1-inch cubes
1/2	cup	Olive oil, treated (See Dietary Tip # 10)
3	tbsp	Lemon juice
1/2	tsp	Ground black pepper
1	tsp	Garlic cloves
1	lb	Italian sausage, turkey, links
18	each	Bay leaves
1	lb	Mushroom caps

Place the lamb in a glass or plastic bowl. Process the oil, lemon juice, pepper and garlic in a food processor or blender until smooth. Pour the pureed sauce over the lamb. Cover and refrigerate 30 minutes.

Remove the lamb from the marinade. Reserve the marinade.

Cut the sausage into eighteen 1-inch pieces. Alternate lamb, sausage, bay leaves and mushroom caps on each of six 10-inch metal skewers, leaving a space between each piece of food.

Cover and grill the kebabs (about 4 inches from hot coals) 10 minutes, turning kebabs and brushing with marinade occasionally, until meat is done. (Do not eat the bay leaves.)

NOTE: To broil, place the kebabs on a rack in a broiler pan. Broil with the tops of the kabobs about 3 inches from the heat for 5 minutes. Turn the kebabs. Brush with the marinade. Broil 5 minutes more. Turn the kebabs. Brush with the marinade. Broil 5 minutes longer or until meat is done

Ingredient	Cal	Fat	Chol	Sod	Prot	Carb	Fiber
LAMB SHOULDER	592	24	288	304	89.6	0	0
OIL	160	18	0	0	0	0	0
LEMON JUICE	9	0	0	0	1.5	3	0
BLACK PEPPER	3	0.1	0	1	0.1	0.7	0.2
GARLIC CLOVE	4	0	0	2	0.2	1	0
SAUSAGE, TURKEY	800	64	0	4000	64	14.4	0
BAY LEAF	0	0	0	0	0	0	0
MUSHROOM CAPS	112	1.6	0	16	9.6	20.8	6.4
Totals Per Serving:	280	17.9	48	721	27.5	6.7	1.1

LAMB CHOPS W/GARLIC AND ROSEMARY
4 servings (22 mcg of VITAMIN K per serving)

1/4	cup	Butter
3	each	Green onions sliced
1	tsp	Garlic Powder
1	cup	Dry red wine
10	each	Mushrooms sliced
1	lb	Lamb shoulder arm chops (4 - 4 ounces each)
1/8	tsp	Pepper
1/2	tsp	Rosemary

Melt half of the butter in a large skillet over medium high heat. Add the mushrooms and onions and sauté until tender, about 5 to 10 minutes. remove from the pan and keep them warm.

Melt the remaining butter in the same skillet over medium high heat.

Sprinkle the chops with rosemary, garlic powder and pepper. Add the chops to the skillet and sauté until browned on both sides, about 5 minutes.

Reduce the heat to medium and continue cooking until tender.

Transfer the lamb chops to a heated platter.

Pour the wine into the skillet and cook over medium high heat, scraping up any browned bits clinging to the bottom of pan, until liquid is reduced by about 1/3.

Spoon vegetables over chops and top with sauce.

Ingredient	Cal	Fat	Chol	Sod	Prot	Carb	Fiber
BUTTER	400	46	140	360	0	0	0
GREEN ONIONS	27	0	0	15	3	3	1.5
GARLIC POWDER	5	0	0	1	0.3	1	0.1
DRY RED WINE	176	0	0	8	0	0	0
MUSHROOMS	70	1	0	10	6	13	4
LAMB CHOPS	592	24	288	304	89.6	0	0
ROSEMARY	0	0	0	0	0	0	0
PEPPER, BLACK	1	0	0	0	0	0.2	0
Totals Per Serving:	**318**	**17.8**	**107**	**175**	**24.7**	**4.3**	**1.4**

PORK

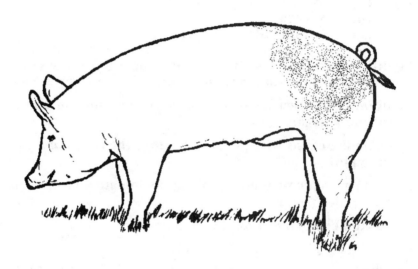

PEACHY PORK CHOPS
6 servings (8 mcgs of VITAMIN K per serving)

1 1/2	lb	Pork chops, boneless
5	tbsp	Brown sugar
1/2	tsp	Cinnamon, ground
1/4	tsp	Cloves, ground
8	oz	Tomato sauce
4	cups	Peaches, fresh, peeled, pit removed
1/4	cup	Water
1/4	cup	Vinegar
1/4	tsp	Ground black pepper

Lightly brown the pork chops on both sides in a large skillet or slow-cooking pot with a browning unit. Pour off any excess fat.

Combine the brown sugar, cinnamon, cloves, tomato sauce, water and vinegar.

Sprinkle the chops with pepper. Arrange the chops in a slow cooking pot.

Place the peach halves on top. Pour the tomato mixture over all.

Cover and cook on low for 4 to 6 hours.

Ingredient	Cal	Fat	Chol	Sod	Prot	Carb	Fiber
PORK CHOPS	1320	48	432	456	124.8	0	0
SUGAR, BROWN	258	0	0	0	0	66.8	0
CINNAMON	3	0.5	0	1	0.1	0.8	0.3
CLOVES	2	0.1	0	1	0	0.3	0.2
TOMATO SAUCE	88	0	0	1320	4	17.6	0
PEACHES	288	0	0	0	6.4	76.8	12.8
WATER	0	0	0	0	0	0	0
VINEGAR	8	0	0	12	0	0	0
BLACK PEPPER	1	0	0	0	0.1	0.4	0.1
Totals Per Serving:	**328**	**8.1**	**72**	**298**	**22.6**	**27.1**	**2.2**

PORK CHOPS BRAISED WITH CIDER AND APPLES
4 servings (1 mcg of VITAMIN K per serving)

1	lb	Pork chops, boneless, lean, 3/4 inch thick
1	tbsp	Canola oil, treated (See Dietary Tip # 10)
2	tbsp	Butter
1	cup	Onion, thinly sliced
1/2	cup	Apple, peeled, cored and chopped*
1/2	cup	Apple cider
1 1/2	tbsp	Apple cider vinegar
1	each	Bay leaf
1/2	tsp	Ground black pepper

*A tart apple like a Granny Smith is best.

Season the pork chops with pepper. Heat the oil in a heavy, large skillet over medium-high heat. Add the pork to the skillet and cook until brown and cooked through, about 10 to 15 minutes per side. Transfer the pork to a platter. Tent with foil to keep warm.

Drain off all but 1 tablespoon drippings from the skillet. Add the butter to the skillet and melt it over medium heat. Add the onion and apple to the skillet and sauté until onion is almost soft, about 5 minutes. Mix in the cider, vinegar and bay leaf.

Cover the skillet and cook until the onions and apples are tender, about 10 minutes. Discard the bay leaf. Add any accumulated juices from the pork chop platter to the skillet. Increase the heat and cook until the sauce thickens slightly, about three minutes. Spoon the sauce over the pork chops and serve.

Ingredient	Cal	Fat	Chol	Sod	Prot	Carb	Fiber
PORK CHOPS	880	32	288	304	83.2	0	0
OIL	120	13.5	0	0	0	0	0
BUTTER	200	23	70	180	0	0	0
ONION	88	0	0	8	0	16	0.8
APPLE	64	0	0	0	0.4	16	4
APPLE CIDER	56	0	0	0	0	13.2	0
CIDER VINEGAR	3	0	0	0	0	1.5	0
BAY LEAF	0	0	0	0	0	0	0
BLACK PEPPER	3	0.1	0	1	0.1	0.7	0.2
Totals Per Serving:	354	17.1	90	123	20.9	11.9	1.3

NEAPOLITAN PORK CHOPS
6 servings (6 mcgs of VITAMIN K per serving)

2	tbsp	Olive oil, treated (See Dietary Tip # 10)
1	tsp	Garlic cloves
1 1/2	lb	Pork chops, boneless, lean
1/4	tsp	Ground black pepper
3	tbsp	Tomato paste
3	tbsp	Water
3/4	cup	Bell pepper, green, chopped
1	cup	Mushrooms, sliced

In a skillet, heat the oil, add the garlic and cook until browned. Discard garlic.

Add the chops and brown them.

Add the pepper, and remaining ingredients. Cover and simmer over low heat 30 to 35 minutes until done. Serve.

Ingredient	Cal	Fat	Chol	Sod	Prot	Carb	Fiber
OIL	240	27	0	0	0	0	0
PORK CHOPS	1320	48	432	456	124.8	0	0
BLACK PEPPER	1	0	0	0	0.1	0.4	0.1
TOMATO PASTE	34	0	0	38	1.5	7.5	1.5
WATER	0	0	0	0	0	0	0
BELL PEPPER	42	0	0	0	0.6	0.6	0.6
MUSHROOMS	56	0	0	8	4.8	10.4	3.2
GARLIC	0	0	0	0	0	0	0
Totals Per Serving:	**282**	**12.5**	**72**	**84**	**22**	**3.1**	**0.9**

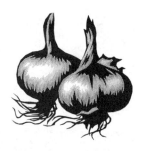

BAKED PORK CHOPS

6 servings (The pork itself contains little vitamin k. The mixture on top of the pork chops contains 20 micrograms of VITAMIN K per cup. If you do not use green peppers, this recipe contains almost no VITAMIN K.)

3	lb	Pork sirloin chops with bone
1	cup	Onion, finely chopped
1	cup	Bell pepper, green, chopped
1/4	tsp	Ground black pepper

Remove the fat from the pork chops and discard. Place the chops in a baking pan.

Mix all the other ingredients together and spread on the chops.

Bake at 350 degrees Fahrenheit until pork chops are cooked, approximately 30 to 40 minutes.

Ingredient	Cal	Fat	Chol	Sod	Prot	Carb	Fiber
PORK	1824	67.2	864	864	278.4	0	0
ONION	88	0	0	8	2.4	19.2	40
BELL PEPPER	56	0	0	0	0.8	0.8	0.8
BLACK PEPPER	1	0	0	0	0.1	0.4	0.1
Totals Per Serving:	328	11.2	144	145	46.9	3.4	6.8

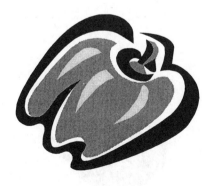

GLAZED PORK LOIN ROAST
8 servings (2 mcgs of VITAMIN K per serving)

2 1/2	lb	Pork loin roast, boneless
1	tsp	Garlic cloves, cut into slivers
1	tbsp	Orange marmalade
1	tsp	Mustard
1	tsp	Thyme leaves, fresh

Preheat the oven to 350 degrees Fahrenheit.

Make slits in the fat on the pork roast with the tip of a sharp knife. Insert a piece of garlic in each slit.

Mix the marmalade, mustard and thyme together and spread on the roast. Place the roast in a roasting pan.

Cover the pan with a lid or foil. Place in the oven and roast for 1 1/2 hours or until the roast registers 170 degrees Fahrenheit on a meat thermometer. Serve with the meat juices.

Ingredient	Cal	Fat	Chol	Sod	Prot	Carb	Fiber
PORK LOIN	1800	80	720	760	248	0	0
GARLIC	4	0	0	2	0.2	1	0
MARMALADE	54	0	0	0	0	12	0
MUSTARD	3	0.2	0	60	0.3	0.3	0
THYME	1	0	0	0	0	0	0
Totals Per Serving:	233	10	90	103	31.1	1.7	0.1

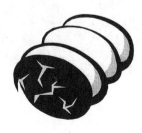

LEMON PECAN PORK CHOPS
4 servings (1 mcg of VITAMIN K per serving)

1	lb	Pork chops, boneless, lean
2	tbsp	Pecans, finely chopped
1/4	tsp	Garlic powder
3	tbsp	Lemon juice
1/4	tsp	Lemon pepper seasoning, salt free
1	tbsp	Canola oil, treated (See Dietary Tip # 10)
		Fresh lemon slices optional

Sprinkle both sides of the chops with the garlic and lemon pepper.

Heat the butter or oil in a large skillet over medium heat. Add the chops and brown 5 to 7 minutes per side or until pork is tender.

Remove the chops to a serving plate, sprinkle with the pecans and keep warm.

Stir the lemon juice into the drippings in the skillet, heat for one minute, stirring constantly. Spoon over the cooked chops. Garnish with lemon slices.

Ingredient	Cal	Fat	Chol	Sod	Prot	Carb	Fiber
PORK CHOPS	880	32	288	304	83.2	0	0
PECANS	99	10	0	0	1.2	2.8	1
GARLIC POWDER	2	0	0	0	0.1	0.5	0
LEMON JUICE	9	0	0	0	1.5	3	0
LEMON PEPPER	0	0	0	0	0	0	0
OIL	120	14	0	0	0	0	0
LEMON SLICES	0	0	0	0	0	0	0
Totals Per Serving:	**278**	**14**	**72**	**76**	**21.5**	**1.6**	**0.3**

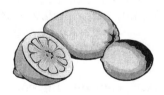

PORK PINWHEELS WITH APRICOT STUFFING
4 servings (5 mcgs of VITAMIN K per serving)

1	lb	Pork tenderloin
	SAUCE	
1 1/2	tsp	Cornstarch
1/8	tsp	Nutmeg (a pinch)
1	cup	Apricot nectar
	APRICOT STUFFING	
2/3	cup	Chicken broth
1/3	cup	Apricots, dried
2	tbsp	Celery, chopped
2	tbsp	Onion, chopped
1	tbsp	Butter
1/8	tsp	Cinnamon, ground
1/8	tsp	Ground black pepper
2	cups	Bread cubes

Split the tenderloin lengthwise, cutting to, but not through, the opposite side. Open out flat. Pound the tenderloin lightly with a meat mallet to a 10x6 rectangle.

APRICOT STUFFING - Chop the apricots very fine. Heat the chicken stock and pour it over the apricots. Let stand 5 minutes. Cook the celery and onion in butter until tender but not brown. Remove from the heat and stir in the cinnamon and pepper. In a large bowl, mix the bread cubes, onion mixture, and apricot mixture and toss lightly to moisten.

Spread the stuffing evenly over the tenderloin. Roll up jelly-roll style, starting from short side. Secure the meat roll with wooden toothpicks or tie with string at 1-inch intervals.

Cut the meat roll into six 1-inch slices. Place the slices on the rack of unheated broiler pan, cut side down. Broil 4 inches from the heat for 12 minutes. Turn and broil 11 to 13 minutes more or until done. Remove toothpicks or string and transfer the meat to a serving platter.

Meanwhile, for the SAUCE, combine the cornstarch and nutmeg. Stir in apricot nectar. Cook over medium heat and stir until the mixture is bubbly. Cook and stir 2 minutes more.

Serve the sauce with the meat slices.

Ingredient	Cal	Fat	Chol	Sod	Prot	Carb	Fiber
PORK TENDERLOIN	544	16	288	224	94.4	0	0
SAUCE							
CORNSTARCH	27	0	0	1	0	6.5	0
NUTMEG	2	0.1	0	0	0	0.1	0.1
APRICOT NECTAR	128	0	0	8	0	32	0
APRICOT STUFFING							
CHICKEN BROTH	21	0	0	880	1.1	3.7	0
APRICOTS, DRIED	179	0	0	8	2.7	48	8
CELERY	2	0	0	13	0.1	0.6	0.1
ONION	8	0	0	0	0.2	1.7	0.3
BUTTER	100	11.5	35	90	0	0	0
CINNAMON	1	0.1	0	0	0	0.2	0.1
BLACK PEPPER	1	0	0	0	0	0.2	0.1
BREAD CUBES	240	4.8	0	416	6.4	48	3.2
Totals Per Serving:	**313**	**8.1**	**81**	**410**	**26.2**	**35.3**	**3**

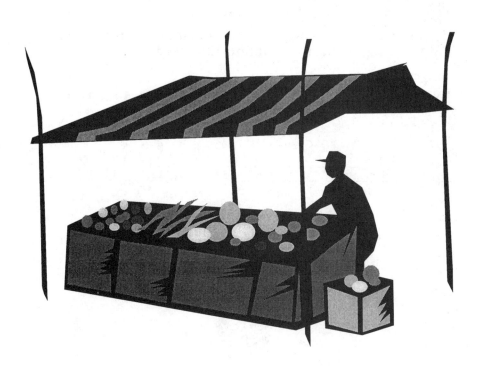

BAKED HAM WITH PINEAPPLE
12 servings (Less than 1 mcg of VITAMIN K per serving)

2	lb	Smoked ham, fully cooked, boneless*
20	each	Cloves, whole
8	oz	Pineapple slices packed in juice, drained (about 4 slices)
1/2	cup	Ginger ale**
1	tsp	Cinnamon, ground

*Try to find a low sodium ham and you will drastically reduce the sodium content.

**You can use diet ginger ale and reduce the calorie and carbohydrate count.

Remove and discard the casing from the ham. Score the top of the ham in a diamond design, and stud with cloves. Place the ham in a shallow baking dish, and arrange the pineapple slices over the top. Pour the ginger ale over the ham, and sprinkle each pineapple slice with cinnamon.

Bake the ham at 325 degrees Fahrenheit for 45 to 60 minutes until thoroughly heated. Cut into 12 slices and serve.

Ingredient	Cal	Fat	Chol	Sod	Prot	Carb	Fiber
SMOKED HAM	1760	76.8	640	24448	252.8	3.2	0
CLOVES	0	0	0	0	0	0	0
PINEAPPLE	280	4	0	40	4	72	1.6
GINGER ALE	40	0	0	8	0	8	0
CINNAMON	6	1	0	1	0.1	1.7	0.6
Totals Per Serving:	**174**	**6.8**	**53**	**2041**	**21.4**	**7.1**	**0.2**

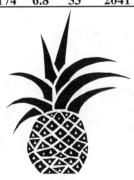

GRILLED BRATWURST

6 servings (Less than 1 mcg of VITAMIN K per serving)

1 1/2	lb	Bratwursts, (about 6)
12	oz	Beer
1/2	cup	Onion, chopped
6	each	Peppercorns
4	each	Cloves
6	each	Hard rolls

Place the Bratwursts, beer, onion, peppercorns, and cloves in a 3-quart saucepan. Simmer for 20 minutes. Drain. Discard the spices.

Grill the Bratwursts 2 to 5 inches from charcoal about 10 minutes, until browned. Sprinkle with water, while cooking, to form a crisp skin.

Serve in hard rolls with mustard.

The onion, peppercorns and cloves are used to flavor only. Since they are discarded they are not added to the nutrition totals.

Ingredient	Cal	Fat	Chol	Sod	Prot	Carb	Fiber
BRATWURSTS	2160	192	192	6648	96	24	0
HARD ROLLS	498	6	0	924	18	90	6
Totals Per Serving:	443	33	32	1262	19	19	1

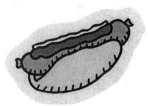

PEANUT PORK CHOPS
4 servings (1 mcg of VITAMIN K per serving)

1	large	Egg
1/4	cup	Water
1/2	cup	Peanuts, oil roasted w/salt, ground
1	lb	Pork chops, boneless, lean (4 per pound)

Beat the egg with the water. Place in a shallow bowl. Place ground peanuts in another shallow bowl.

Remove and discard any excess fat from the chops. Dip chops first into the egg, shaking off excess, then into the ground peanuts, covering each chop.

Grill the chops on medium-high for 8-10 minutes on each side.

Ingredient	Cal	Fat	Chol	Sod	Prot	Carb	Fiber
EGG	75	5	213	63	6.3	0.6	0
PEANUTS	424	36	0	320	20.8	12.8	2
PORK CHOPS	656	27.2	272	240	96	0	0
Totals Per Serving:	289	17.1	121	156	30.8	3.4	0.5

CITRUS-MARINATED PORK ROAST
8 servings (12.2 mcg of VITAMIN K per serving)

1 1/2	cups	Orange juice
1/4	cup	Lime juice
3	lb	Pork boneless loin roast
3	clove	Garlic, finely minced
1	tsp	Oregano leaves, fresh, minced
1/2	tsp	Coarsely ground pepper
1	lg	Onion, chopped
1	cup	Celery, sliced
1	lg	Carrot, sliced

Mix together 1 cup of the orange juice and all the lime juice.

Pour over the pork roast in a glass or plastic bowl. Cover and refrigerate, turning pork occasionally, at least 4 hours.

Remove the pork from the juices and reserve the juices. Pat the pork dry.

Mix together the garlic, oregano and pepper. Rub evenly over the pork.

Place the onion, celery and carrot in a shallow roasting pan. Pour the reserved juice over the vegetables. Place the pork on top of the vegetables. Insert a meat thermometer so the tip is in the center of the thickest part of the pork and does not rest in fat. Roast, uncovered, at 325F, spooning the reserved juices over the pork occasionally, until the thermometer registers 170F, about 2 1/2 hours. Remove the pork from the oven. Cover with foil and let stand 15 to 20 minutes before carving.

Place the vegetable mixture and the 1/2 cup orange juice in a blender container. Cover and blend on medium-high speed, stopping blender occasionally to scrape sides, until well blended, about 1 minute. Heat to boiling. Serve with pork.

Ingredient	Cal	Fat	Chol	Sod	Prot	Carb	Fiber
ORANGE JUICE	204	0	0	0	2.4	38.4	1.2
LIME JUICE	16	0	0	0	0.4	5.6	0
PORK ROAST	1968	81.6	816	720	288	0	0
GARLIC	72	0.3	0	36	2.7	18	0
OREGANO LEAVES	1	0	0	1	0	0	0
PEPPER, BLACK	3	0.1	0	1	0.1	0.7	0.2
ONION	8	0	0	0	0.2	1.7	0.3
CELERY	4	0	0	26	0.2	1.2	0.2
CARROT, SLICED	6	0.1	0	5	0.1	1.5	0.1
Totals Per Serving:	**285**	**10.3**	**102**	**99**	**36.8**	**8.4**	**0.2**

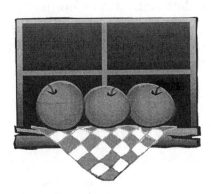

GRILLED PORK TENDERLOIN WITH MUSTARD CREAM
6 servings (Less than 1 mcg of VITAMIN K per serving)

1 1/2	lb	Pork tenderloin, trimmed
3/4	cup	Oil, Canola or olive, treated (See Dietary Tip # 10)
1/2	cup	Dry white wine
1	tbsp	Garlic cloves, crushed
	SAUCE	
1/4	cup	Dry white wine
1	tbsp	Shallots, minced
1	cup	Heavy cream
3	tbsp	Dijon mustard
1/8	tsp	White pepper

In a small deep dish just large enough to hold the pork, combine the oil, 1/2 cup wine and garlic. Add the pork, turning it to coat thoroughly and let it marinate, covered and chilled, overnight.

Drain the pork and discard the marinade.

Grill the pork on an oiled rack set about 6 inches over glowing coals. Turn it frequently for about 25 minutes, or until a meat thermometer registers 155 degrees Fahrenheit, for meat that is just cooked through but still juicy.

Transfer the pork to a cutting board and let it stand while making the sauce.

SAUCE: In a small heavy saucepan, boil the 1/4 cup white wine with the shallots until it is reduced to about 2 tablespoons.

Add the cream, bring the mixture just to a boil and simmer for 2 minutes, or until it is thickened slightly. Strain the sauce through a fine sieve into a bowl and whisk in the mustard and white pepper.

Cut the pork diagonally into 1/2 inch slices and serve it with the mustard cream sauce.

(Because you discard the marinade, it is not added to the nutrition totals for the dish.)

Ingredient	Cal	Fat	Chol	Sod	Prot	Carb	Fiber
PORK TENDERLOIN	984	40.8	408	360	144	0	0
OIL	40	4.5	0	0	0	0	0
SAUCE							
DRY WHITE WINE	44	0	0	2	0	1.4	0
GARLIC	12	0.1	0	6	0.5	3	0
SHALLOTS	7	0.1	0	1	0.4	1.7	0.1
HEAVY CREAM	824	88	328	88	4.8	6.4	0
DIJON MUSTARD	45	0	0	1080	0	1.5	0
WHITE PEPPER	2	0	0	0	0.1	0.4	0.1
Totals Per Serving:	**326**	**22.2**	**123**	**256**	**24.9**	**2.4**	**0**

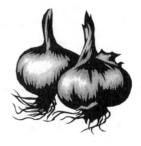

HAM IN ZIPPY CREAM SAUCE
4 servings (1 mcg of VITAMIN K per serving)

1	lb	Ham, smoked, in cubes
		CREAM SAUCE
3	tbsp	All purpose flour
3	tbsp	Butter
1 1/2	cups	Milk, skim
1	tsp	Dijon mustard
1	tsp	Horseradish, fresh

Sauté the ham cubes in a non-stick pan until lightly browned. Remove from the pan and keep warm.

Melt the butter in a sauce pan, add the flour and mix thoroughly. Add the milk and stir continuously until the sauce thickens and comes to just bubbling. Add the mustard and horseradish, stir and allow to heat through.

Add the ham cubes and allow to heat through. To serve over noodles, add more milk to make the sauce thinner.

Don't forget to change the nutrition values to include whatever you put the sauce over.

Ingredient	Cal	Fat	Chol	Sod	Prot	Carb	Fiber
HAM	736	38.4	240	5792	83.2	11.2	0
CREAM SAUCE							
FLOUR	75	0.3	0	0	2.1	16.5	0
BUTTER	300	34.5	105	270	0	0	0
MILK, SKIM	132	1.2	12	192	12	18	0
DIJON MUSTARD	5	0	0	120	0	0.2	0
HORSERADISH	2	0	0	0	0.1	0.5	0.1
Totals Per Serving:	**313**	**18.6**	**89**	**1594**	**24.3**	**11.6**	**0**

MUSHROOM SAUSAGE PIE
8 servings (5 mcgs of VITAMIN K per serving)

1	each	PIE CRUST, single crust (See Recipe Index)
1	lb	Turkey sausage, spicy*
1/4	cup	Butter
12	oz	Mushrooms, sliced
1	cup	Whipping cream, not whipped**
2	each	Egg yolks, beaten
1	tbsp	All purpose flour
1	tbsp	Butter, melted

1	tbsp	Lemon juice
1/2	tsp	Ground black pepper
2	oz	Parmesan cheese, freshly grated

*Pork sausage may be substituted. (Adjust the nutrition values accordingly.)

**You could substitute evaporated skim milk. (Adjust the nutrition values accordingly.)

Preheat the oven to 450 degrees Fahrenheit. Roll out and fit the pastry into a 9-inch pie plate. Without pricking, bake the crust about 8 to 10 minutes, until lightly brown. As it bakes, air pockets underneath the pastry can cause it to puff up and crack. So, check the pastry every 2 or 3 minutes and push it down to fit the shape of the pie plate. (Or use some dried beans in the shell to weight the pastry down while it is cooking.) Remove the pie shell from the oven and let stand while making the filling.

In a large skillet, fry the sausage and drain. In the same skillet, melt the butter, add the mushrooms, and cook briefly. Spread the sausage and mushrooms evenly in the pastry.

In a medium mixing bowl, whisk together, thoroughly, the heavy cream, egg yolks, flour, melted butter, lemon juice and pepper. Pour this mixture evenly over the pie filling.

Bake the pie for 30 or 40 minutes at 375 degrees Fahrenheit, until rich brown and set. As you remove from the oven, sprinkle the Parmesan cheese over the top. Serve warm.

Ingredient	Cal	Fat	Chol	Sod	Prot	Carb	Fiber
PIE CRUST	699	15.3	105	501	0	26.6	2.7
TURKEY SAUSAGE	1568	144	352	3312	64	1.6	0
BUTTER	400	46	140	360	0	0	0
MUSHROOMS	84	1.2	0	12	7.2	15.6	4.8
WHIPPING CREAM	824	88	328	88	4.8	6.4	0
EGG YOLKS	202	17.6	726	24	9.6	1	0
FLOUR	25	0.1	0	0	0.7	5.5	0
BUTTER	100	11.5	35	90	0	0	0
LEMON JUICE	3	0	0	0	0.5	1	0
BLACK PEPPER	3	0.1	0	1	0.1	0.7	0.2
PARMESAN	222	15	48	908	20.2	1.8	0
Totals Per Serving:	516	42.3	217	662	13.4	7.5	1

HAM AND CHEESE PIE
6 servings (21 mcgs of VITAMIN K per serving)

2	tsp	Canola oil (See Dietary Tip # 10)
12	oz	Cottage cheese, lowfat, creamed, drained
3	oz	Cream cheese, softened*
4	oz	Cheddar cheese shredded (about 1 cup)
2	large	Eggs
1	cup	Ham, cooked and chopped
1	cup	Bisquick, reduced fat
1/4	cup	Milk, skim
2	large	Eggs
1/4	cup	Green onions, sliced
1	tbsp	Sesame seeds, toasted

*Non-fat or low-fat cream cheese may be used.

Preheat the oven to 375 degrees Fahrenheit. Lightly grease a 9 inch pie plate with the 2 teaspoons of Canola oil.

Mix the cheeses, 2 eggs and the ham, reserve.

Mix the Bisquick, milk, 2 eggs and onions together. Beat vigorously for about 20 strokes. Spread half of the batter in the pie plate. Spoon reserved cheese mixture evenly over batter. Carefully spread remaining batter over cheese mixture. Sprinkle with sesame seed.

Bake until a knife inserted halfway between the center and the edge comes out clean, 35 to 40 minutes. Let stand 5 minutes before cutting.

Ingredient	Cal	Fat	Chol	Sod	Prot	Carb	Fiber
CANOLA OIL	80	9.3	0	0	0	0	0
COTTAGE CHEESE	348	13.2	36	1272	42	12	0
CREAM CHEESE	297	29.7	90	255	6	3	0
CHEDDAR	440	36	120	800	28	4	0
EGGS	150	11.2	426	126	12.6	1.2	0
HAM	368	19.2	120	2896	41.6	5.6	0
BISQUICK	448	8	0	1376	8.8	84	1.6
MILK, SKIM	22	0.2	2	32	2	3	0
EGGS	150	11.2	426	126	12.6	1.2	0
GREEN ONIONS	18	0	0	10	2	2	1
SESAME SEEDS	47	4.4	0	3	2.1	0.8	0.2
Totals Per Serving:	**395**	**23.7**	**203**	**1149**	**26.3**	**19.5**	**0.5**

PORK LOIN WITH MUSTARD CRUST
6 servings (6 mcgs of VITAMIN K per serving)

2	lb	Pork tenderloin or loin
1/4	tsp	Ground black pepper
1 1/2	cups	Bread crumbs, dry, plain
1	tbsp	Basil, fresh, chopped
1/4	cup	Shallots, minced
1	tsp	Garlic, minced
1/2	cup	Mustard, grainy

Trim away any fat and season the pork loin with pepper.

Lightly toast the bread crumbs in a 400 degree Fahrenheit oven but do not let them brown too much. (You can toast them at a lower heat, it will just take longer.)

Mince the basil, shallot and garlic together and stir into the bread crumbs.

Using a pastry brush, paint the pork all over with the mustard and then dredge it in the crumb mixture. Place the loin in an oiled roasting pan.

Bake at 400 degrees Fahrenheit 30 minutes, or until internal temperature reaches 150 degrees Fahrenheit. Let the roast stand 5 minutes before carving. Cut into 1/2 inch slices and serve at once.

Ingredient	Cal	Fat	Chol	Sod	Prot	Carb	Fiber
PORK TENDERLOIN	1312	54.4	544	480	192	0	0
BLACK PEPPER	1	0	0	0	0.1	0.4	0.1
BREAD CRUMBS	636	8.4	0	1392	18	115.2	6
BASIL	0	0	0	0	0.1	0.1	0.1
SHALLOTS	28	0.2	0	4	1.4	6.8	0.4
GARLIC	4	0	0	2	0.2	1	0
MUSTARD, GRAINY	80	4.8	0	1440	7.2	8	0
Totals Per Serving:	344	11.3	91	553	36.5	21.9	1.1

PORK CHOPS PARMESAN
4 servings (3 mcg of VITAMIN K per serving)

3	tbsp	Cornmeal*
1/4	oz	Parmesan cheese, grated (about 1 tablespoon)
1/2	tsp	Pepper, black
1/2	tsp	Basil, fresh, chopped
1	lb	Pork chops, boneless, lean about 1/2-inch thick
1	tbsp	Olive oil, treated (See Dietary Tip # 10)
1/2	cup	Onion, chopped
1	tsp	Garlic cloves, minced
1/4	tsp	Fennel seeds, crushed

*Flour or bread crumbs may be substituted. (Change the nutrition values accordingly.)

Combine the cornmeal, Parmesan cheese, black pepper and basil.

Trim the pork chops of all visible fat, pat them dry, and dredge them in the cornmeal mixture.

Heat a skillet over medium heat, and add the oil. When the oil is hot, place the chops in the skillet and reduce the heat to low.

Fry the chops for 10 minutes on each side. Then add the onions, garlic, fennel, and continue frying for another 10 minutes, turning as necessary to keep from sticking.

Ingredient	Cal	Fat	Chol	Sod	Prot	Carb	Fiber
CORNMEAL	114	1.5	0	10	3	22.5	0.8
PARMESAN CHEESE	28	1.9	6	114	2.5	0.2	0
PEPPER, BLACK	3	0.1	0	1	0.1	0.7	0.2
BASIL	0	0	0	0	0	0	0
PORK CHOPS	656	27.2	272	240	96	0	0
OIL	120	13.5	0	0	0	0	0
ONION, CHOPPED	32	0	0	0	0.8	6.8	1.2
GARLIC CLOVE	4	0	0	2	0.2	1	0
FENNEL SEEDS	4	0.2	0	1	0.2	0.6	0.5
Totals Per Serving:	**240**	**11.1**	**70**	**92**	**25.7**	**8**	**0.6**

PORK CHOPS IN TOMATO SAUCE WITH OREGANO
4 servings (20 mcgs of VITAMIN K per serving)

2	cups	Plum tomatoes, diced
1/4	cup	Water
1/4	tsp	Ground black pepper
1	lb	Pork chops, boneless, lean
2	tbsp	Olive oil, treated (See Dietary Tip # 10)
2	tsp	Garlic, chopped
1 1/2	cups	Mushrooms, thin sliced
1 1/2	cups	Bell pepper, green, cut in 1 inch cubes
1/2	cup	Dry white wine
1	tsp	Oregano leaves, fresh, minced

Put the tomatoes and water into a pot and bring to a boil, stirring occasionally.

Sprinkle the chops with pepper. Heat the oil in the skillet and add the chops. Brown on both sides, about 5 minutes to a side.

Add the garlic, bell pepper and mushrooms. Stir in the wine, tomatoes and oregano. Cover closely and cook 35 to 40 minutes.

Serve with pasta.

Ingredient	Cal	Fat	Chol	Sod	Prot	Carb	Fiber
PLUM TOMATOES	96	0	0	48	3.2	20.8	6.4
BLACK PEPPER	1	0	0	0	0.1	0.4	0.1
PORK CHOPS	656	27.2	272	240	96	0	0
OIL	238	27	0	0	0	0	0
GARLIC	8	0	0	4	0.3	2	0.1
MUSHROOMS	84	1.2	0	12	7.2	15.6	4.8
BELL PEPPER	84	0	0	0	1.2	1.2	1.2
DRY WHITE WINE	88	0	0	4	0	2.8	0
OREGANO	1	0	0	1	0	0	0
Totals Per Serving:	**314**	**13.9**	**68**	**77**	**27**	**10.7**	**3.1**

PORK MARENGO
6 servings (8 mcg of VITAMIN K per serving)

2	lb	Pork shoulder, lean boneless, cut in 1 inch cubes
1/2	cup	Onion, chopped
2	tbsp	Canola oil, treated (See Dietary Tip # 10)
16	oz	Tomatoes, canned, 'No Salt Added', peeled and chopped
1	tsp	Chicken bouillon granules, instant, low sodium
1	tsp	Marjoram leaves, fresh, minced
1	tsp	Thyme leaves, fresh, minced
1/8	tsp	Ground black pepper
3	oz	Mushrooms, chopped
1/3	cup	Water
3	tbsp	All purpose flour
2	cups	Rice, white, cooked

In a skillet, brown half of the pork cubes and half of the chopped onion, in the hot oil. Drain off fat. Transfer meat and onion to a crock pot. Do the same with the remaining pork and onion.

In the same skillet combine the undrained tomatoes, bouillon granules, marjoram, thyme and pepper. Stir together, scraping browned bits from the bottom of the skillet. Pour over the pork.

Cover, cook on LOW for 4 to 6 hours. Turn to HIGH. Stir in the drained mushrooms. Blend the cold water slowly into the flour and stir into the pork mixture. Cook, uncovered, on HIGH until thickened, 15 to 20 minutes, stirring occasionally.

Serve over rice.

Ingredient	Cal	Fat	Chol	Sod	Prot	Carb	Fiber
PORK SHOULDER	1312	54.4	544	480	192	0	0
ONION	32	0	0	0	0.8	6.8	1.2
OIL	241	28	0	0	0	0	0
TOMATOES	128	0	0	880	4.8	19.2	0
CHICKEN BOUILLON	12	0.8	0	5	0.3	2	0
MARJORAM	0	0	0	0	0	0	0
THYME LEAVES	1	0	0	0	0	0	0
BLACK PEPPER	1	0	0	0	0	0.2	0.1
MUSHROOMS	21	0.3	0	3	1.8	3.9	1.2
FLOUR	75	0.3	0	0	2.1	16.5	0
RICE	784	22.4	0	16	52.8	208	1.6
Totals Per Serving:	**435**	**17.7**	**91**	**231**	**42.4**	**42.8**	**0.7**

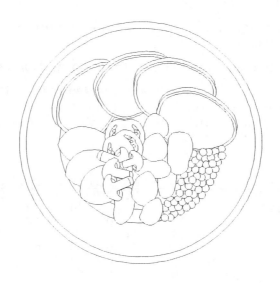

PORK CHOPS WITH ONIONS
4 servings (Less than 1 mcg of VITAMIN K per serving)

1	lb	Pork chops, boneless, lean
1/4	tsp	Ground black pepper
1 1/2	tbsp	All purpose flour
1 1/2	tbsp	Canola oil, treated (See Dietary Tip # 10)
1	cup	Onion, thinly sliced
1/2	cup	Beer
1/2	cup	Beef broth, hot
1	tsp	Cornstarch

Season the pork chops with the pepper and coat with the flour.

Heat the oil in a heavy frying pan. Add the pork chops and fry for 3 minutes on each side.

Add the onions and cook for another 5 minutes, turning the chops once.

Pour in the beer and beef broth, cover and simmer 15 minutes.

Remove the pork chops to a preheated platter. Blend the cornstarch with a small amount of cold water. Stir into the pan sauce and cook until thick and bubbly. Pour over the pork chops.

Ingredient	Cal	Fat	Chol	Sod	Prot	Carb	Fiber
PORK CHOPS	656	27.2	272	240	96	0	0
BLACK PEPPER	1	0	0	0	0.1	0.4	0.1
FLOUR	38	0.2	0	0	1.1	8.3	0
OIL	180	20.4	0	0	0	0	0
ONION	88	0	0	8	0	16	0.8
BEER	48	0	0	4	0.4	4	0
BEEF BROTH	20	0	0	872	4	0	0
CORNSTARCH	18	0	0	1	0	4.3	0
Totals Per Serving:	262	11.9	68	281	25.4	8.2	0.2

SEAFOOD

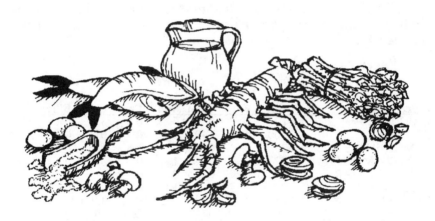

SAUTÉED GARLIC SHRIMP
2 servings (1 mcg of VITAMIN K per serving)

3	tsp	Garlic cloves minced
1/4	cup	Butter
3	tbsp	Lemon juice, fresh
2	tbsp	Dry vermouth
2	tsp	Wine vinegar
1/8	tsp	Hot Sauce
1	lb	Shrimp, peeled, deveined and drained
1	cup	Rice, white, cooked, hot

Sauté the garlic in the butter in a skillet. Combine the next 7 ingredients, and slowly add this mixture to the skillet, add the shrimp. Sauté 5 minutes or until the shrimp are done, stirring frequently.

Serve over rice.

Ingredient	Cal	Fat	Chol	Sod	Prot	Carb	Fiber
GARLIC	12	.1	0	6	0.5	3	0
BUTTER	400	46	140	360	0	0	0
LEMON JUICE	33	0.5	0	3	1.8	13.1	0
DRY VERMOUTH	22	0	0	1	0	0.7	0
WINE VINEGAR	1	0	0	2	0	0	0
HOT SAUCE	0	0	0	14	0	0	0
SHRIMP	480	8	688	672	91.2	3.2	0
RICE	392	11.2	0	8	26.4	104	0.8
Totals Per Serving:	**670**	**32.9**	**414**	**533**	**59.9**	**62**	**.4**

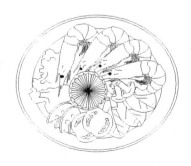

PAN FRIED TUNA

4 servings (26 mcgs of VITAMIN K per serving. If you omit the
parsley, the VITAMIN K per serving is 3 mcg)

24	oz	Tuna, fresh, Bluefin steaks (six or so)
1/2	cup	All purpose flour
1/2	cup	Olive oil, treated (See Dietary Tip # 10)
1	cup	Onion, thinly sliced
1/4	cup	Chicken broth
1 1/2	tbsp	White wine vinegar
1	tbsp	Parsley, fresh, chopped
1/2	tsp	Black pepper, freshly ground

Roll the tuna steaks in flour and pat off the excess. Discard the
remaining flour.

Heat a large frying pan and add the oil. Pan-fry the fish over
medium heat, about 1 to 2 minutes per side, and remove to a
warm plate. Do not overcook.

Discard half the oil and return the pan to the heat. Add the
onion, chicken stock, vinegar, and black pepper. Sauté for
about 5 minutes until the onion just becomes tender and the
sauce reduces a bit. Add the parsley.

Spoon the sauce over the warm fish and serve.

Ingredient	Cal	Fat	Chol	Sod	Prot	Carb	Fiber
TUNA	984	24	264	264	168	0	0
FLOUR	100	0.4	0	0	52.8	22	0
OIL	476	54	0	0	0	0	0
ONION	88	0	0	8	0	16	0.8
CHICKEN BROTH	8	0	0	330	0.4	1.4	0
VINEGAR	3	0	0	4	0	0	0
VINEGAR	3	0	0	4	0	0	0
PARSLEY, FRESH	2	0.1	0	2	0.1	0.3	0
BLACK PEPPER	3	0.1	0	1	0.1	0.7	0.2
Totals Per Serving:	416	19.6	66	152	42.9	10.1	0.2

PEPPER GRILLED SALMON
4 servings (2 mcgs of VITAMIN K per serving)

1	lb	Salmon fillets
1	tsp	Black peppercorns
1	tsp	Anise seed
1/2	tsp	Salt, Coarse (kosher)
1	tbsp	Canola oil for grill rack, treated (See Dietary Tip # 10)

Coat a grill rack with oil. Place the grill rack 5 inch from the coals.

In a clean coffee grinder or spice mill, grind the peppercorns, anise seeds and salt until coarsely ground. Sprinkle over the salmon.

Grill the salmon 4 to 5 minutes on each side or until cooked through. Serve hot.

Ingredient	Cal	Fat	Chol	Sod	Prot	Carb	Fiber
SALMON FILLETS	656	27.2	176	208	121.6	0	0
PEPPERCORNS	5	0.1	0	1	0.2	1.4	0.3
ANISE SEED	8	0.4	0	0	0.4	1.1	0.1
SALT	0	0	0	940	0	0	0
Totals Per Serving:	**167**	**6.9**	**44**	**287**	**30.6**	**0.6**	**0.1**

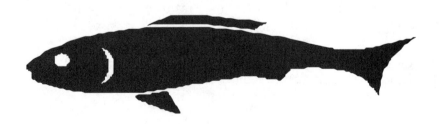

BAKED HALIBUT

4 servings (VITAMIN K content = 10 mcg per cup of mixture on top of fish. Add 5 mcg VITAMIN K for every 100 grams of fish ONLY if mackerel is used.)

1 1/4	lb	Halibut (or any other fish)
3	tbsp	Lime juice or lemon juice
1/2	cup	Onion, chopped
1	cup	Tomato, finely chopped
1/2	tsp	Canola oil, treated (See Dietary Tip # 10)
1/2	tsp	Ground black pepper

Place the fish in a baking dish.

Mix the remaining ingredients and pour over the fish.

Bake at 350 degrees Fahrenheit until fish is cooked (usually 10 to 20 minutes).

Ingredient	Cal	Fat	Chol	Sod	Prot	Carb	Fiber
HALIBUT	620	12	180	300	118	0	0
LIME JUICE	33	0.5	0	3	1.8	13.1	0
ONION	32	0	0	0	0.8	6.8	1.2
TOMATO	40	0.8	0	16	1.6	8	2.4
OIL	21	2.3	0	0	0	0	0
BLACK PEPPER	3	0.1	0	1	0.1	0.7	0.2
Totals Per Serving:	**187**	**3.9**	**45**	**80**	**30.6**	**7.1**	**1**

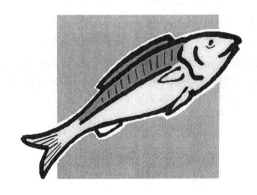

MEDITERRANEAN BAKED FISH

4 servings (VITAMIN K content of SAUCE ONLY = 7 mcg per cup)

This recipe can be used with any of the types of fish we know have a very low amount of VITAMIN K. These include butterfly bream, eel, mackerel, salmon, tuna, and yellowtail (snapper). However, it will probably taste best with bream, tuna, or yellowtail.

It is very likely that other fish will be added to this list when more data regarding the VITAMIN K content of various fish species is determined.

Also, since the above fish contains little VITAMIN K, the amount of fish you use in this recipe will not significantly change the VITAMIN K intake. The only possible exception to this is mackerel, which contains 5 mcg of VITAMIN K per 100 grams or about 22 1/2 mcgs of VITAMIN K per pound.

1	lb	Tuna (or any other fish)
2	tsp	Olive oil, treated (See Dietary Tip # 10)
1	cup	Onion, sliced or diced
2	cups	Tomato, chopped, plus juice
1	tsp	Garlic cloves, minced
1	cup	White wine
1/2	cup	Lemon juice or lime juice
1/2	tsp	Oregano leaves, fresh, minced
1/4	tsp	Ground black pepper

Sauté the onion and garlic in the olive oil.

Add all the remaining ingredients, except the tuna, and cook on low heat for 30 minutes to make a sauce.

Meanwhile, heat the oven to 350 degrees Fahrenheit. Cover approximately 1 pound of fish with the sauce and bake until the fish is cooked. The fish will easily flake apart with a fork when it is done.

Ingredient	Cal	Fat	Chol	Sod	Prot	Carb	Fiber
OIL	79	9	0	0	0	0	0
ONION	88	0	0	8	2.4	19.2	40
TOMATO	80	1.6	0	32	3.2	16	4.8
GARLIC	4	0	0	2	0.2	1	0
WHITE WINE	176	0	0	8	0	1.6	0
LEMON JUICE	88	1.2	0	8	4.8	34.8	0
OREGANO	1	0	0	0	0	0	0
BLACK PEPPER	1	0	0	0	0.1	0.4	0.1
TUNA	656	16	176	176	112	0	0
Totals Per Serving:	**293**	**7**	**44**	**59**	**30.7**	**18.2**	**11.2**

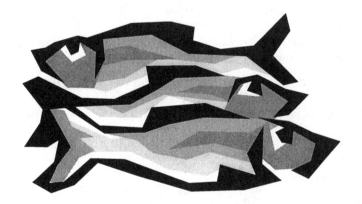

ARTICHOKE BOTTOMS WITH SHRIMP SAUTÉ
6 servings (9 mcgs of VITAMIN K per serving)

6	each	Artichoke bottoms, frozen (approximately 1 cup)
1	quart	Water
3	oz	Butter
1	tbsp	Onion, minced
1	tsp	Garlic cloves, minced
1	tbsp	Bell pepper, minced
1	tbsp	Pimiento, minced
1/4	lb	Mushrooms, sliced
1/4	tsp	Thyme, fresh
1/2	tsp	Dill weed, fresh
1 1/2	lb	Shrimp, peeled, deveined and chopped
1/4	tsp	Ground black pepper

Bring the water to a boil and add the artichoke bottoms. Cook for 5 minutes or until tender. Drain and keep warm.

Melt the butter in a skillet and add the onion, garlic, bell pepper and pimento. Cook over moderate heat for 5 minutes. Add the mushrooms, thyme, dill weed and black pepper.

Sauté for 3 minutes and add the shrimp. Toss for 4 minutes over high heat. Spoon over artichokes. Serve.

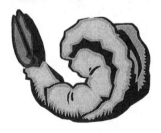

Ingredient	Cal	Fat	Chol	Sod	Prot	Carb	Fiber
ARTICHOKES	78	0	0	162	6	18	12
BUTTER	600	69	210	540	0	0	0
ONION	4	0	0	0	0.1	0.9	0.2
GARLIC	4	0	0	2	0.2	1	0
BELL PEPPER	15	0.3	0	3	0.6	4.2	0.9
PIMIENTO	3	0.1	0	2	0.1	0.6	0.1
MUSHROOMS	28	0.4	0	4	2.4	5.2	1.6
THYME LEAVES	0	0	0	0	0	0	0
DILL WEED	0	0	0	0	0	0	0
SHRIMP	720	12	1032	1008	136.8	4.8	0
BLACK PEPPER	1	0	0	0	0.1	0.4	0.1
Totals Per Serving:	**242**	**13.6**	**207**	**287**	**24.4**	**5.8**	**2.5**

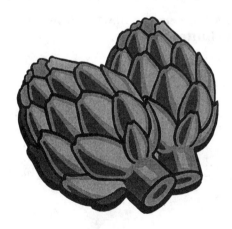

SALMON GRILL DIABLE
6 servings (1 mcg of VITAMIN K per serving)

1/3	cup	Butter, soft
2	tbsp	Lemon juice
2	tsp	Dijon mustard
2	lb	Salmon steaks or fillets, 1 inch thick, 6 pieces
1	tbsp	Olive oil, treated (See Dietary Tip # 10)
1/4	tsp	Ground black pepper

Beat the butter until creamy, gradually adding the lemon juice until the mixture is fluffy. Beat in the mustard. (Cover and chill if you are making it ahead.) Bring the butter mixture to room temperature before using.

Lightly coat the salmon steaks with olive oil, using a pastry brush or spray. Sprinkle with pepper.

Set the salmon on the grill 6 inches above hot gray coals. Cook, turning once with a wide spatula, until the fish flakes in the center when prodded with a fork, about 10 minutes.

Place the steaks on a hot serving platter, topping each with an equal portion of the butter mixture.

Ingredient	Cal	Fat	Chol	Sod	Prot	Carb	Fiber
BUTTER	533	61.3	187	480	0	0	0
LEMON JUICE	6	0	0	0	1	2	0
DIJON MUSTARD	10	0	0	240	0	0.3	0
SALMON	1312	54.4	352	416	243.2	0	0
OIL	119	13.5	0	0	0	0	0
BLACK PEPPER	1	0	0	0	0.1	0.4	0.1
Totals Per Serving:	**330**	**21.5**	**90**	**189**	**40.7**	**0.4**	**0**

SHRIMP WITH TOMATO SAUCE
6 servings (24 mcgs of VITAMIN K per serving)

1 1/2	lb	Shrimp, large
1/4	tsp	Crushed dried red pepper
2	tbsp	Olive oil, treated (See Dietary Tip # 10)
2	tbsp	Ginger root, chopped
1	tsp	Garlic, chopped
1/4	tsp	Ground black pepper
1 1/2	cups	Tomatoes, diced
1/4	cup	Scallions, chopped

Peel and de-vein the shrimp.

Heat 1 tablespoon of the oil in a frying pan and add the garlic. Cook briefly. Add the tomatoes, hot pepper flakes and 1 tablespoon of the ginger. Cook, reducing the liquid, for 5 minutes. Set aside and keep warm.

Heat the remaining tablespoon of oil in a nonstick frying pan and add the shrimp and ground pepper. Sauté over high heat for 1 minute on each side.

Add the remaining ginger and the scallions. Blend well, cooking for 1 minute.

Place the shrimp over the tomato mixture and serve.

Ingredient	Cal	Fat	Chol	Sod	Prot	Carb	Fiber
SHRIMP, LARGE	720	12	1032	1008	136.8	4.8	0
DRIED RED PEPPER	2	0.1	0	0	0	0	0
OIL	238	27	0	0	0	0	0
GINGER ROOT	20	0.2	0	4	0.5	4.3	0.3
GARLIC	4	0	0	2	0.2	1	0.1
BLACK PEPPER	1	0	0	0	0.1	0.4	0.1
TOMATOES	60	1.2	0	24	2.4	12	3.6
SCALLIONS	8	0.2	0	4	0.4	1.6	0.4
Totals Per Serving:	176	6.8	172	174	23.4	4	0.7

SEAFOOD STROGANOFF
6 servings (2 mcgs of VITAMIN K per serving)

1 1/2	lb	Salmon. fillets
2	tbsp	Butter
3/4	cup	Onion, sliced thin
8	oz	Mushrooms, sliced
14	oz	Tomatoes, crushed, canned
1	tsp	Worcestershire Sauce
1	tbsp	Lime juice
1	tbsp	Catsup
1/2	lb	Shrimp, raw, medium
1	cup	Sour cream, nonfat
2	tbsp	All purpose flour
1	lb	Egg noodles, uncooked

Bone, skin, and cut the fish into bite size pieces and set aside.

Melt the butter in a large frying pan and sauté the onion over medium heat until golden. Add the mushrooms. Mix until they are butter-coated. Add the tomatoes, Worcestershire Sauce, lime juice, and catsup. Cook, stirring, until liquid is reduced to the consistency of thick cream.

Stir in the shrimp. Cover and simmer for 1 minute.

Stir in the fish and simmer for 2 minutes more.

Blend the sour cream with the flour until smooth, stir into the fish mixture and cook, stirring, until it boils and thickens.

Meanwhile, cook the egg noodles according to package directions and drain.

Serve the Stroganoff over the egg noodles.

Ingredient	Cal	Fat	Chol	Sod	Prot	Carb	Fiber
SALMON. FILLETS	984	40.8	264	312	182.4	0	0
BUTTER	200	23	70	180	0	0	0
ONION	66	0	0	6	1.8	14.4	30
MUSHROOMS	56	0.8	0	8	4.8	10.4	3.2
TOMATOES	126	0	0	518	0	28	14
WORCESTERSHIRE	3	0	0	67	0	0.7	0
LIME JUICE	4	0	0	0	0.1	1.4	0
CATSUP	14	0.1	0	168	0.2	4	0
SHRIMP	240	4	344	336	45.6	1.6	0
SOUR CREAM	120	0	0	120	24	8	0
FLOUR	50	0.2	0	0	1.4	11	0
EGG NOODLES	1728	19.2	432	96	64	323.2	12.8
Totals Per Serving:	**599**	**14.7**	**185**	**302**	**54.1**	**67.1**	**10**

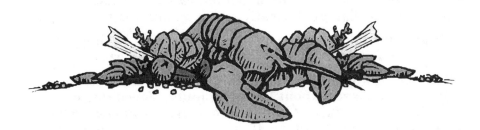

BALSAMIC-GLAZED SALMON FILLETS
6 servings (5 mcgs of VITAMIN K per serving)

1	tsp	Garlic, thinly sliced
2	tbsp	Olive oil, treated (See Dietary Tip # 10)
1	tsp	Dijon mustard
1	tbsp	Honey
1/3	cup	Balsamic vinegar
1/4	tsp	Ground black pepper
2	lb	Salmon fillets, (about 6 pieces) washed and patted dry with paper towels
2	tbsp	Basil, fresh, julienne cut (in thin strips)

In a small saucepan, sauté the garlic in 1 tablespoon of the olive oil over medium heat until the garlic is tender, about 3 minutes. Stir often. Do not brown.

Add the remaining tablespoon of olive oil, mustard, honey, vinegar and pepper. Stir well to combine. Simmer, uncovered, until slightly thickened, about 3 minutes. Can be made 2 days ahead and refrigerated. Gently reheat before using.

Arrange the salmon fillets in a single layer on a baking pan lined with foil. Brush the fillets with the warm glaze.

Bake on the upper oven rack at 475 degrees Fahrenheit until sizzling and glazed, about 10 to 14 minutes, depending on thickness of the fillets. Use a fork to pierce the thickest part of the fillets to see if it is done. If the fork is hot, the salmon is done! Do not overcook.

Brush with the remaining glaze. Use a spatula to transfer to a warm serving platter.

Garnish the fillets with julienned basil.

Ingredient	Cal	Fat	Chol	Sod	Prot	Carb	Fiber
GARLIC	4	0	0	2	0.2	1	0
OIL	238	27	0	0	0	0	0
DIJON MUSTARD	5	0	0	120	0	0.2	0
HONEY	44	0	0	0	0.1	11.8	0
VINEGAR	11	0	0	16	0	0	0
BLACK PEPPER	1	0	0	0	0.1	0.4	0.1
SALMON FILLETS	1312	54.4	352	416	243.2	0	0
BASIL, FRESH	1	0	0	0	0.1	0.2	0.1
Totals Per Serving:	**269**	**13.6**	**59**	**92**	**40.6**	**2.2**	**0**

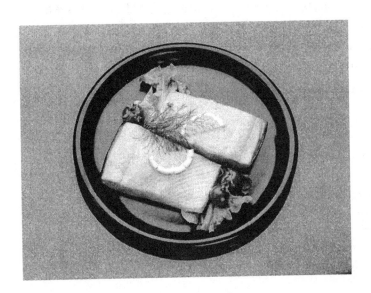

SCALLOPED OYSTERS
8 servings (1 mcg VITAMIN K per serving)

1/2	cup	Butter
4	oz	Saltine crackers, crushed (about 1 1/2 cups)
1 1/2	pints	Oysters
1/4	tsp	Ground black pepper
1/4	tsp	Tabasco Sauce
1/2	cup	Oyster liquor
1/2	cup	Heavy cream
1/2	cup	Bread crumbs, dry, plain
2	tsp	Butter, melted

Butter a 1 1/2 to 2 quart baking dish. Cover with a layer of cracker crumbs. Add a layer of half the oysters and another of cracker crumbs. Dot with the butter and pepper.

Make another layer of oysters and another of cracker crumbs. Dot again with the butter and pepper.

Combine the Tabasco Sauce, cream and 1/2 cup of oyster liquor and pour over the top.

Toss the bread crumbs with the melted butter and sprinkle over the top.

Bake 25 minutes at 400 degrees Fahrenheit.

Ingredient	Cal	Fat	Chol	Sod	Prot	Carb	Fiber
BUTTER	800	92	280	720	0	0	0
SALTINE CRACKERS	492	12	0	720	12	80	4
OYSTERS	456	16.8	384	768	48	26.4	0
BLACK PEPPER	1	0	0	0	0.1	0.4	0.1
TABASCO SAUCE	0	0	0	0	0	0	0
OYSTER LIQUOR	0	0	0	24	0	0	0
HEAVY CREAM	412	44	164	44	2.4	3.2	0
BREAD CRUMBS	212	2.8	0	464	6	38.4	2
BUTTER, MELTED	67	7.7	23	60	0	0	0
Totals Per Serving:	**305**	**21.9**	**106**	**350**	**8.6**	**18.5**	**0.8**

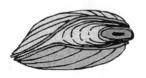

SALMON WITH PISTACHIO-BASIL BUTTER
6 servings (13 mcg of VITAMIN K per serving)

1/4	cup	Pistachio nuts (about 1 ounce)
6	large	Whole fresh basil leaves
1	tsp	Garlic cloves
1/2	cup	Butter (room temperature)
1	tsp	Lime juice
2	lb	Salmon filets, 1-1/2 inch thick (6 pieces)
1/2	cup	Dry white wine

Process the pistachios, 6 basil leaves and garlic clove in a food processor until finely chopped. Add 1/2 cup butter and 1 teaspoon lime juice and process until incorporated into the mixture. Transfer the butter mixture to a small bowl and refrigerate until well chilled (Pistachio butter can be prepared up to 4 days ahead.)

Preheat the oven to 400 degrees Fahrenheit. Butter a 9 by 13 inch baking dish. Place the salmon fillets in the dish in a single layer. Pour the white wine over salmon. Bake the salmon until almost opaque on top, about 10 minutes.

Place 2 tablespoons pistachio butter on top of each salmon piece. Continue baking until the salmon fillets are just opaque in the center, about 5 minutes.

Ingredient	Cal	Fat	Chol	Sod	Prot	Carb	Fiber
PISTACHIO NUTS	344	30	0	442	8	16	6
BASIL	6	0	0	0	0.6	1.2	0.6
GARLIC	4	0	0	2	0.2	1	0
BUTTER	800	92	280	720	0	0	0
LIME JUICE	1	0	0	0	0	0.5	0
SALMON FILETS	1312	54.4	352	416	243.2	0	0
DRY WHITE WINE	88	0	0	4	0	2.8	0
Totals Per Serving:	426	29.4	105	264	42	3.6	1.1

BAKED SALMON WITH FETA VINAIGRETTE
4 servings (5 mcg of VITAMIN K per serving)

20	oz	Salmon filets cut into 5 ounce portions
1	oz	Cheese, Feta, crumbled
2 1/2	tbsp	Lemon juice
1 1/2	tbsp	Orange juice
1	tbsp	Water
2	tsp	Dijon mustard
2	tsp	Oil, olive or Canola, treated (See Dietary Tip # 10)
1	tbsp	Oil, olive or Canola for coating the salmon
1/8	tsp	Tabasco sauce
1/2	cup	Bell pepper, red, diced

Preheat the oven to 500 degrees Fahrenheit.

Combine cheese, lemon juice, orange juice, water, Dijon mustard, oil and hot sauce. Stir with a wire whisk.

Coat each piece of salmon with oil. Place on an oiled, foil lined pan. Place in the oven at 500 degrees Fahrenheit for 10 to 12 minutes or until a fork, inserted in the thickest part of the filet, feels 'warm to hot,' to the touch.

Top each serving of roasted salmon with 2 tablespoons feta dressing and 2 tablespoons bell pepper.

Ingredient	Cal	Fat	Chol	Sod	Prot	Carb	Fiber
SALMON FILETS	820	34	220	260	152	0	0
CHEESE, FETA	38	3	12	158	2	0.6	0
LEMON JUICE	8	0	0	0	1.3	2.5	0
ORANGE JUICE	13	0	0	0	0.2	2.4	0.1
DIJON MUSTARD	10	0	0	240	0	0.3	0
OIL	80	9.1	0	0	0	0	0
OIL	120	13.6	0	0	0	0	0
TABASCO SAUCE	0	0	0	0	0	0	0
BELL PEPPER	120	2.4	0	24	4.8	33.6	7.2
Totals Per Serving:	**302**	**15.5**	**58**	**171**	**40.1**	**9.9**	**1.8**

GRILLED FISH IN FOIL

4 servings (9 mcg of VITAMIN K per serving for the sauce.
Remember to add the VITAMIN K content for the type of fish
you are using.)
This recipe can be used with any of the types of fish we know
have a very low amount of VITAMIN K. These include
butterfly bream, eel, mackerel, salmon, tuna, and yellowtail
(snapper.) However, it will probably taste best with bream,
tuna, or yellowtail.

1	lb	Sole fillets (or any other fish)
2	tbsp	Butter
1/4	cup	Lemon juice
1	tsp	Dill weed, fresh
1/4	tsp	Ground black pepper
1/4	tsp	Paprika (or more)
4	oz	Onion, thinly sliced (about 2/3 cup)

On 4 large buttered squares of heavy-duty aluminum foil,
place equal amounts of fish.

In a small saucepan, melt the butter, add the lemon juice, dill
weed and pepper and combine thoroughly.

Pour equal amounts of the sauce over the fish. Sprinkle with
paprika, top with onion slices.

Wrap foil securely around the fish, leaving space for the fish to
expand. Grill 5 to 7 minutes on each side or until the fish flakes
when tested with a fork.

Ingredient	Cal	Fat	Chol	Sod	Prot	Carb	Fiber
FISH, SOLE FILET	400	6.4	224	368	84.8	0	0
BUTTER	200	23	70	180	0	0	0
LEMON JUICE	12	0	0	0	2	4	0
DILL WEED	0	0	0	0	0	0	0
BLACK PEPPER	1	0	0	0	0.1	0.4	0.1
PAPRIKA	2	0.1	0	0	0.1	0.3	0.1
ONION	44	0	0	4	1.2	9.6	20
Totals Per Serving:	165	7.4	74	138	22	3.6	5.1

SCALLOPS OREGANATA
2 servings (31.6 mcg of VITAMIN K per serving)

3	tbsp	Bread crumbs; dried
1	tsp	Fresh parsley
1	tsp	Oregano, fresh chopped
1	tsp	Lemon peel; grated
1/2	tsp	Butter
8	oz	Scallops; sea scallops
1	tbsp	Lemon juice; freshly squeezed
1	tbsp	Dry vermouth
1	tbsp	Butter
1	clove	Garlic; minced

In a mixing bowl, combine the crumbs, parsley, oregano and lemon peel; add 1/2 tsp butter and mix thoroughly. Set aside.

Preheat broiler.

In a shallow, flameproof, 1 1/2 cup casserole, arrange the scallops in a single layer. Mix together the remaining ingredients and arrange over the scallops.

Broil 6 inches from the heat until the scallops are opaque, 4 to 5 minutes.

Sprinkle the crumb mixture evenly over the scallops and broil until crisp and lightly browned, about 1 minute longer.

Ingredient	Cal	Fat	Chol	Sod	Prot	Carb	Fiber
BREAD CRUMBS	96	0	0	0	0	0	0
PARSLEY	1	0	0	1	0	0.1	0
OREGANO	0	0	0	0	0	0	0
LEMON PEEL	4	0.1	0	0	0.2	1.5	0
BUTTER	17	1.9	6	15	0	0	0
SCALLOPS	200	1.6	72	368	36	50.4	0
LEMON JUICE	11	0.2	0	1	0.6	4.4	0
DRY VERMOUTH	11	0	0	0	0	0.4	0
BUTTER	100	11.5	35	90	0	0	0
GARLIC; MINCED	24	0.1	0	12	0.9	6	0
Totals Per Serving:	232	7.7	57	244	18.9	31.3	0

EGGS & CHEESE

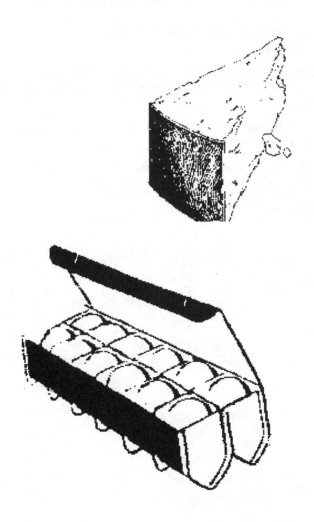

SAUSAGE & EGG CASSEROLE
8 servings (1 mcg of VITAMIN K per serving)

1	lb	Turkey kielbasa
1	tbsp	Canola oil (See Dietary Tip # 10)
4	cups	Bread cubes, fresh
8	large	Eggs
2	cups	Milk, skim
1	tsp	Mustard, powdered
4	oz	Cheddar cheese, sharp, grated (about 1 cup)

Sauté 1 pound of turkey kielbasa in a non-stick pan until lightly browned.

Grease a 9x13 casserole dish with the Canola oil and put the cubed bread in the bottom of the dish. Crumble the sausage over the bread.

Beat eggs, milk, and dry mustard together and pour over sausage. Sprinkle with cheese.

Cover and refrigerate overnight or freeze.

Bake 1 hour at 350 degrees Fahrenheit. Takes about 1 hour cooking time whether frozen or not.

Ingredient	Cal	Fat	Chol	Sod	Prot	Carb	Fiber
KIELBASA	896	64	368	4560	80	16	0
CANOLA OIL	120	14	0	0	0	0	0
BREAD CUBES	480	9.6	0	832	12.8	96	6.4
EGGS	600	44.8	1704	504	50.4	4.8	0
MILK, SKIM	176	1.6	16	256	16	24	0
MUSTARD	19	0	0	0	0	0	0
CHEDDAR	440	36	120	800	28	4	0
Totals Per Serving:	**341**	**21.3**	**276**	**869**	**23.4**	**18.1**	**0.8**

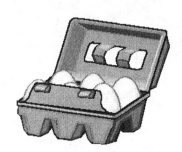

SCOTCH EGGS

12 servings (Less than 2 mcg of VITAMIN K per serving)

1 1/2	lb	Sausage, pork
1/2	cup	Onion, chopped
2	tbsp	Steak sauce
1/4	cup	Milk, skim
1/2	cup	Bread crumbs, dry, plain
1	each	Egg white, beaten until frothy
6	large	Eggs, hard cooked, shelled (7 eggs if they are small)
1	each	Egg, beaten slightly
2/3	cup	Bread crumbs, dry, plain
1/4	tsp	Ground black pepper
1/4	cup	All purpose flour
		Canola oil, treated (See Dietary Tip # 10)

Lightly mix the first six ingredients. Divide into 6 or 7 lumps. Shape each around a hard cooked egg, making an oval shape. Roll in flour, then the beaten egg and then the crumbs.

Put enough oil in a fry pan to make a 2 inch depth. Heat to 325 degrees Fahrenheit.

Fry meat rolls, turning once or twice, for five minutes, or until crispy brown. Discard the remaining oil.

Arrange the fried eggs on a cookie sheet. Put in a 325 degree Fahrenheit oven for about 10 to 15 minutes to finish them off. Then drain on paper towels.

Cut in half and serve hot or cold.

Ingredient	Cal	Fat	Chol	Sod	Prot	Carb	Fiber
SAUSAGE, PORK	2520	211.2	576	8808	134.4	7.2	0
ONION	32	0	0	0	0.8	6.8	1.2
STEAK SAUCE	32	0.3	0	380	0	8	0
MILK, SKIM	22	0.2	2	32	2	3	0
BREAD CRUMBS	212	2.8	0	464	6	38.4	2
EGG WHITE	14	0	0	46	3	3	0
EGGS	450	33.6	1278	378	37.8	3.6	0
EGG, BEATEN	75	5.6	213	63	6.3	0.6	0
BREAD CRUMBS	283	3.7	0	619	8	51.2	2.7
BLACK PEPPER	1	0	0	0	0.1	0.4	0.1
FLOUR	100	0.4	0	0	2.8	22	0
CANOLA OIL	964	112	0	0	0	0	0
Totals Per Serving:	**392**	**30.8**	**172**	**899**	**16.8**	**12**	**0.5**

BRUNCH ENCHILADAS

3 servings (2 mcgs of VITAMIN K per serving)   (If salsa is used, add the VITAMIN K content of the salsa.)

3	each	Tortillas, flour, 7 inch diameter
1	tbsp	Olive oil, treated (See Dietary Tip # 10)
3/4	cup	Ham, diced
2	large	Eggs
1/2	cup	Onion, diced
1/4	tsp	Ground black pepper
2	tbsp	Butter
1/4	cup	All purpose flour
2	oz	Cheese, Colby, shredded (about 1/2 cup)
3/4	cup	Milk, skim
2/3	cup	SALSA (See Recipe Index)

Sauté the ham and onion in the olive oil. Add the two eggs and scramble.

In a small pan, heat the butter, and whisk in the flour. Slowly add the milk, while whisking. Heat until thickened and bubbly. Add pepper.

Heat the tortillas on a griddle until soft and pliable, but do not allow to harden.

Divide the egg mixture into the three tortillas and roll up the tortillas. Pour the white sauce over and top with the cheese.

Serve with salsa on the side.

Ingredient	Cal	Fat	Chol	Sod	Prot	Carb	Fiber
TORTILLAS	240	6	0	330	6	42	0
OIL	119	12.5	0	0	0	0	0
HAM, DICED	276	14.4	90	2172	31.2	4.2	0
EGGS	150	11.2	426	126	12.6	1.2	0
ONION, DICED	32	0	0	0	0.8	6.8	1.2
BLACK PEPPER	1	0	0	0	0.1	0.4	0.1
BUTTER	200	23	70	180	0	0	0
FLOUR	100	0.4	0	0	2.8	22	0
CHEESE, COLBY	224	18	54	342	14	2	0
MILK, SKIM	66	0.6	6	96	6	9	0
SALSA	32	0.5	0	43	0.5	6.9	1.6
Totals Per Serving:	**480**	**29.2**	**215**	**1096**	**24.7**	**31.5**	**1**

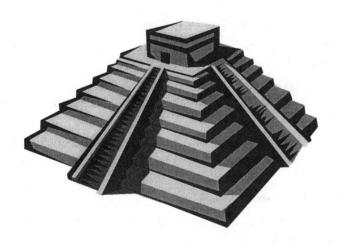

SPICY BREAKFAST SAUSAGE CASSEROLE
12 servings (Less than 2 mcgs of VITAMIN K per serving)

6	slices	Bread, Sourdough
8	oz	Cheddar cheese, shredded (about 2 cups)
1/2	lb	Italian sausage, turkey, spicy, cooked and drained
1	cup	Ham
1	cup	Mushrooms sliced
1/2	cup	Onion, chopped
10	large	Eggs
2 1/2	cup	Milk, skim
1/2	tsp	Paprika
1	tsp	Oregano leaves, fresh, minced
1/2	tsp	Ground black pepper
1/4	tsp	Garlic, finely minced
1/2	tsp	Mustard, powdered
1	tbsp	Butter

Grease a 9 by 13 inch pan with butter.

Slice the bread into one inch cubes. Put a single, crowded layer of bread into the pan. Dot with butter.

Sprinkle the shredded cheddar on top of the bread. Crumble cooked, drained sausage on top of the cheese. Sprinkle with turkey ham, onions, and mushrooms.

Beat eggs and milk together, add paprika, oregano, pepper, garlic and dry mustard. Mix and pour over the cheese in the pan.

Chill at least 12 hours.

Bake uncovered at 325 degrees Fahrenheit for 50 minutes. Let stand for 10 minutes before serving.

Ingredient	Cal	Fat	Chol	Sod	Prot	Carb	Fiber
BREAD	462	6	0	996	12	84	6
CHEDDAR	880	72	240	1600	56	8	0
SAUSAGE	784	71.2	176	1656	32	1.6	0
HAM	368	19.2	120	2896	41.6	5.6	0
MUSHROOMS	56	0.8	0	8	4.8	10.4	3.2
ONION	32	0	0	0	0.8	6.8	1.2
EGGS	750	56	2130	630	63	6	0
MILK, SKIM	220	2	20	320	20	30	0
PAPRIKA	3	0.2	0	1	0.2	0.6	0.2
OREGANO	1	0	0	1	0	0	0
BLACK PEPPER	3	0.1	0	1	0.1	0.7	0.2
GARLIC	1	0	0	1	0	0.3	0
MUSTARD	10	0	0	0	0	0	0
BUTTER	100	11.5	35	90	0	0	0
Totals Per Serving:	**306**	**19.9**	**227**	**683**	**19.2**	**12.8**	**0.9**

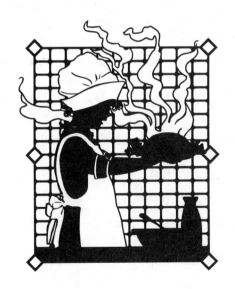

ITALIAN EGGS
8 servings (2 mcg of VITAMIN K per serving)

1	tbsp	Olive oil, treated (See Dietary Tip # 10)
1	tbsp	Butter
1	tsp	Garlic cloves, smashed
3/4	cup	Onion, diced
1/2	lb	Italian sausage, turkey, sweet or spicy
1/2	lb	Beef, ground extra lean
1	cup	Potato, peeled and diced
1	cup	Tomato, sliced thin
1/2	tsp	Ground black pepper
8	large	Eggs*

*Using an egg substitute will greatly reduce the cholesterol and fat in this recipe.

Combine olive oil and butter in a skillet and heat. Add onion and garlic and cook until medium brown.

Remove the casing from the sausages and cut the meat into small pieces. Add both the sausage and the beef to the onion. Add the diced potato.

Cover and cook slowly for 20 minutes. Add tomato and black pepper and stir. Cook for 15 minutes.

Beat all the eggs together and pour over the top. Cook to taste for 8 to 10 minutes.

Serve with toasted slices of Italian bread.

Ingredient	Cal	Fat	Chol	Sod	Prot	Carb	Fiber
OIL	119	13.5	0	0	0	0	0
BUTTER	100	11.5	35	90	0	0	0
GARLIC	4	0	0	2	0.2	1	0
ONION, DICED	48	0	0	0	1.2	10.2	1.8
SAUSAGE	784	71.2	176	1656	32	1.6	0
BEEF, GROUND	528	40	160	152	40	0	0
POTATO	120	0	0	8	3.2	27.2	2.4
TOMATOES	40	0.8	0	16	1.6	8	2.4
BLACK PEPPER	3	0.1	0	1	0.1	0.7	0.2
EGGS	600	44.8	1704	504	50.4	4.8	0
Totals Per Serving:	293	22.7	259	304	16.1	6.7	0.9

SOUPS

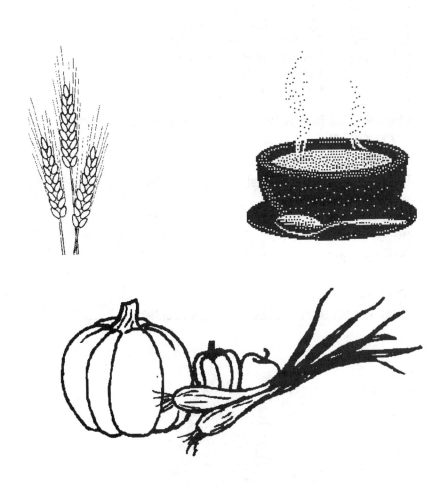

GAZPACHO
6 servings (VITAMIN K content = 13 mcg per cup)

2	cups	Tomato, chopped
1/2	cup	Bell pepper, green, finely chopped
2	cups	Tomato juice
1/2	cup	Basil, fresh, minced
1	tsp	Garlic cloves, minced
1/2	cup	Cucumber, peeled, chopped
1 1/2	cups	Onion, finely chopped
1	tbsp	Lemon juice
1/4	tsp	Ground black pepper

Combine all ingredients in a mixing bowl and refrigerate. Serve chilled.

Ingredient	Cal	Fat	Chol	Sod	Prot	Carb	Fiber
TOMATO	80	1.6	0	32	3.2	16	4.8
BELL PEPPER	28	0	0	0	0.4	0.4	0.4
TOMATO JUICE	80	0	0	48	0	16	0
BASIL	4	0	0	0	0.4	0.8	0.4
GARLIC	4	0	0	2	0.2	1	0
CUCUMBER	12	0	0	4	0.4	1.2	0.4
ONION	132	0	0	12	3.6	28.8	60
LEMON JUICE	3	0	0	0	0.5	1	0
BLACK PEPPER	1	0	0	0	0.1	0.4	0.1
Totals Per Serving:	**57**	**0.3**	**0**	**16**	**1.5**	**10.9**	**11**

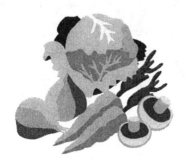

GOULASH SOUP

8 servings (6 mcgs of VITAMIN K per serving)

2	tbsp	Olive oil, treated (See Dietary Tip # 10)
1	lb	Sirloin OR round steak, lean, cut in cubes
1/2	cup	Onion, sliced
2	tsp	Garlic cloves, minced
1/4	tsp	Ground black pepper
3 3/4	cup	Beef broth*
3	cups	Tomato juice
1	tsp	Paprika
1/2	cup	Bell pepper, green, sliced
8	oz	Noodles, uncooked extra wide

*If you can find a salt free beef broth you will reduce your sodium intake considerably.

In a large kettle or Dutch oven, heat the oil. Add meat, onion, garlic and pepper. Cook and stir until meat is browned.

Add beef broth, tomato juice and paprika. Simmer covered 20 to 30 minutes until meat is tender. Bring mixture to a boil. Stir in the bell peppers and noodles.

Cook on a low boil (high simmer) 10 minutes until noodles are tender.

Ingredient	Cal	Fat	Chol	Sod	Prot	Carb	Fiber
OIL	238	27	0	0	0	0	0
STEAK, LEAN,	864	32	352	288	128	0	0
ONION	44	0	0	4	1.2	9.6	20
GARLIC	8	0	0	4	0.3	2	0
BLACK PEPPER	1	0	0	0	0.1	0.4	0.1
BEEF BROTH	150	0	0	6540	30	0	0
TOMATO JUICE	120	0	0	72	0	24	0
PAPRIKA	6	0.3	0	1	0.3	1.2	0.4
BELL PEPPER	28	0	0	0	0.4	0.4	0.4
NOODLES	864	8	216	48	32	160	8
Totals Per Serving:	290	8.4	71	870	24	24.7	3.8

SHERRIED CHICKEN SOUP
6 servings (2 mcg of VITAMIN K per serving)

6	oz	Chicken breast, skinless, boneless
1	cup	Water
1	piece	Celery
1	piece	Onion
1/2	cup	Bell pepper, green cut in thin strips
2	oz	Mushrooms, sliced (about 1/2 to 1/3 cup)
1/4	cup	All purpose flour
4	tbsp	Butter
2 1/2	cup	Half-and-half (cream)
1/2	cup	Sherry

Poach chicken in one cup water, with a piece of celery and onion, for flavor, until done. Approximately 15 to 30 minutes, depending on the thickness of the breasts.

Reserve broth, discard celery and onion, and cut chicken into bite size pieces. Add enough water to the reserved broth to make 1 cup.

Sauté green pepper and mushrooms lightly in a bit of the butter.

Make a white sauce with the rest of the butter (melted), flour and half and half. Thin with broth and add mushrooms, green pepper and chicken.

Heat without boiling, add sherry and serve. This is equally good chilled.

Note: Since the celery and onion are discarded, they are not included in the nutrition totals.

Ingredient	Cal	Fat	Chol	Sod	Prot	Carb	Fiber
CHICKEN BREAST	186	0	96	108	42	0	0
BELL PEPPER	28	0	0	0	0.4	0.4	0.4
MUSHROOMS	14	0.2	0	2	1.2	2.6	0.8
FLOUR	100	0.4	0	0	2.8	22	0
BUTTER	200	23	70	180	0	0	0
HALF-AND-HALF	740	68	200	240	16	24	0
SHERRY	160	0	0	368	0	20	0
Totals Per Serving:	**238**	**15.3**	**61**	**150**	**10.4**	**11.5**	**0.2**

BAKED POTATO CHICKEN SOUP
6 servings (6 mcgs of VITAMIN K per serving)

2	lb	Baking potatoes, cooked and cooled
1/2	cup	Ham, diced (Prosciutto would be good here.)
2	tbsp	Olive oil, treated (See Dietary Tip # 10)
1/2	cup	Onion, chopped
4	cups	Chicken broth
1 1/2	cups	Chicken, cooked (skin and bones removed)
1/4	tsp	Ground black pepper, to taste
2	tbsp	Yogurt, plain, lowfat
1	tbsp	Chives, fresh, snipped

Cut the potatoes into quarters lengthwise, do not remove the skins. Cut each quarter into 1/4-inch thick slices and set the potatoes aside.

Sauté the ham in the oil in a deep saucepan over medium heat until crisp and slightly browned. Remove the ham with a slotted spoon and drain on paper towels. Pour off all but 1 tablespoon of the oil.

Add the onion to the saucepan and sauté until translucent. Add the stock and bring to boiling. Add the potatoes and the chicken.

Simmer the soup for 5 minutes, stirring once or twice, to heat the chicken and the potatoes. Season the soup with pepper. Garnish the soup with the ham, yogurt and chives.

Ingredient	Cal	Fat	Chol	Sod	Prot	Carb	Fiber
BAKING POTATOES	704	3.2	0	64	19.2	163.2	16
HAM, DICED	184	9.6	60	1448	20.8	2.8	0
OIL	238	27	0	0	0	0	0
ONION	32	0	0	0	0.8	6.8	1.2
CHICKEN BROTH	128	0	0	5280	6.4	22.4	0
CHICKEN	376	16	168	168	56	0	0
BLACK PEPPER	1	0	0	0	0.1	0.4	0.1
YOGURT	16	0.5	2	25	2	2	0
CHIVES	4	0	0	0	0.5	0.5	0.5
Totals Per Serving:	**281**	**9.4**	**38**	**1164**	**17.6**	**33**	**3**

OLD-FASHIONED CHICKEN SOUP
8 servings (16 mcgs of VITAMIN K per serving)

2 1/2	lb	Chicken, fryer, cut into serving pieces
1/4	tsp	Ground black pepper
1/4	tsp	Paprika
1/4	tsp	Onion powder
1	cup	Leek, white and 1 1/2 inch green part, thinly sliced
1	cup	Onion, chopped
4	tsp	Garlic cloves, minced
1	lb	Tomatoes, stewed, chopped, undrained
1 1/2	cups	Carrots, peeled, thinly sliced
1/2	cup	Celery, thinly sliced
6	cups	Chicken broth
1/8	tsp	White pepper
2	cups	Potatoes, peeled, cubed and cooked
2	tbsp	Chives, fresh, chopped

Sprinkle the chicken pieces with the pepper, paprika and onion powder. Arrange in a 9x13-inch baking pan.

Bake chicken at 350-degrees Fahrenheit for 40 minutes. (This seals in the juices and replaces browning the chicken in oil, reducing the amount of oil needed. It will also de-fat the chicken).

Meanwhile, in a Dutch oven casserole, cook together the next 8 ingredients for 40 minutes.

Add the chicken to the casserole, discarding the skin, bones and fat in the pan.

Continue cooking for 15 minutes, or until chicken is tender. Add the potatoes and heat through. Sprinkle with chives.

Ingredient	Cal	Fat	Chol	Sod	Prot	Carb	Fiber
CHICKEN	1360	40	800	880	240	0	0
BLACK PEPPER	1	0	0	0	0.1	0.4	0.1
PAPRIKA	2	0.1	0	0	0.1	0.3	0.1
ONION POWDER	4	0	0	1	0.1	1	0.1
LEEK	136	0.8	0	48	3.2	32	2.4
ONION	64	0	0	0	1.6	13.6	2.4
GARLIC	16	0.1	0	8	0.6	4	0
TOMATOES	128	0	0	1008	0	32	0
CARROTS	72	1.2	0	60	1.2	18	1.2
CELERY	8	0	0	52	0.4	2.4	0.4
CHICKEN BROTH	192	0	0	7920	9.6	33.6	0
WHITE PEPPER	2	0	0	0	0.1	0.4	0.1
POTATOES	240	0	0	16	6.4	56	4.8
CHIVES, FRESH	9	0	0	1	1	1	1
Totals Per Serving:	**279**	**5.3**	**100**	**1249**	**33**	**24.3**	**1.6**

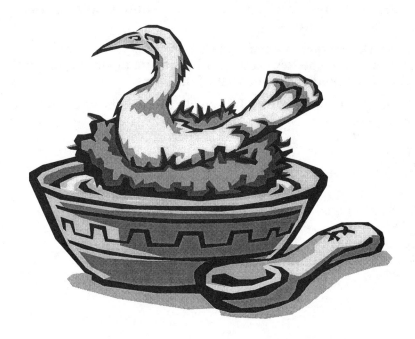

CHICKEN AND RICE SOUP
4 servings (Less than 1 mcg of VITAMIN K per serving)

2	cups	Chicken broth
3	cups	Water
1	tbsp	Lemon juice
1	tsp	Garlic cloves
1/2	cup	Rice, white dry, long-grain
1	lb	Chicken breast, skinless, boneless
1/4	tsp	Ground black pepper

Combine chicken broth, water and lemon juice in a saucepan. Peel the garlic and drop it in. Cover the pan and bring to a boil over high heat.

Add the rice, cover, and simmer over medium heat until rice is soft, about 15 minutes.

Meanwhile cut the chicken into thin shreds. When rice is tender, add the chicken, cover and continue to simmer until the chicken is cooked through, about 5 minutes.

Fish out the garlic clove and discard. Season the soup to taste with pepper.

Ingredient	Cal	Fat	Chol	Sod	Prot	Carb	Fiber
CHICKEN BROTH	64	0	0	2640	3.2	11.2	0
LEMON JUICE	3	0	0	0	0.5	1	0
GARLIC	4	0	0	2	0.2	1	0
RICE	412	0.8	0	4	8	90.8	1.2
CHICKEN BREAST	496	0	256	288	112	0	0
BLACK PEPPER	1	0	0	0	0.1	0.4	0.1
Totals Per Serving:	245	0.2	64	734	31	26.1	0.3

CHICKEN SOUP
8 servings (5 mcgs of VITAMIN K per serving)

3	lb	Chicken, fryer, cut up
1	lb	Potatoes, peeled
1	cup	Carrots, peeled and diced .
1	cup	Celery, chopped with leaves
1	cup	Onion, chopped
6	cups	Water
6	each	Peppercorns
1	each	Bay leaf

Remove any visible fat from the chicken pieces.

Layer the chicken and potatoes, carrots, celery and onion in crock pot. Add water.

Tie peppercorns and bay leaf in a piece of cheesecloth. Push under the liquid.

Cook on low 8 hours, or high 4 hours, until chicken is tender. Remove chicken skin and cheesecloth with spices, before serving.

Ingredient	Cal	Fat	Chol	Sod	Prot	Carb	Fiber
CHICKEN	1632	48	960	1056	288	0	0
POTATOES	352	0	0	32	9.6	81.6	8
CARROTS	48	0.8	0	40	0.8	12	0.8
CELERY	16	0	0	104	0.8	4.8	0.8
ONION	64	0	0	0	1.6	13.6	2.4
Totals Per Serving:	264	6.1	120	154	37.6	14	1.5

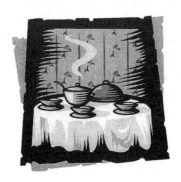

ITALIAN VEGETABLE SOUP WITH PROSCIUTTO
10 servings (76 mcgs of VITAMIN K per serving)

2	tbsp	Olive oil, treated (See Dietary Tip # 10)
3/4	cup	Onion, diced
1	tsp	Garlic, minced
6	cups	Water
28	oz	Tomatoes, canned, 'no salt added', chopped (liquid reserved)
1	cup	Carrots, peeled, cut in 1/2 inch slices
1	cup	Celery, sliced
2	cups	Cabbage, sliced
4	oz	Prosciutto, diced very fine
1/2	cup	Dry red wine
1/4	tsp	Ground black pepper
16	oz	Kidney beans, canned, drained
1	cup	Zucchini, peeled and sliced
4	oz	Pasta, Pennette or other tube shaped pasta
4	oz	Parmesan cheese, grated, (about 1 cup)

Heat oil in heavy large saucepan over high heat.

Add onion and garlic and sauté until garlic is brown, about 45 seconds.

Add next 8 ingredients. Season with pepper.

Bring mixture to boil. Reduce heat and simmer, stirring occasionally for 1 hour.

Mix the beans, zucchini and pasta into the soup. Simmer until pasta and zucchini are tender, about 15 minutes.

Serve hot, passing cheese separately.

Ingredient	Cal	Fat	Chol	Sod	Prot	Carb	Fiber
OLIVE OIL	238	27	0	0	0	0	0
ONION, DICED	48	0	0	0	1.2	10.2	1.8
GARLIC	4	0	0	2	0.2	1	0
TOMATOES	224	0	0	1540	8.4	33.6	0
CARROTS	48	0.8	0	40	0.8	12	0.8
CELERY	16	0	0	104	0.8	4.8	0.8
CABBAGE	32	0	0	32	1.6	8	3.2
PROSCIUTTO	360	28	0	2008	28	0	0
DRY RED WINE	88	0	0	4	0	0	0
BLACK PEPPER	1	0	0	0	0.1	0.4	0.1
KIDNEY BEANS	528	8	0	1312	32	96	19.2
ZUCCHINI	40	0	0	8	1.6	8	0.8
PASTA, DRY	440	4	0	40	16	80	0
PARMESAN CHEESE	444	30	96	1816	40.4	3.6	0
Totals Per Serving:	**251**	**9.8**	**10**	**691**	**13.1**	**25.8**	**2.7**

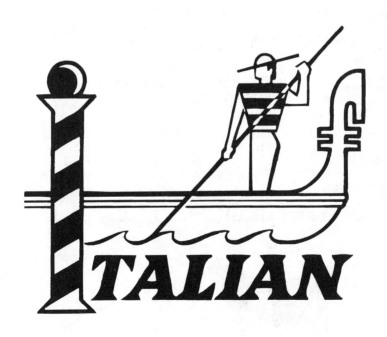

TOMATO-BEEF SOUP
8 servings (8 mcgs of VITAMIN K per serving)

1	lb	Beef, ground extra lean
1	cup	Onion, chopped
1/2	cup	Celery, chopped
1	tbsp	Butter
3	cups	Tomatoes, canned, 'No Salt Added'
2	tsp	Beef bouillon granules, instant, low sodium
1/3	cup	Rice, white uncooked, long grain
1/2	tsp	Chili powder
1	each	Bay leaf
3 1/2	cup	Water

Sauté beef, onion and celery in melted butter until meat is browned.

Stir in the remaining ingredients. Bring to a boil. Reduce heat, cover and simmer for 20 minutes.

Remove bay leaf.

Makes 2 quarts of hearty soup.

Ingredient	Cal	Fat	Chol	Sod	Prot	Carb	Fiber
BEEF	1056	80	320	304	80	0	0
ONION	64	0	0	0	1.6	13.6	2.4
CELERY	8	0	0	52	0.4	2.4	0.4
BUTTER	100	11.5	35	90	0	0	0
TOMATOES	216	0	0	120	7.2	48	0
BEEF BOUILLON	24	1.7	0	10	0.7	4	0
RICE	275	0.5	0	3	5.3	60.5	0.8
CHILI POWDER	3	0	0	0	0	0	0
BAY LEAF	0	0	0	0	0	0	0
Totals Per Serving:	218	11.7	44	72	11.9	16.1	0.5

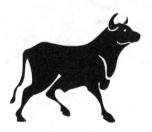

TEX-MEX BEEF SOUP
4 servings (18 mcgs of VITAMIN K per serving)

1/2	lb	Beef, round, steak, boneless, cut into 1/2 inch cubes
1	cup	Onion, chopped
1	tsp	Garlic cloves, minced
2	cups	Water
16	oz	Tomatoes, canned, 'No Salt Added', chopped
1	cup	Carrot, peeled and chopped
8	oz	Kidney beans, canned, low-salt, drained
1/2	cup	Green pepper, chopped
1/2	cup	Tomato puree
1	tbsp	Chili powder
2	tsp	Beef bouillon granules, instant, low sodium
1/4	tsp	Ground black pepper
1	tbsp	Canola oil for pan, treated (See Dietary Tip # 10)

Oil a large saucepan with Canola oil. Preheat over medium-high heat.

Add beef, onion, and garlic. Cook and stir about 3 minutes or until meat is brown.

Stir in remaining ingredients

Cover and simmer about 30 minutes or until meat is tender.

Serve

Ingredient	Cal	Fat	Chol	Sod	Prot	Carb	Fiber
BEEF,	640	80	192	152	67.2	0	0
ONION	64	0	0	0	1.6	13.6	2.4
GARLIC	4	0	0	2	.2	1	0
TOMATOES	128	0	0	880	4.8	19.2	0
CARROT	48	0.8	0	40	0.8	12	0.8
KIDNEY BEANS	264	4	0	656	16	48	9.6
GREEN PEPPER	32	0.4	0	0	1.2	7.2	2
TOMATO PUREE	44	0	0	40	0	12	4
CHILI POWDER	16	0	0	0	0	0	0
BEEF BOUILLON	24	1.7	0	10	0.7	4	0
BLACK PEPPER	1	0	0	0	0.1	0.4	0.1
OIL FOR PAN	120	14	0	0	0	0	0
Totals Per Serving:	346	25.2	48	445	23.1	29.3	4.7

VEGETABLE-BEEF SOUP
16 cup servings (31 mcgs of VITAMIN K per serving)

8	cups	Beef broth*
1 1/2	lb	Beef chuck, boneless, fat removed, cut into 1 inch cubes
1	tsp	Ground black pepper
1 1/4	lb	Potatoes, peeled and cubed (about 4 medium potatoes)
1	cup	Carrots, peeled and cubed
1	cup	Onion, coarsely chopped
16	oz	Tomato sauce
1	cup	Cabbage, coarsely chopped
17	oz	Corn, fresh or frozen
2	cups	Peas, green, fresh or frozen

*If you can find salt free beef broth you will lower the sodium count of this recipe considerably. You can also make your beef broth by buying beef bones and boiling them in eight cups of water for an hour. Strain and use broth.

Combine beef broth, beef cubes and pepper, cover and simmer one hour.

Add potatoes, carrots, onions, tomato sauce, hot pepper, and cabbage, cover and simmer 40 minutes.

Add corn and peas, simmer, uncovered, 30 minutes.

Ingredient	Cal	Fat	Chol	Sod	Prot	Carb	Fiber
BEEF BROTH	320	0	0	13952	64	0	0
BEEF CHUCK	1584	72	672	432	213.6	0	0
BLACK PEPPER	5	0.1	0	1	0.2	1.4	0.4
POTATOES	440	2	0	40	12	102	10
CARROTS	48	0.8	0	40	0.8	12	0.8
ONION	88	0	0	8	2.4	19.2	40
TOMATO SAUCE	176	0	0	2640	8	35.2	0
CABBAGE	16	0	0	16	0.8	4	1.6
CORN	408	5.1	0	68	15.3	91.8	15.3
PEAS	368	1.6	0	16	24	65.6	16
Totals Per Serving:	**216**	**5.1**	**42**	**1076**	**21.3**	**20.7**	**5.3**

CREAMY BEEF-NOODLE COMBO
5 servings (11 mcgs of VITAMIN K per serving)

1	lb	Beef, ground extra lean
1/2	cup	Onion, chopped (about 1 medium onion)
4	oz	Mushrooms, chopped
1 1/4	cups	MUSHROOM CREAM SAUCE (See Recipe Index)
1	cup	Celery, sliced, 2 stalks
1/2	cup	Green pepper, chopped
1/4	cup	Pimiento, sliced
1 1/4	cups	Milk, skim
1	tbsp	Worcestershire Sauce
4	oz	Noodles, uncooked (about 2 cups)

Cook and stir the meat and onion in a large skillet until the meat is brown. Drain off any excess fat.

Stir in the mushroom pieces and the remaining ingredients. Heat to boiling then reduce the heat and simmer, covered, stirring occasionally, until the noodles are tender, about 25 minutes.

A small amount of water can be added if necessary. Serve hot.

Ingredient	Cal	Fat	Chol	Sod	Prot	Carb	Fiber
BEEF	1056	80	320	304	80	0	0
ONION	44	0	0	4	1.2	9.6	20
MUSHROOMS	28	0.4	0	4	2.4	5.2	1.6
MSHRM CRM SAUCE	70	1	0	10	6	13	4
CELERY	16	0	0	104	0.8	4.8	0.8
GREEN PEPPER	32	0.4	0	0	1.2	7.2	2
PIMIENTO	12	0.2	0	8	0.4	2.4	0.2
MILK, SKIM	110	1	10	160	10	15	0
WORCESTERSHIRE	10	0	0	200	0	2	0
NOODLES	432	4	108	24	16	80	4
Totals Per Serving:	362	17.4	88	164	23.6	27.8	6.5

RED FISH CHOWDER
6 servings (7 mcgs of VITAMIN K per serving)

2	tbsp	Butter,
1	tsp	Garlic cloves, minced
4	oz	Onion, diced (about 1/2 cup)
1/2	cup	Green pepper, diced
1/2	cup	Celery, diced
1	cup	Tomatoes, crushed, canned
1	cup	Dry red wine
1	lb	Haddock
3	cups	Potatoes, peeled and diced
6	cups	Water
1/4	tsp	Ground black pepper
1/8	tsp	Tabasco sauce
1/8	tsp	Worcestershire Sauce

Melt butter in stock pot and sauté garlic, onion, green pepper and celery until tender, stirring often.

Add water, fish, tomatoes, wine and potatoes. Add seasonings, bring to a boil and cook until the potatoes and fish are tender.

Ingredient	Cal	Fat	Chol	Sod	Prot	Carb	Fiber
BUTTER,	200	23	70	180	0	0	0
GARLIC	4	0	0	2	0.2	1	0
ONION	44	0	0	4	1.2	9.6	20
GREEN PEPPER	32	0.4	0	0	1.2	7.2	2
CELERY, DICED	8	0	0	52	0.4	2.4	0.4
TOMATOES	72	0	0	296	0	16	8
DRY RED WINE	176	0	0	8	0	0	0
HADDOCK	400	3.2	256	304	86.4	0	0
POTATO	360	0	0	24	9.6	81.6	7.2
BLACK PEPPER	1	0	0	0	0.1	0.4	0.1
TABASCO SAUCE	0	0	0	0	0	0	0
WORCESTERSHIRE	0	0	0	8	0	0.1	0
Totals Per Serving:	**216**	**4.4**	**54**	**146**	**16.5**	**19.7**	**6.3**

SOPA DE PESCADO (FISH)
8 servings (5 mcgs of VITAMIN K per serving)

2	quarts	Fish stock*
1	cup	Shrimp, cooked pieces
2	tbsp	Lemon juice
1/2	lb	Vermicelli noodles, uncooked
1	each	Egg, hard boiled and cubed
1	each	GREEN CHILE SAUCE (See Recipe Index)
1/2	cup	Croutons, plain, or other garnish

*Can be liquid from boiled fish, seasoned with a few drops of olive oil, onion and bay leaf.

Heat the broth. Add the shellfish, lemon juice and vermicelli noodles, simmer until heated through and pasta is al dente.

Serve with a small dollop of GREEN CHILE SAUCE (See Recipe Index) in each dish. To be stirred in by the diner.

Garnish with the egg and croutons

Ingredient	Cal	Fat	Chol	Sod	Prot	Carb	Fiber
FISH STOCK	320	0	0	2816	64	0	0
SHRIMP	152	2.4	224	216	28.8	1.6	0
LEMON JUICE	6	0	0	0	1	2	0
VERMICELLI	800	4	0	0	28	168	0
EGG	75	5	213	63	6.3	0.6	0
GRN CHILE SAUCE	392	37.6	2	479	27.7	0	9.6
CROUTONS	60	1	0	104	1.8	11.2	0.8
Totals Per Serving:	**226**	**6.3**	**55**	**460**	**19.7**	**22.9**	**1.3**

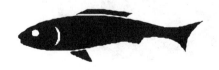

GREEN CHILE SAUCE
8 servings (3 mcgs of VITAMIN K per serving)

2	tbsp	Oil, olive or Canola treated (See Dietary Tip # 10)
1	tsp	Garlic cloves
1/2	cup	Onion, minced
1	tbsp	All purpose flour
1	cup	Water
1	cup	Green chili, diced

Sauté garlic and onion in oil in a heavy saucepan,

Blend in flour with a wooden spoon.

Add the water and green chili.

Bring to a boil and simmer, stirring frequently, for 5 minutes.

Ingredient	Cal	Fat	Chol	Sod	Prot	Carb	Fiber
OIL	240	27.2	0	0	0	0	0
GARLIC	4	0	0	2	0.2	1	0
ONION	32	0	0	0	0.8	6.8	1.2
FLOUR	25	0.1	0	0	0.7	5.5	0
GREEN CHILI	88	0	0	16	8	24	0
Totals Per Serving:	**49**	**3.4**	**0**	**2**	**1.2**	**4.7**	**0.2**

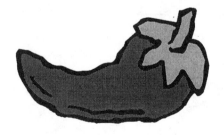

QUICK FISH CHOWDER
4 servings (8 mcgs of VITAMIN K per serving)

3	tbsp	Olive oil, treated (See Dietary Tip # 10)
1/2	cup	Onion, chopped
3/4	cup	Celery, sliced, about 2 stalks
1	tsp	Chili powder
1	lb	Tomatoes, stewed and juice
1	cup	Fish stock*
1	tsp	Sugar
1	tsp	Worcestershire Sauce
1	lb	Haddock, snapper or bream, cut into chunks
1/2	cup	Croutons for garnish, garlic flavored

*Water may be substituted.

Heat oil in a saucepan. Pitch in the onion, celery, and chili powder. Sauté over medium heat for 10 minutes.

Stir in the tomatoes, water, sugar, and Worcestershire Sauce. Bring to a rolling boil and add the fish. Reduce heat and simmer, covered, for about 15 minutes.

Sprinkle with garlic croutons.

Ingredient	Cal	Fat	Chol	Sod	Prot	Carb	Fiber
OIL	357	40.5	0	0	0	0	0
ONION	32	0	0	0	0.8	6.8	1.2
CELERY	12	0	0	78	0.6	3.6	0.6
CHILI POWDER	6	0	0	0	0	0	0
TOMATOES	128	0	0	1008	0	32	0
FISH STOCK	40	0	0	352	8	0	0
SUGAR	16	0	0	0	0	4.2	0
WORCESTERSHIRE	3	0	0	67	0	0.7	0
HADDOCK	400	3.2	256	304	86.4	0	0
CROUTONS	92	3.6	0	248	2	16.8	1.2
Totals Per Serving:	272	11.8	64	514	24.5	16	.8

TOMATO BISQUE
6 cups (17 mcgs of VITAMIN K per serving)

1	cup	Onion, white, diced
1	tsp	Garlic, minced
3	tbsp	Olive oil, treated (See Dietary Tip # 10)
1	cup	Eggplant, diced
1	cup	Squash, zucchini, peeled and diced
1	cup	Squash, yellow summer, peeled and diced
1	cup	Green pepper, diced Bell peppers
1/4	cup	Tomato puree
1 1/3	cups	Tomato juice
1 1/3	cups	Chicken broth
6	leaves	Whole fresh basil, chopped
1/4	tsp	Ground black pepper

Cook the onion and garlic in hot oil for 2 minutes.

Add the eggplant, zucchini and peppers. Cook 5 minutes.

Add tomato paste and cook 5 minutes on low heat. Stir in tomato juice and stock. Simmer until vegetables are just tender, about 8 to 10 minutes.

Stir in basil and season with pepper.

Ingredient	Cal	Fat	Chol	Sod	Prot	Carb	Fiber
ONION	88	0	0	8	2.4	19.2	40
GARLIC	7	0	0	1	0.3	1.6	0.1
OIL	357	40.5	0	0	0	0	0
EGGPLANT	56	0	0	8	0.8	2.4	3.2
SQUASH	48	0.8	0	8	2.4	9.6	2.4
SQUASH	48	0.8	0	8	2.4	9.6	2.4
GREEN PEPPER	64	0.8	0	0	2.4	14.4	4
TOMATO PUREE	22	0	0	20	0	6	2
TOMATO JUICE	53	0	0	32	0	10.7	0
CHICKEN BROTH	43	0	0	1760	2.1	7.5	0
BASIL	6	0	0	0	0.6	1.2	0.6
BLACK PEPPER	1	0	0	0	0.1	0.4	0.1
Totals Per Serving:	132	7.2	0	308	2.2	13.7	9.1

CARROT VICHYSSOISE
10 servings (less than 12 mcgs of VITAMIN K per serving)

2	cups	Potatoes, peeled and chopped
1 1/2	cups	Carrots, peeled and thinly sliced
3	cups	Leeks, white part and green part, sliced
5	cups	Chicken broth
1/8	tsp	Pepper, white
1	cup	Milk, evaporated skim*
6	tbsp	Sour cream, lowfat

*If you do not need to watch your fat intake you can substitute Half & Half.

Combine the potatoes, carrots, leeks and broth in a large saucepan. Bring to a boil, then simmer, uncovered, 25 minutes or until vegetables are tender.

Puree the vegetables and liquid, half at a time, in a blender. Pour mixture into a mixing bowl.

Stir in the white pepper and half and half. Chill well.

Serve in cups or mugs, garnished with a dollop of sour cream.

Ingredient	Cal	Fat	Chol	Sod	Prot	Carb	Fiber
POTATOES	240	0	0	16	6.4	64	4.8
CARROTS	72	1.2	0	60	1.2	18	1.2
LEEKS	408	2.4	0	144	9.6	96	7.2
CHICKEN BROTH	160	0	0	6600	8	28	0
PEPPER, WHITE	2	0	0	0	0.1	0.4	0.1
MILK, EVAP SKIM	200	0.8	8	296	19.2	13.6	0
SOUR CREAM	120	6	15	105	6	12	0
Totals Per Serving:	**120**	**1**	**2**	**722**	**5**	**23.2**	**1.3**

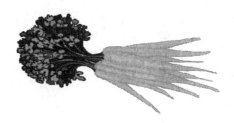

VEGETABLE SOUP

16 servings (12 mcgs of VITAMIN K per serving)

8	cups	Chicken broth
1	cup	Carrots, peeled and diced
1	cup	Celery, chopped
1	cup	Onion, sliced
3	tsp	Garlic cloves, minced
1	tbsp	Basil, fresh, chopped
2	cups	Beans, green snap (fresh or frozen)
2	cups	Squash, yellow summer squash, peeled and diced
2	cups	Squash, Zucchini, peeled and diced
1	cup	Navy beans, cooked
1	cup	Corn kernels, fresh or frozen
1/8	tsp	Ground black pepper

Please note: This may be made ahead and frozen.

Combine the broth, carrots, celery, onion, garlic, and basil in a large pot. Bring to a boil and simmer for 30 minutes.

Add the green beans, yellow squash, zucchini and beans. Simmer for 30 minutes.

Add the corn and cook 20 minutes longer.

Variations: Add 1 cup pasta along with the corn, or add 1 cup barley in the beginning.

Ingredient	Cal	Fat	Chol	Sod	Prot	Carb	Fiber
CHICKEN BROTH	256	0	0	10560	12.8	44.8	0
CARROTS	48	0.8	0	40	0.8	12	0.8
CELERY	16	0	0	104	0.8	4.8	0.8
ONION	88	0	0	8	2.4	19.2	40
GARLIC	12	0.1	0	6	0.5	3	0
BASIL	0	0	0	0	0.1	0.1	0.1
BEANS	144	0	0	32	16	32	32
SQUASH, YELLOW	96	1.6	0	16	4.8	19.2	4.8
SQUASH, ZUCCHIN	96	1.6	0	16	4.8	19.2	4.8
NAVY BEANS	320	0.8	0	0	20	59.2	8
CORN KERNELS	192	2.4	0	32	7.2	43.2	7.2
BLACK PEPPER	1	0	0	0	0	0.2	0.1
Totals Per Serving:	79	0.5	0	676	4.4	16.1	6.2

BEEF AND LENTIL STEW
6 servings (14 mcgs of VITAMIN K per serving)

1	lb	Beef, lean, ground
1/2	cup	Onion, chopped (about 1 medium)
1	tsp	Garlic cloves, minced
4	oz	Mushroom stems and pieces
16	oz	Tomatoes, stewed, 'No Salt Added'
1/2	cup	Celery, sliced
1/2	cup	Carrot, peeled and cut in 1/2 inch slices
1	cup	Lentils, uncooked
3	cups	Water
1/4	cup	Dry red wine
1	each	Bay leaf
1	tsp	Beef bouillon granules (instant), low sodium
1/4	tsp	Ground black pepper

Cook and stir the meat, onion and garlic in a Dutch oven until the meat is brown. Drain off any excess fat.

Stir in the undrained mushrooms, and the remaining ingredients. Heat to boiling, then reduce the heat, cover, and simmer, stirring occasionally, until the lentils are tender, about 40 minutes.

Remove the bay leaf and serve.

Ingredient	Cal	Fat	Chol	Sod	Prot	Carb	Fiber
BEEF GROUND	1056	80	320	304	80	0	0
ONION	44	0	0	4	1.2	9.6	20
GARLIC	4	0	0	2	1	0.2	0
MUSHROOMS	28	0.4	0	4	2.4	5.2	1.6
TOMATOES	128	0	0	1008	0	32	0
CELERY	8	0	0	52	0.4	2.4	0.4
CARROT	24	0.4	0	20	0.4	6	0.4
LENTILS	768	0	0	24	64	128	72
DRY RED WINE	44	0	0	2	0	0	0
BAY LEAF	0	0	0	0	0	0	0
BEEF BOUILLON	12	.8	0	5	0.3	2	0
BLACK PEPPER	1	0	0	0	0.1	0.4	0.1
Totals Per Serving:	353	13.6	53	238	24.8	31.1	15.8

PUREE OF CARROT SOUP
6 servings (4 mcgs of VITAMIN K per serving)

1	lb	Carrots, peeled and thinly sliced
1	cup	Onion, chopped
1	tbsp	Oil, olive or Canola, treated (See Dietary Tip # 10)
2	tbsp	Butter
4	cups	Chicken broth
1/4	tsp	Ground black pepper

Heat a large saucepan. Add the butter and oil and sauté onions until golden.

Add the carrots and chicken broth and simmer gently until carrots are tender.

Puree in a blender, return to pan and thin (or not) with additional chicken broth. You could add some heavy cream or evaporated skim milk if you wanted a creamed soup.

Bring to a boil, garnish with a sprig of dill and serve.

Ingredient	Cal	Fat	Chol	Sod	Prot	Carb	Fiber
CARROTS	96	1.6	0	80	1.6	24	1.6
ONION	64	0	0	0	1.6	13.6	2.4
OIL	120	13.6	0	0	0	0	0
BUTTER	200	23	70	180	0	0	0
CHICKEN BROTH	128	0	0	5280	6.4	22.4	0
BLACK PEPPER	1	0	0	0	0.1	0.4	0.1
Totals Per Serving:	102	6.4	12	923	1.6	10.1	0.7

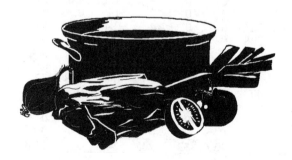

CARROT HORSERADISH SOUP
4 servings (6 mcgs of VITAMIN K per serving)

2	tbsp	Oil, olive or Canola, treated (See Dietary Tip # 10)
4	oz	Onion, minced (about 1 small onion)
1/2	cup	Celery, minced
1	tsp	Garlic cloves, minced
1	cup	Carrots, peeled and diced
20	oz	Beef broth
6	oz	Water
1	tbsp	Horseradish
2	tsp	Butter
2	tsp	All purpose flour
1/8	tsp	Ground black pepper

In a saucepan, heat the oil and add onions, celery, and garlic. Lightly sauté until onion is transparent, about 5 minutes.

Add the carrots, beef broth and water. Cover tightly, bring to a boil, reduce heat and simmer until carrots are tender, about 15 minutes.

Add horseradish.

Combine the butter and flour into a paste. Drop (in small bits) into the gently simmering soup. Cook, stirring, until the mixture is absorbed and very lightly thickened.

Taste for seasoning and add pepper. Serve hot.

Ingredient	Cal	Fat	Chol	Sod	Prot	Carb	Fiber
OIL	240	27.2	0	0	0	0	0
ONION	44	0	0	4	1.2	9.6	20
CELERY	8	0	0	52	0.4	2.4	0.4
GARLIC	4	0	0	2	0.2	1	0
CARROTS	48	0.8	0	40	0.8	12	0.8
BEEF BROTH	100	0	0	4360	20	0	0
HORSERADISH	6	0.1	0	0	0.2	1.4	0.2
BUTTER	67	7.7	23	60	0	0	0
FLOUR	17	0.1	0	0	0.5	3.7	0
BLACK PEPPER	1	0	0	0	0	0.2	0.1
Totals Per Serving:	134	8.9	6	1130	5.8	7.5	5.3

CARROT POTATO CHOWDER

6 servings (2 mcgs of VITAMIN K per serving)

3/4	cup	Onion, white, minced
1/4	cup	Butter
2	cups	Potatoes, peeled and diced, raw
3	cups	Boiling water
1/4	tsp	Paprika
1	tbsp	All purpose flour
2	cups	Milk, skim, heated
3/4	cup	Carrots, peeled and diced (cooked)

Sauté onion in 2 tablespoons of butter in a large saucepan until lightly browned. Add potatoes, boiling water and paprika. Boil about 15 minutes or until potatoes are soft.

Blend flour with remaining butter and gradually add milk, stirring constantly, until smooth and thickened.

Add sauce to the potato mixture. Add carrots. Cook 5 minutes, stirring until smooth.

Ingredient	Cal	Fat	Chol	Sod	Prot	Carb	Fiber
ONION, WHITE	66	0	0	6	1.8	14.4	30
BUTTER	400	46	140	360	0	0	0
POTATO	240	0	0	16	6.4	54.4	4.8
PAPRIKA	2	0.1	0	0	0.1	0.3	0.1
FLOUR	25	0.1	0	0	0.7	5.5	0
MILK, SKIM	176	1.6	16	256	16	24	0
CARROTS	36	0.6	0	30	0.6	9	0.6
Totals Per Serving:	**158**	**8.1**	**26**	**111**	**4.3**	**17.9**	**5.9**

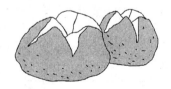

SAUSAGE CHOWDER
6 servings (3 mcgs of VITAMIN K per serving)

1	lb	Smoked sausage, cut in chunks*
1	cup	Onion, chopped
6	cups	Potatoes, peeled and cubed
1	tsp	Basil, fresh, chopped
1/8	tsp	Ground black pepper
2	cups	Water
16	oz	Cream style corn
16	oz	Corn kernels, fresh or frozen
18	oz	Milk, evaporated skim

*Using one of the 'lite' or 'lean' smoked sausages, on the market, will change the nutrition values.

Brown the sausage. Add onion and sauté without browning.

Add potatoes, seasonings and water. Cover, simmer 15 minutes.

Stir in corn and milk. Heat to boiling point. Do not let boil! Serve hot.

Ingredient	Cal	Fat	Chol	Sod	Prot	Carb	Fiber
SMOKED SAUSAGE	1568	144	352	3312	64	1.6	0
ONION	64	0	0	0	1.6	13.6	2.4
POTATOES	720	0	0	48	19.2	192	14.4
BASIL	0	0	0	0	0	0	0
BLACK PEPPER	1	0	0	0	0	0.2	0.1
CREAM STYLE CORN	320	0	0	1296	0	80	0
CORN KERNELS	384	4.8	0	64	14.4	86.4	14.4
MILK, EVAP SKIM	450	1.8	18	666	43.2	30.6	0
Totals Per Serving:	585	25.1	62	898	23.7	67.4	5.2

CORN CHOWDER
11 servings (2 mcgs of VITAMIN K per serving)

3	slices	Bacon, diced
4	cups	Chicken broth
1	lb	Chicken, cut in 1/2 inch cubes
3/4	cup	Onion, minced
3/4	cup	Celery, finely chopped
4	cups	Corn kernels. fresh or frozen (divided)
2	cups	Potatoes, peeled and diced
1	cup	Heavy cream
1/8	tsp	Pepper, white

In a Dutch oven, over medium heat, cook the bacon until crisp. Remove with a slotted spoon and pour off all but 2 tablespoons of the drippings.

Add chicken, onion, celery and cook 10-15 minutes or until tender.

In a blender, combine 1 cup of chicken broth and 2 cups of corn. Blend on high until smooth. Stir into the Dutch oven along with remaining corn, potatoes and chicken broth. Bring to a boil.

Reduce heat and simmer partially covered 20 minutes or until potatoes are tender.

Stir in cream and pepper and simmer 2-3 minutes more. Stir in bacon and serve.

Ingredient	Cal	Fat	Chol	Sod	Prot	Carb	Fiber
BACON, DICED	138	11.7	21	381	6.9	0.3	0
CHICKEN BROTH	128	0	0	5280	6.4	22.4	0
CHICKEN	544	16	320	352	96	0	0
ONION	48	0	0	0	1.2	10.2	1.8
CELERY	12	0	0	78	0.6	3.6	0.6
CORN KERNELS	768	9.6	0	128	28.8	172.8	28.8
POTATO	240	0	0	16	6.4	54.4	4.8
HEAVY CREAM	824	88	328	88	4.8	6.4	0
BACON DRIPPINGS	252	25.6	24	207	0	0	0
PEPPER, WHITE	2	0	0	0	0.1	0.4	0.1
Totals Per Serving:	**269**	**13.7**	**63**	**594**	**13.7**	**24.6**	**3.3**

MUSHROOM SOUP

6 servings (Less than 1 mcg of VITAMIN K per serving)

1	lb	Mushrooms
1/2	cup	Shallots, finely chopped
1	tsp	Lemon juice
4	cups	Chicken broth
1/8	tsp	Ground black pepper
4	tbsp	Butter
6	slices	Bread, Italian or French, dry, crusts removed
1/2	cup	Heavy cream

Wash and dry the mushrooms. Chop about 3/4 pound and slice the rest.

In a soup kettle, melt 3 tablespoons of the butter and sauté the shallots until tender. Add the chopped mushrooms and continue cooking 5 minutes, stirring occasionally.

Pour in the chicken broth, season with pepper and cook slowly for 30 minutes, uncovered.

Meanwhile, with the remaining one tablespoon of butter, sauté the sliced mushrooms on high heat add the teaspoon of lemon juice.

Make bread crumbs with the dry bread. Add the bread crumbs to the soup and continue cooking for 8 more minutes.

When ready to serve, add the cream and the reserved sliced mushrooms to the hot soup.

Ingredient	Cal	Fat	Chol	Sod	Prot	Carb	Fiber
MUSHROOMS	112	1.6	0	16	9.6	20.8	6.4
SHALLOTS	56	0.4	0	8	2.8	13.6	0.8
LEMON JUICE	1	0.0	0	0	0.2	0.3	0
CHICKEN BROTH	128	0	0	5280	6.4	22.4	0
BLACK PEPPER	1	0	0	0	0	0.2	0.1
BUTTER	400	46	140	360	0	0	0
BREAD	462	6	0	996	12	84	6
HEAVY CREAM	412	44	164	44	2.4	3.2	0
Totals Per Serving:	262	16.3	51	1117	5.5	24	2.2

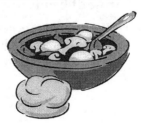

BEAN SOUP
80 servings (5 mcgs of VITAMIN K per serving))

1	lb	Navy beans, dry
1	lb	Pinto beans, dry
1	lb	Green split peas, dry
1	lb	Black-eyed peas, dry
1	lb	Lentils, dry
1	lb	Lima beans, large, dry
1	lb	Red kidney beans, dry
1	lb	Barley, dry

RECIPE CARD FOR JAR

6 3/4	cup	Chicken broth
2	tsp	Garlic cloves
1/4	tsp	Ground black pepper
3	cups	Ham, diced and cooked
1	cup	Onion, chopped
16	oz	Tomatoes, canned, 'No Salt Added' undrained and chopped
3	tbsp	Lime juice

This is a recipe for Bean Soup. (It is meant to be used for gifts.)

One pound each of the seven varieties of beans and the barley are to be mixed together and then divided into 10 (1 1/2 cups) portions.

Each portion is packed for gift giving. (Mason jar, cloth sack, etc.) Include the ingredients listed above (for the card) and the following directions with each gift portion of beans.

DIRECTIONS: Sort and wash the beans. Place the beans in a large pot. Cover with water 2 inches above level of beans and soak overnight.

Drain off the water leaving the beans in the pot. Add broth and pepper. Cover and bring to a boil. Reduce heat and simmer 1 1/2 hours or until beans are tender.

Add remaining ingredients and simmer, uncovered, 30 minutes, stirring occasionally. Serve hot. Yield 2 1/2 quarts.

Ingredient	Cal	Fat	Chol	Sod	Prot	Carb	Fiber
NAVY BEANS, DRIED	1520	6.4	0	64	100.8	275.2	43.2
PINTO BEANS, DRY	1536	4.8	0	48	94.4	288	54.4
GREEN SPLIT PEAS	1552	4.8	0	64	112	273.6	25.6
BLACK-EYED PEAS	1520	6.4	0	80	107.2	272	123.2
LENTILS, DRY	1536	0	0	48	128	256	144
LIMA BEANS	1536	3.2	0	80	97.6	288	86.4
RED KIDNEY BEANS	1504	0	0	112	112	272	112
BARLEY, DRY	1600	11.2	0	48	56	332.8	78.4
RECIPE CARD FOR JAR							
CHICKEN BROTH	216	0	0	8910	10.8	37.8	0
GARLIC	8	0	0	4	0.3	2	0.1
BLACK PEPPER	1	0	0	0	0.1	0.4	0.1
HAM	1104	57.6	360	8688	124.8	16.8	0
ONION	64	0	0	0	1.6	13.6	2.4
TOMATOES	144	0	0	80	4.8	32	0
LIME JUICE	12	0	0	0	0.3	4.2	0
Totals Per Serving:	**327**	**7.5**	**45**	**2217**	**27.2**	**37.4**	**7.7**

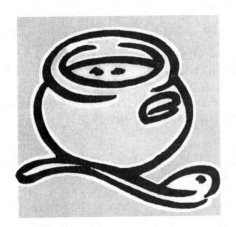

WHITE GAZPACHO
6 servings (4 mcgs of VITAMIN K per serving)

4	tsp	Chicken bouillon granules, instant, low sodium
2	cups	Boiling water
20	oz	Cucumber, peeled (about 3 medium cucumber.)
16	oz	Sour cream, lowfat
2	tbsp	Lemon juice
1/4	tsp	Garlic powder
1/4	tsp	Ground black pepper

Pare and remove the seeds from the cucumbers. Cut into cubes so that you have about 3 cups of cubes.

In a small saucepan, dissolve the bouillon in water. Cool completely.

In a blender or food processor, blend the peeled cucumber with 1/2 cup bouillon liquid until smooth.

In medium bowl, combine the cucumber mixture, remaining bouillon liquid, sour cream, lemon juice, garlic powder and pepper, mix well.

Chill thoroughly. Garnish as desired. Serve with condiments.

SUGGESTED CONDIMENTS: Chopped fresh tomato, chopped red onions, chopped green peppers, toasted slivered almonds or toasted croutons. Use 1/4 cup garnish per serving. Do not forget to add the nutrition information of the condiments to the basic recipe counts.

Ingredient	Cal	Fat	Chol	Sod	Prot	Carb	Fiber
CHICKEN BOUILLON	48	3.3	0	20	1.3	8	0
CUCUMBER	60	0	0	20	2	6	2
SOUR CREAM	640	32	80	560	32	64	0
LEMON JUICE	6	0	0	0	1	2	0
GARLIC POWDER	2	0	0	0	0.1	0.5	0
BLACK PEPPER	1	0	0	0	0.1	0.4	0.1
Totals Per Serving:	126	5.9	13	100	6.1	13.5	0.4

STRAW MUSHROOM SOUP
2 servings (80 mcgs of VITAMIN K per serving)

14	oz	Chicken broth
1/4	cup	Dry sherry
1/8	tsp	White pepper
1/3	cup	Straw mushrooms
1	tsp	Sesame oil
1/3	cup	Green onions, sliced

In a small saucepan, combine the chicken broth, sherry and white pepper.

Bring to a boil, reduce heat and add mushrooms and sesame oil. Heat for a minute.

Just before serving, sprinkle with scallions.

Ingredient	Cal	Fat	Chol	Sod	Prot	Carb	Fiber
CHICKEN BROTH	56	0	0	2310	2.8	9.8	0
DRY SHERRY	60	0	0	0	0	1	0
WHITE PEPPER	2	0	0	0	0.1	0.4	0.1
STRAW MUSHROOMS	24	0	0	291	2.7	2.7	2.7
SESAME OIL	42	4.7	0	0	0	0	0
GREEN ONIONS	24	0	0	13	2.7	2.7	1.3
Totals Per Serving:	104	2.3	0	1307	4.1	8.3	2.1

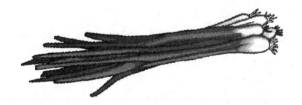

POTATO SOUP
4 servings (10 mcgs of VITAMIN K per serving)

10	oz	Potatoes, peeled (About 2 medium potatoes)
6	oz	Onion, sliced thin (about 1 medium onion)
1 1/2	cups	Celery stalks and leaves
2	tbsp	Olive or Canola oil, treated (See Dietary Tip # 10)
		Boiling water
1		Bay leaf
2	tbsp	Butter
2	cups	Milk, skim, up to 3 cups may be used

Peel and thinly slice potatoes, onion and celery. Sauté for 3 to 5 minutes in hot vegetable oil.

In a large pot, add all the vegetables and cover with just enough boiling water to cover. Place bay leaf in pot and boil vegetables until tender.

Drain vegetables and reserve liquid. Mash the vegetables into the reserved liquid and add butter.

Thin soup with milk, heat until warm. (DO NOT boil.)

Ladle into soup bowls. (The nutrition counts are calculated for 2 cups of milk.)

Ingredient	Cal	Fat	Chol	Sod	Prot	Carb	Fiber
POTATOES	220	0	0	20	6	51	5
ONION	66	0	0	6	1.8	14.4	30
CELERY	24	0	0	156	1.2	7.2	1.2
OIL	251	28	0	0	0	0	0
BAY LEAF	0	0	0	0	0	0	0
BUTTER	200	23	70	180	0	0	0
MILK,SKIM	176	1.6	16	256	16	24	0
Totals Per Serving:	**232**	**13.2**	**22**	**155**	**6.3**	**24.2**	**9.1**

FRUIT SOUP
4 servings (10 mcgs of VITAMIN K per serving)

1 1/3	cups	Apricot nectar
2	tsp	Cornstarch
2	tbsp	Brandy
2	tbsp	Honey
1/8	tsp	Allspice, ground
1 1/2	cups	Plums, pineapples, apricots and peaches

In a nonmetal, microwave safe bowl, stir together the apricot nectar and cornstarch. Stir in brandy, honey, and allspice.

Micro-cook, uncovered, on 100% power for 2 to 3 minutes or until the mixture is thickened and bubbly, stirring every 30 seconds.

Stir in the fruit. Micro-cook, uncovered, on 100% power for 45 seconds to 1 minute or until heated through.

Chill thoroughly, if desired. Serve hot or cold.

Ingredient	Cal	Fat	Chol	Sod	Prot	Carb	Fiber
APRICOT NECTAR	171	0	0	11	0	42.7	0
CORNSTARCH	36	0	0	1	0	8.7	0
BRANDY	65	0	0	0	0	0	0
HONEY	87	0	0	1	0.1	23.5	0
GROUND ALLSPICE	2	0.1	0	0	0	0.1	0.1
FRUIT	192	0	0	0	0	48	0
Totals Per Serving:	**138**	**0**	**0**	**3**	**0**	**30.7**	**0**

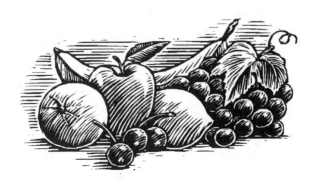

SWEET SQUASH BISQUE
6 servings (6 mcg of VITAMIN K per serving)

1	tsp	Olive oil, treated (See Dietary Tip # 10)
1	cup	Celery, minced
1	cup	Onion, minced
2 1/4	cup	Winter squash, peeled, seeded and diced
2	cups	Potato, peeled and diced
1	each	Whole pear, peeled, cored, diced
1	qt	Vegetable broth
1	cup	Water
1/4	tsp	Cumin, ground
1/4	tsp	Nutmeg, fresh grated is best
1/4	cup	Half-and-half
1/8	tsp	Ground black pepper

Heat oil in a 3 quart pot over medium to high heat.

When hot, add celery and onion. Cook until hot and fragrant, about 3 minutes.

Add squash, potato, pear, broth, water, cumin and nutmeg. Simmer, covered, until squash and potato are soft, about 25 minutes.

Strain vegetables from cooking liquid, reserving both. Puree solids in food processor or in blender until completely smooth, about 2 minutes. Add 1/2 cup reserved liquid to the food processor to make the mixture smoother.

Return the pureed mixture and reserved liquid to the pot. Add half-and-half. Heat through. Season with pepper.

Can be made 3 days ahead and refrigerated, or frozen as long as 4 months. Gently reheat. Serve hot.

Ingredient	Cal	Fat	Chol	Sod	Prot	Carb	Fiber
OIL	40	4.5	0	0	0	0	0
CELERY	16	0	0	104	0.8	4.8	0.8
ONION	64	0	0	0	1.6	13.6	2.4
WINTER SQUASH	180	0	0	18	0	36	0
POTATO	240	0	0	16	6.4	54.4	4.8
WHOLE PEAR	100	1	0	1	1	25	4
VEGETABLE BROTH	32	0	0	2944	0	0	0
CUMIN	2	0	0	1	0.1	0.2	0.1
NUTMEG	3	0.2	0	0	0	0.3	0.1
HALF-AND-HALF	74	6.8	20	24	1.6	2.4	0
BLACK PEPPER	1	0	0	0	0	0.2	0.1
Totals Per Serving:	**125**	**2.1**	**3**	**518**	**1.9**	**22.8**	**2**

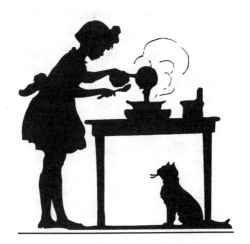

TOMATO SOUP
8 servings (10 mcgs of VITAMIN K per serving)

1/2	cup	Onion, chopped
1	tbsp	Olive oil, treated (See Dietary Tip # 10)
3	tsp	Garlic cloves, chopped
4	oz	Butter
1/2	cup	All purpose flour
28	oz	Tomatoes, crushed, canned
1	cup	Tomato, chopped fine
1	quart	Chicken broth, heated
2	cups	Half-and-half or milk
1/4	tsp	Ground black pepper
1	cup	Croutons, plain for garnish

Sauté the onions in olive oil until translucent. Add the garlic and butter. When butter is melted, add flour and stir until smooth.

Add crushed tomatoes with juice, fresh tomatoes and heated stock, bring to a boil, reduce heat and simmer 5 minutes.

Heat cream or milk. (In a heavy saucepan, heat the cream or milk gently, just until bubbles are seen at the edge of the pan, do not allow to boil). Stir heated milk into soup and add pepper. Garnish with croutons.

Ingredient	Cal	Fat	Chol	Sod	Prot	Carb	Fiber
ONION	32	0	0	0	0.8	6.8	1.2
OIL	119	13.5	0	0	0	0	0
GARLIC	12	.1	0	6	0.5	3	0
BUTTER	800	92	280	720	0	0	0
FLOUR	200	0.8	0	0	5.6	44	0
TOMATOES	252	0	0	1036	0	56	28
TOMATO	40	0.8	0	16	1.6	8	2.4
CHICKEN BROTH	128	0	0	5280	6.4	22.4	0
HALF-AND-HALF	592	54.4	160	192	12.8	19.2	0
BLACK PEPPER	1	0	0	0	0.1	0.4	0.1
CROUTONS	120	2.4	0	208	4	22.4	1.6
Totals Per Serving:	**287**	**20.5**	**55**	**932**	**4**	**22.8**	**4.2**

FRENCH ONION SOUP
6 servings (Less than 1 mcg of VITAMIN K per serving)

1 1/2	lb	Onion, thinly sliced (about 4 medium onions)
4	tbsp	Butter
1	tbsp	Olive oil, treated (See Dietary Tip # 10)
1	tbsp	Sugar, granulated
3	tbsp	All purpose flour
1	quart	Beef broth
1	tbsp	Beef bouillon granules, instant, low sodium
1	cup	Dry white wine
1/2	cup	Brandy
1/2	tsp	Ground black pepper
4	cups	Water

To caramelize the onions, place onions, butter, and oil in a large saucepan over medium heat. Cover and cook, stirring occasionally, 20 minutes.

Stir in the sugar, and flour. Cook uncovered 40 minutes, stirring frequently.

Stir in the beef broth, bouillon granules, wine, brandy, pepper, and water. Bring to a boil, reduce heat, and simmer for 40 minutes.

Ladle the soup into oven-proof serving bowls, top with a slice of toasted French bread and grated Swiss cheese (Gruyere is best). Place under broiler just until cheese is melted and bubbly.

Ingredient	Cal	Fat	Chol	Sod	Prot	Carb	Fiber
ONION	264	0	0	24	7.2	57.6	120
BUTTER	400	46	140	360	0	0	0
OIL	119	13.5	0	0	0	0	0
SUGAR	48	0	0	0	0	12.5	0
FLOUR	75	0.3	0	0	2.1	16.5	0
BEEF BROTH	160	0	0	6976	32	0	0
BEEF BOUILLON	36	2.5	0	15	1	6	0
DRY WHITE WINE	176	0	0	8	0	5.6	0
BRANDY	260	0	0	0	0	0	0
BLACK PEPPER	3	0.1	0	1	0.1	0.7	0.2
Totals Per Serving:	257	10.4	23	1231	7.1	16.5	20

HUNGARIAN STYLE SOUP
10 servings (3.6 mcgs of VITAMIN K per serving)

1/4	lb	Bacon, in 1 inch pieces
1 1/2	lb	Onion, chopped (about 4 medium onions)
1	lb	Beef, lean, cut into 1/2 inch cubes
6	cups	Beef broth
16	oz	Tomatoes, canned 'No Salt Added', chopped
1/4	cup	Red wine
1	tbsp	Tomato paste
1	tsp	Garlic cloves minced
2	tsp	Paprika
1/2	tsp	Caraway seeds
1/4	tsp	Marjoram leaves, fresh chopped
1/4	tsp	Ground black pepper
1/2	tsp	Sugar
1	lb	Potatoes, peeled and diced
3/4	lb	Kielbasa, knockwurst, etc., sliced

Cook the bacon until transparent. Add the onion and cook until golden. Add the beef and cook until it's lost its red color.

Add the remaining ingredients except for the potatoes and sausage. Bring to a boil. Simmer covered for 30 minutes.

Add the potatoes and sliced sausage. Cook for about 30 minutes until potatoes are tender.

Skim off fat. Serve hot.

Ingredient	Cal	Fat	Chol	Sod	Prot	Carb	Fiber
BACON	184	15.60	28	508	9.2	0.4	0
ONION	264	0	0	24	7.2	57.6	120
BEEF	1280	160	384	304	134.4	0	0
BEEF BROTH	240	0	0	10464	48	0	0
TOMATOES	144	0	0	80	4.8	32	0
RED WINE	44	0	0	2	0	0.2	0
TOMATO PASTE	12	0	0	12	0.5	2.5	0.5
GARLIC	4	0	0	2	0.2	1	0
PAPRIKA	12	0.6	0	2	0.6	2.4	0.8
CARAWAY SEEDS	4	0.2	0	0	0.2	0.6	0.2
MARJORAM LEAVES	0	0	0	0	0	0	0
BLACK PEPPER	1	0	0	0	0.1	0.4	0.1
SUGAR	8	0	0	0	0	2.1	0
POTATOES	352	0	0	32	9.6	81.6	8
KIELBASA	876	75.6	96	2688	48	12	0
Totals Per Serving:	**343**	**25.2**	**51**	**1412**	**26.3**	**19.3**	**13**

HEARTY CHICKEN AND RICE SOUP
8 servings (6 mcgs of VITAMIN K per serving)

10	cups	Chicken broth
1/2	cup	Onion, chopped
1	cup	Celery, sliced
1	cup	Carrots, peeled and thinly sliced
1/4	tsp	Ground black pepper
1/2	tsp	Thyme leaves, fresh
1	each	Bay leaf
1 1/2	cups	Chicken, cubed - (3/4 pound)
2	cups	Rice, white, cooked
2	tbsp	Lime juice
		Lime slices, for garnish

Combine the broth, onion, celery, carrots, pepper, thyme, and bay leaf in a large pot. Bring to a boil, stir once or twice. Reduce heat and simmer, uncovered, 10 to 15 minutes.

Add the chicken and simmer, uncovered, 5 to 10 minutes or until chicken is cooked.

Remove and discard the bay leaf.

Stir in rice and lime juice just before serving.

Garnish with lime slices.

Ingredient	Cal	Fat	Chol	Sod	Prot	Carb	Fiber
CHICKEN BROTH	320	0	0	13200	16	56	0
ONION	32	0	0	0	0.8	6.8	1.2
CELERY	16	0	0	104	0.8	4.8	0.8
CARROTS	48	0.8	0	40	0.8	12	0.8
BLACK PEPPER	1	0	0	0	0.1	0.4	0.1
THYME	0	0	0	0	0	0	0
BAY LEAF	0	0	0	0	0	0	0
CHICKEN	408	12	240	264	72	0	0
RICE	784	22.4	0	16	52.8	208	1.6
LIME JUICE	8	0	0	0	0.2	2.8	0
LIME SLICES	0	0	0	0	0	0	0
Totals Per Serving:	**202**	**4.4**	**30**	**1703**	**17.9**	**36.3**	**0.6**

MINESTRONE SOUP
15 servings (VITAMIN K content = 68 mcg per cup)

1	tsp	Garlic cloves, minced
1/4	cup	Olive oil, treated (See Dietary Tip # 10)
1 1/2	cups	Onion, chopped
10	cup	Water
6	oz	Tomato paste
1 1/2	cups	Celery, chopped
1	tsp	Parsley, fresh, chopped
1	cup	Carrots, peeled and chopped
4 1/2	cup	Cabbage, shredded
2	cups	Tomato, chopped
1	cup	Kidney beans
1 1/2	cups	Peas, green, fresh or frozen
1 1/2	cups	Beans, green, fresh or frozen
2	cups	Pasta, uncooked plain

Sauté garlic and onions in olive oil. Add all remaining ingredients except pasta. Bring to boil and cover.

Cook on low heat, for 45 minutes to an hour, until vegetables are at desired tenderness.

Add uncooked pasta and cook until pasta is al dente.

Ingredient	Cal	Fat	Chol	Sod	Prot	Carb	Fiber
GARLIC	7	0.4	0	5	0.1	1.3	0.8
OIL	476	54	0	0	0	0	0
ONION	96	0	0	0	2.4	20.4	3.6
TOMATO PASTE	138	0	0	150	6	30	6
CELERY	24	0	0	156	1.2	7.2	1.2
PARSLEY	1	0	0	1	0	0.1	0
CARROTS	48	0.8	0	40	0.8	12	0.8
CABBAGE	72	0	0	72	3.6	18	7.2
TOMATO	80	1.6	0	32	3.2	16	4.8
KIDNEY BEANS	264	4	0	656	16	48	9.6
PEAS	276	1.2	0	12	18	49.2	12
BEANS	108	0	0	24	12	24	24
PASTA, DRY	1760	16	0	160	64	320	0
Totals Per Serving:	223	5.2	0	87	8.5	36.4	4.7

WINTER SQUASH, APPLE AND WALNUT SOUP
6 servings (5 mcgs of VITAMIN K per serving)

24	oz	Butternut squash, peeled, cooked and pureed
2	tbsp	Butter
1	cup	Applesauce, unsweetened
1	cup	Light cream
1 1/2	cups	Chicken broth
1/4	cup	Walnuts, ground and toasted
1/2	tsp	Ground mace
1/8	tsp	White pepper
1/4	cup	Walnuts pieces, toasted, for garnish

Combine all the ingredients (except the walnut pieces) in a large saucepan and stir to blend well. Cook the soup over medium heat until warmed through, about 6 to 8 minutes.

Ladle the soup into bowls and add a few chopped walnut pieces in the center.

Ingredient	Cal	Fat	Chol	Sod	Prot	Carb	Fiber
SQUASH	312	0	0	24	0	72	0
BUTTER	200	23	70	180	0	0	0
APPLESAUCE	96	0	0	8	1.6	0	0
LIGHT CREAM	440	44	152	88	6.4	8	0
CHICKEN BROTH	48	0	0	1980	2.4	8.4	0
WALNUTS	122	12	0	0	4	2	1
GROUND MACE	4	0.3	0	0	0.1	0.5	0.2
WHITE PEPPER	2	0	0	0	0.1	0.4	0.1
WALNUT PIECES	192	18.6	0	4	4.2	5.6	1.4
Totals Per Serving:	**236**	**16.3**	**37**	**381**	**3.1**	**16.1**	**0.5**

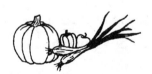

GOLDEN MUSTARD SQUASH SOUP
6 servings (8 mcgs of VITAMIN K per serving. 11 mcgs of
VITAMIN K per serving with chives)

1/4	cup	Butter
1	cup	Onion, chopped
1/2	cup	Carrots, peeled and chopped
1/3	cup	Celery stalk, chopped
3	cups	Chicken broth*
2	cups	Beef broth*
1 1/2	lb	Squash, yellow summer, peeled and diced
1/2	cup	Potato, peeled and diced
3/4	cup	Whipping cream
1 1/2	tbsp	Dijon mustard
1/2	tsp	Nutmeg, fresh grated is best
1/8	tsp	Pepper, white
1/3	cup	Carrot, peeled and grated for garnish and
2	tsp	Chives, snipped fresh for garnish

*Find no salt broth and save on the sodium.

Melt butter in a large, heavy saucepan over low heat. Add onion, carrot and celery. Cover and cook until onion is translucent, about 10 minutes, stir occasionally.

Add chicken and beef broth, squash and potato. Increase heat to high and bring to simmer. Let simmer until vegetable mixture is very tender, about 30 minutes.

Transfer the mixture to a food processor, or blender, in batches and puree until smooth. Pour into a bowl. (For a finer texture, strain the soup.) Stir in the cream, mustard, nutmeg and pepper.

Cover and refrigerate. Taste and adjust seasoning.

Garnish with carrot and chives just before serving.

Ingredient	Cal	Fat	Chol	Sod	Prot	Carb	Fiber
BUTTER	400	46	140	360	0	0	0
ONION	64	0	0	0	1.6	13.6	2.4
CARROTS	24	0.4	0	20	0.4	6	0.4
CELERY STALK	5	0	0	35	0.3	1.6	0.3
CHICKEN BROTH	96	0	0	3960	4.8	16.8	0
BEEF BROTH	80	0	0	3488	16	0	0
SQUASH, YELLOW	144	2.4	0	24	7.2	28.8	7.2
POTATO	60	0	0	4	1.6	13.6	1.2
WHIPPING CREAM	618	66	246	66	3.6	4.8	0
DIJON MUSTARD	22	0	0	540	0	0.8	0
NUTMEG	6	0.4	0	0	0.1	0.6	0.3
PEPPER, WHITE	2	0	0	0	0.1	0.4	0.1
CARROT	16	0.3	0	13	0.3	4	0.3
CHIVES	3	0	0	0	0.3	0.3	0.3
Totals Per Serving:	**257**	**19.3**	**64**	**1418**	**6**	**15.2**	**2.1**

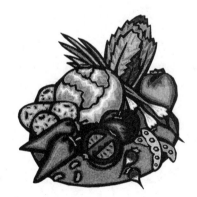

RICE, PASTA & POTATOES

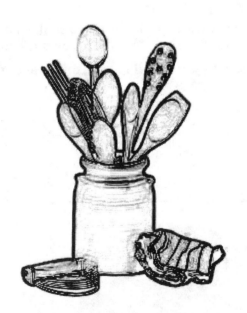

TASTY WHITE RICE WITH CORN

8 servings (This recipe essentially contains no vitamin K. The corn is optional.)

4	cups	Water
2	cups	Rice, white uncooked
1	tbsp	Canola oil, treated (See Dietary Tip # 10)
2	tsp	Garlic cloves, minced
1/2	cup	Corn kernels, frozen or fresh

Sauté onion and garlic.

Add rice, 4 cups of water and bring to a boil. Reduce heat. Cover and simmer for 15 to 25 minutes or until rice is cooked.

Cook corn separately and add to rice, onion and garlic mixture.

Ingredient	Cal	Fat	Chol	Sod	Prot	Carb	Fiber
RICE	1648	3.2	0	16	32	363.2	4.8
OIL	126	14	0	0	0	0	0
GARLIC	8	0	0	4	0.3	2	0
CORN KERNELS	96	1.2	0	16	3.6	21.6	3.6
Totals Per Serving:	**234**	**2.3**	**0**	**5**	**4.5**	**48.4**	**1.1**

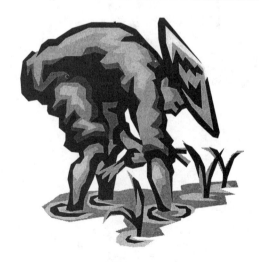

BAKED POTATOES STUFFED WITH COTTAGE CHEESE
4 servings (VITAMIN K content = less than 1 mcg per 1/2 potato, with or without skin)

1 1/4	lb	Potatoes, baking variety (4 potatoes)
3/4	cup	Cottage cheese
1/4	cup	Milk, skim
1	tbsp	Butter
2	tsp	Parmesan cheese, grated
1	tsp	Dill weed, fresh

Bake the potatoes in the oven for 1 hour at 400 degrees Fahrenheit or until tender.

Remove the potatoes from the oven and cut in half. Remove the potato flesh, leaving the skins intact, and put into a bowl.

Add all other ingredients to the potato flesh to make a stuffing mixture. Mix well. Place the mixture back into the potato skins.

Bake for 15 minutes until top is golden brown.

Ingredient	Cal	Fat	Chol	Sod	Prot	Carb	Fiber
POTATOES	440	0	0	40	12	102	10
COTTAGE CHEESE	174	6.6	18	636	21	6	0
MILK, SKIM	22	0.2	2	32	2	3	0
BUTTER	100	11.5	35	90	0	0	0
PARMESAN	14	0.9	3	57	1.3	0.1	0
DILL WEED	0	0	0	0	0	0	0
Totals Per Serving:	**188**	**4.8**	**15**	**214**	**9.1**	**27.8**	**2.5**

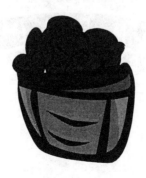

RAW POTATO LOAF
4 servings (14 mcgs of vitamin K per serving)

4	cups	Potatoes, peeled and grated (raw)
1	cup	Onion grated with the potatoes
1/2	cup	All purpose flour
4	tbsp	Milk, evaporated skim, canned
1	each	Egg (beaten into the canned milk)
1 1/2	tsp	Baking powder
1/4	tsp	Ground black pepper
2	tbsp	Butter

Mix all the ingredients together. Place the mixture into a loaf pan. Put dabs of butter on top of the potatoes. Put them in the oven and bake 60 minutes at 350 degrees Fahrenheit.

You can also use the mixture for potato pancakes instead of the loaf.

Ingredient	Cal	Fat	Chol	Sod	Prot	Carb	Fiber
POTATOES	640	0	0	64	16	144	12.8
ONION	88	0	0	8	2.4	19.2	40
FLOUR	200	0.8	0	0	5.6	44	0
MILK, EVAP SKIM	50	0.2	2	74	4.8	3.4	0
EGG	75	5.6	213	63	6.3	0.6	0
BAKING POWDER	3	0	0	306	0	0.7	0
BLACK PEPPER	1	0	0	0	0.1	0.4	0.1
BUTTER	200	23	70	180	0	0	0
Totals Per Serving:	**210**	**4.9**	**48**	**116**	**5.9**	**35.4**	**8.8**

MACARONI AND CHEESE
4 servings (VITAMIN K content = 2 mcg per cup)

8	oz	Macaroni, elbow (2 cups)
1	tsp	Canola or olive oil (See Dietary Tip # 10)
1/2	cup	Milk, evaporated skim
1	large	Egg, beaten
1/4	tsp	Ground black pepper
5	oz	Cheddar cheese, shredded, sharp white (about 1 1/4 cups)

Cook macaroni, drain, and set aside.

Grease baking pan with Canola or olive oil.

Combine all ingredients, including macaroni, in a mixing bowl. Mix thoroughly, place in the baking dish and bake for 25 minutes.

Ingredient	Cal	Fat	Chol	Sod	Prot	Carb	Fiber
MACARONI	840	4	0	0	28	168	8
OIL	40	4.7	0	0	0	0	0
MILK, EVAP SKIM	100	0.4	4	148	9.6	6.8	0
EGG, BEATEN	75	5.6	213	63	6.3	0.6	0
BLACK PEPPER	1	0	0	0	0.1	0.4	0.1
CHEDDAR	550	45	150	1000	35	5	0
Totals Per Serving:	402	14.9	92	303	19.7	45.2	2

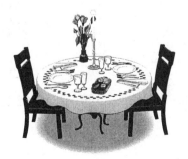

PASTA AND TURKEY RED SAUCE

4 servings (VITAMIN K content = 12 mcg per cup of sauce. The pasta contains insignificant amounts of vitamin K.)

1	lb	Ground turkey
28	oz	Tomatoes, canned, 'no salt added', chopped
1	cup	Green pepper, finely chopped
1	cup	Onion, chopped
2	tsp	Garlic cloves, minced
1/2	tsp	Oregano leaves, fresh, minced
1/2	tsp	Basil, fresh, chopped
8	oz	Dry Spaghetti, plain*
1	tsp	Olive oil, treated (See Dietary Tip # 10)

*Or other plain pasta.

Cook ground turkey in olive oil. Drain and throw away any fat. Add remaining ingredients, except pasta, and bring to a boil. Cook on low heat for at least one hour.

Cook the spaghetti.

Serve sauce over spaghetti.

Ingredient	Cal	Fat	Chol	Sod	Prot	Carb	Fiber
GROUND TURKEY	640	32	432	240	116.8	0	0
TOMATOES	252	0	0	140	8.4	56	0
GREEN PEPPER	64	0.8	0	0	2.4	14.4	4
ONION	64	0	0	0	1.6	13.6	2.4
GARLIC	8	0	0	4	0.3	2	0
OREGANO	1	0	0	0	0	0	0
BASIL	0	0	0	0	0	0	0
DRY SPAGHETTI	848	3.2	0	16	28.8	170.4	0.8
OIL	40	4.5	0	0	0	0	0
Totals Per Serving:	479	10.1	108	100	39.6	64.1	1.8

POLISH NOODLES AND CABBAGE
4 servings (90 mcgs of vitamin K per serving)

1/4	cup	Butter
1/2	cup	Onion, chopped
1/2	lb	Cabbage, sliced thin
1	tsp	Caraway seeds or fennel seed
8	oz	Noodles, uncooked
1/2	cup	Sour cream, lowfat
1/8	tsp	Black pepper, freshly ground

Melt the butter in a large skillet. Add the onion and sauté until transparent.

Add the cabbage and sauté 5 minutes or until tender but still crisp.

Stir in the caraway seeds and pepper.

Meanwhile, cook the noodles in water as directed on package. Do not overcook. Drain well.

Stir the noodles into the cabbage and add the sour cream. Cook 5 minutes longer, stirring frequently.

Ingredient	Cal	Fat	Chol	Sod	Prot	Carb	Fiber
BUTTER	400	46	140	360	0	0	0
ONION	32	0	0	0	0.8	6.8	1.2
CABBAGE	16	0	0	16	0.8	4	1.6
CARAWAY SEEDS	7	0.3	0	0	0.4	1.1	0.3
NOODLES	864	8	216	48	32	160	8
SOUR CREAM	160	8	20	140	8	16	0
BLACK PEPPER	1	0	0	0	0	0.2	0
Totals Per Serving:	370	15.6	94	141	10.5	47	2.8

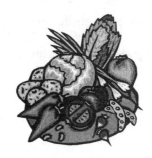

MEAT PASTA SAUCE
6 servings (11 mcgs of vitamin K per serving)

2	tbsp	Olive oil, extra-virgin, treated (See TIP # 10)
1/2	cup	Carrots, peeled and diced
1/2	cup	Onion, diced
1/2	cup	Celery, diced
1	tsp	Garlic, minced
1	lb	Italian sausage, turkey*
1/3	lb	Ground beef
6 1/2	oz	Prosciutto, diced
1/2	tsp	Ground black pepper
1/4	tsp	Nutmeg, freshly grated
1/2	cup	Dry red wine
3/4	cup	Tomato puree
1	cup	Plum tomatoes, chopped
1/2	oz	Mushrooms, dried porcini mushrooms (soaked in warm water for at least 1/2 hour)

*You can substitute Italian pork sausage. (Nutrition values will change.)

Remove the Porcini from the water, squeeze dry and finely chop.

Meanwhile, in a large saucepan or flameproof casserole, heat the olive oil over moderate heat. Add the carrot, onion and celery and sauté until the onion is golden, about 4 minutes.

Add the garlic and cook until fragrant, about 1 minute.

Add the sausage, ground beef and prosciutto to the pan. Cook over moderate heat, stirring to break up the meat, until the beef and sausage are no longer pink. Drain off any fat. Season with the pepper and nutmeg.

Pour in the red wine and cook, stirring occasionally, until it evaporates, about 5 minutes. Add the tomato puree, tomatoes, porcini and 1/4 cup of warm water. Simmer for 30 minutes. If the sauce gets too thick, add a little more water.

Serve hot over polenta or pasta. (This can be made up to 2 days ahead. Cover and refrigerate. Reheat before serving.)

Ingredient	Cal	Fat	Chol	Sod	Prot	Carb	Fiber
OIL	240	27	0	0	0	0	0
CARROTS	24	0.4	0	20	0.4	6	0.4
ONION, DICED	32	0	0	0	0.8	6.8	1.2
CELERY, DICED	8	0	0	52	0.4	2.4	0.4
GARLIC	4	0	0	2	0.2	1	0
SAUSAGE	800	64	0	4000	64	14.4	0
BEEF	464	40	128	101	24	0	0
PROSCIUTTO	585	45.5	0	3263	45.5	0	0
BLACK PEPPER	3	0.1	0	1	0.1	0.7	0.2
NUTMEG	3	0.2	0	0	0	0.3	0.1
DRY RED WINE	88	0	0	4	0	0	0
TOMATO PUREE	66	0	0	60	0	18	6
PLUM TOMATOES	48	0	0	24	1.6	10.4	3.2
MUSHROOMS	4	0.1	0	0	0.3	0.7	0.2
Totals Per Serving:	**395**	**29.5**	**21**	**1255**	**22.9**	**10.1**	**2**

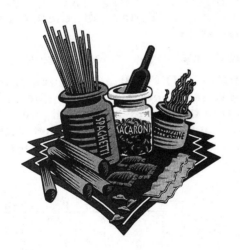

MY RICE-A-RONI
6 servings (4 mcgs of vitamin K per serving)

1/2	cup	Wild rice
1	cup	Rice, white uncooked
2	oz	Vermicelli noodles, broken (about 1 cup)
3	cups	Water
1	tbsp	Chicken bouillon granules, instant low sodium
1/4	cup	Onion
1	tsp	Garlic cloves
4	oz	Mushrooms, chopped or sliced
3/4	cup	Bell pepper
3	tbsp	Parmesan cheese, grated (or more according to your taste.)
2	tbsp	Olive oil, treated (See Dietary Tip # 10)
1	tbsp	Butter

Sauté onion and green pepper in butter and oil.

Add white rice and vermicelli. Sauté, stirring often, until brown.

Add the rest of the ingredients. Bring to a boil, reduce heat and simmer for 30 to 35 minutes. Periodically check the water level and add more if necessary.

Serve hot. Add the Parmesan just before serving.

MICROWAVE DIRECTIONS: Bring the mixture to a boil. Put it in a microwave safe container that is quite a bit larger than the mix. Put it in the microwave on full power for 13 minutes. Check the liquid level and rice for doneness. Add more liquid if necessary and cook on full power for another 5 minutes.

Ingredient	Cal	Fat	Chol	Sod	Prot	Carb	Fiber
WILD RICE	404	1.2	0	8	16.8	84.8	6
RICE	824	1.6	0	8	16	181.6	2.4
VERMICELLI	200	1	0	0	7	42	0
CHICKEN BOUILLON	36	2.5	0	15	1	6	0
ONION	22	0	0	2	0.6	4.8	10
GARLIC	4	0	0	2	0.2	1	0
MUSHROOMS	28	0.4	0	4	2.4	5.2	1.6
BELL PEPPER	180	3.6	0	36	7.2	50.4	10.8
PARMESAN	62	4.2	12	255	5.7	0.6	0
OIL	240	27.2	0	0	0	0	0
BUTTER	100	11.5	35	90	0	0	0
Totals Per Serving:	350	8.8	8	70	9.5	62.7	5.1

QUICK TOMATO SAUCE FOR PASTA
8 servings (38 mcgs of vitamin K per serving)

3/4	cup	Onion, chopped fine
5	tsp	Garlic cloves, crushed
10	tbsp	Olive oil, treated (See Dietary Tip # 10)
28	oz	Plum tomatoes, cut in small pieces
2	tbsp	Basil, fresh, chopped
1/4	tsp	Ground black pepper
1	tbsp	Sugar

To make sauce, sauté onion and garlic in olive oil until golden.

Add undrained tomatoes and basil. Season with pepper to taste.

Bring to boil and simmer 15 minutes. Add sugar at the last minute.

Serve over pasta or polenta.

Ingredient	Cal	Fat	Chol	Sod	Prot	Carb	Fiber
ONION	66	0	0	6	1.8	14.4	30
GARLIC	20	0.1	0	10	0.8	5	0
OIL	1190	135	0	0	0	0	0
PLUM TOMATOES	168	0	0	84	5.6	36.4	11.2
BASIL	1	0	0	0	0.1	0.2	0.1
BLACK PEPPER	1	0	0	0	0.1	0.4	0.1
SUGAR	48	0	0	0	0	12.5	0
Totals Per Serving:	187	16.9	0	13	1	8.6	5.2

POLENTA
4 servings (Less than 7 mcgs of vitamin K per serving)

1	cup	Cornmeal
1	cup	Cold water
3	cups	Boiling water
1/4	tsp	Salt
2	tbsp	Butter
1/4	cup	Parmesan cheese, grated

Mix the Cornmeal and salt with the cup of cold water.

Slowly whisk this mixture into the boiling water. Reduce heat to medium. Cook for about 15 minutes, stirring frequently.

Mix in butter and cheese. Pour into a serving dish. Serve hot with your favorite Italian sauce.

You can make this ahead and reheat in a microwave or regular oven. Also, if you add some low sodium chicken bouillon to the boiling water it will give the polenta a deeper flavor.

Ingredient	Cal	Fat	Chol	Sod	Prot	Carb	Fiber
CORNMEAL	608	8	0	56	16	120	4
SALT	0	0	0	575	0	0	0
BUTTER	200	23	70	180	0	0	0
PARMESAN	82	5.6	16	340	7.6	0.8	0
Totals Per Serving:	223	9.2	22	288	5.9	30.2	1

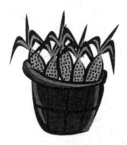

SHRIMP AND WINE-SAUCED SPAGHETTI
2 servings (18 mcgs of vitamin K per serving)

2	tsp	Olive oil, treated (See Dietary Tip # 10)
2	each	Green onions, chopped (about 1/4 cup)
1	tsp	Garlic cloves, minced
3	cups	Tomatoes, canned, not drained
2	tbsp	White wine

1	tsp	Sugar
1	tsp	Basil, fresh, minced
1/4	tsp	Oregano leaves, fresh, minced
1/8	tsp	Ground black pepper
8	oz	Shrimp, peeled and cleaned (You could substitute chicken breast)
1	tbsp	Cornstarch
1	tbsp	Cold water
4	oz	Dry Spaghetti, cooked and hot
1	tbsp	Romano cheese, grated

Sauté onion and garlic in oil.

Add undrained tomatoes, wine, sugar and seasonings. Cover and simmer 25 minutes.

Add shrimp (or chicken), return to simmer and cook about 5 minutes until cooked through (if using chicken cook a little longer).

Blend cornstarch in 1 tablespoon cold water and stir into the shrimp mixture. Cook until bubbly.

Serve over the hot spaghetti and sprinkle with cheese. Serve immediately. This is wonderful with a good French bread.

Ingredient	Cal	Fat	Chol	Sod	Prot	Carb	Fiber
OIL	79	9	0	0	0	0	0
GREEN ONIONS	18	0	0	10	2	2	1
GARLIC	4	0	0	2	0.2	1	0
TOMATOES	120	0	0	1008	0	24	0
WHITE WINE	22	0	0	1	0	0.2	0
SUGAR	16	0	0	0	0	4.2	0
BASIL	0	0	0	0	0	0	0
OREGANO	0	0	0	0	0	0	0
BLACK PEPPER	1	0	0	0	0	0.2	0.1
SHRIMP	240	4	344	336	45.6	1.6	0
CORNSTARCH	54	0	0	2	0	13	0
DRY SPAGHETTI	424	1.6	0	8	14.4	85.2	0.4
ROMANO CHEESE	23	2	6	70	2	0.5	0
Totals Per Serving:	501	8.3	175	719	32.1	65.9	0.8

PASTA JAMBALAYA
4 servings (33 mcgs of vitamin K per serving)

2	tsp	Olive oil, treated (See Dietary Tip # 10)
8	oz	Italian sausage, turkey, spicy, cut in 1 inch pieces
8	oz	Chicken breasts, skinless, boneless, cut in 1 inch pieces
1/2	lb	Shrimp, medium, shelled and deveined
2	cups	Bell pepper, green, cut in strips
1	cup	Onion, chopped
3	tsp	Garlic cloves, minced
2	cups	Tomatoes, crushed, canned (or Plum tomatoes)
1/2	cup	Clam broth or juice
1/4	cup	Chicken broth
1/2	tsp	Basil, fresh, chopped
1/4	tsp	Garlic powder
1/8	tsp	Ground red pepper
6	oz	Fettuccine

In a large non-stick skillet, heat the oil.

Add the sausage and cook, stirring often, for 6-8 minutes or until brown.

Add chicken and cook, stirring often, for 5 minutes.

Add shrimp and cook 3 minutes longer or until chicken is brown and shrimp is pink. Move meat to a plate.

Add green peppers, onions and garlic to skillet, cook, stirring often, 3 minutes or until tender.

Add tomatoes and remaining ingredients except pasta. Bring to boil and add the meat back to the pan. Reduce to low and simmer 15 minutes.

Meanwhile cook pasta, drain, add to skillet, toss and serve.

Ingredient	Cal	Fat	Chol	Sod	Prot	Carb	Fiber
OIL	79	9	0	0	0	0	0
SAUSAGE	400	32	0	2000	32	7.2	0
CHICKEN	248	0	128	144	56	0	0
SHRIMP	240	4	344	336	45.6	1.6	0
BELL PEPPER	64	0	0	0	1.6	17.6	3.2
ONION	64	0	0	0	1.6	13.6	2.4
GARLIC	21	1.3	0	16	0.4	4	2.3
TOMATOES	96	0	0	48	3.2	20.8	6.4
CLAM BROTH	4	0	4	244	0	0	0
CHICKEN BROTH	8	0	0	330	0.4	1.4	0
BASIL	0	0	0	0	0	0	0
GARLIC POWDER	2	0	0	0	0.1	0.5	0
RED PEPPER	1	0	0	0	0	0.2	0
FETTUCCINE	630	6	0	102	24	120	0
Totals Per Serving:	**462**	**12.8**	**119**	**803**	**41.3**	**46.5**	**3**

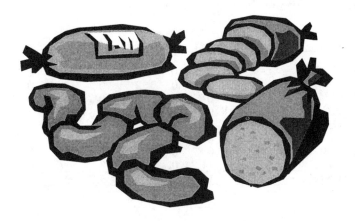

HERBED RICE TOSS
4 servings (6 mcgs of vitamin K per serving)

3	tbsp	Butter
1/2	cup	Onion, chopped
1	tsp	Garlic cloves, minced
1	cup	Celery, chopped
1/2	lb	Mushrooms, chopped
1/2	tsp	Sage, fresh, chopped
1/2	tsp	Thyme leaves, fresh, chopped
1	tsp	Chicken bouillon granules, instant, low sodium
2	cups	Brown rice, cooked*

*2 cups of cooked rice.

Melt butter in a large nonstick skillet over medium heat.

Add onions, garlic, and celery. Sauté until tender, about 10 minutes.

Add mushrooms, spices, and bouillon. Cook, stirring occasionally, 10 more minutes, until mushrooms are tender. Add small amounts of water, if necessary, to prevent drying.

Add rice. Toss until heated through. This goes especially well with baked chicken or fish.

Ingredient	Cal	Fat	Chol	Sod	Prot	Carb	Fiber
BUTTER	300	34.5	105	270	0	0	0
ONION	32	0	0	0	0.8	6.8	1.2
GARLIC	4	0	0	2	0.2	1	0
CELERY	16	0	0	104	0.8	4.8	0.8
MUSHROOMS	56	0.8	0	8	4.8	10.4	3.2
SAGE, FRESH	1	0	0	0	0	0	0
THYME	0	0	0	0	0	0	0
CHICKEN BOUILLON	12	0.8	0	5	.3	2	0
BROWN RICE	448	11.2	0	64	8	86.4	0
Totals Per Serving:	217	11.8	26	113	3.7	27.9	1.3

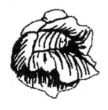

CHEESY RICE AND HAM
6 servings (9 mcgs of vitamin K per serving)

1 1/2	cups	CHEDDAR CHEESE SAUCE (See Recipe Index.)
2	cups	Rice, cooked
2	cups	Ham, diced
1	cup	Corn kernels, fresh or frozen
4	oz	Cheese, Colby, shredded (about 1 cup)
1/2	cup	Green onions, chopped

In a large bowl, combine the CHEDDAR CHEESE SAUCE, rice, ham and corn. Turn the mixture into a 10 by 6 inch baking pan. Sprinkle with cheese.

Bake at 350 degrees Fahrenheit for 30 minutes.

MICROWAVE: Cook on HIGH for 7-10 minutes, or until heated through, stirring once. Then top with shredded cheese and cook on HIGH for 2 minutes or until cheese is melted.

Ingredient	Cal	Fat	Chol	Sod	Prot	Carb	Fiber
CHEDDAR SAUCE	576	42	144	1200	25.2	28.8	0
RICE	784	22.4	0	16	52.8	208	1.6
HAM	736	38.4	240	5792	83.2	11.2	0
CORN KERNELS	192	2.4	0	32	7.2	43.2	7.2
CHEESE, COLBY	448	36	108	684	28	4	0
GREEN ONIONS	36	0	0	20	4	8	4
Totals Per Serving:	462	23.5	82	1291	33.4	50.5	2.1

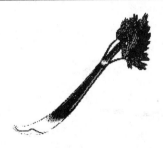

CANDIED SWEET POTATOES
6 servings (VITAMIN K content = 10 mcg per cup)

1 1/2	lb	Sweet potatoes, peeled
1	tsp	Cinnamon, ground
1/2	cup	Brown sugar
2	tsp	All purpose flour
1	cup	Orange juice
1	tsp	Butter

Cut sweet potatoes into pieces of desired size (usually halves or quarters) and boil until mildly tender. Place sweet potatoes in a baking dish.

Mix together the cinnamon, sugar, flour and orange juice.

Pour the mixture over the sweet potatoes and place a teaspoon of butter on top.

Bake uncovered at 350 degrees Fahrenheit for 20 to 25 minutes, or until sweet potatoes are at desired tenderness.

Ingredient	Cal	Fat	Chol	Sod	Prot	Carb	Fiber
SWEET POTATOES	696	2.4	0	72	9.6	189.6	12.6
CINNAMON	6	1	0	1	0.1	1.7	0.6
BROWN SUGAR	412	0	0	0	0	106.8	0
FLOUR	17	0.1	0	0	0.5	3.7	0
ORANGE JUICE	136	0	0	0	1.6	25.6	0.8
BUTTER	33	3.8	12	30	0	0	0
Totals Per Serving:	217	1.2	2	17	2	54.6	3.8

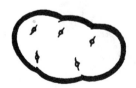

LEMON HERB ROASTED POTATOES
6 servings (15 mcgs of vitamin K per serving)

2 1/2	lb	Red potatoes, small size
1/4	cup	Olive oil, treated (See Dietary Tip # 10)
2	tbsp	Lemon juice, fresh
1	tsp	Oregano leaves, fresh, minced
1/2	tsp	Thyme leaves, fresh minced
1/4	tsp	Paprika
1/4	tsp	Ground black pepper

Preheat the oven to 425 degrees Fahrenheit.

Wash the potatoes, rinse, and pat dry. Cut each into 3/4 inch dice.

Combine the olive oil, lemon juice, oregano, thyme, paprika, and pepper in a large bowl and mix well.

Add the potatoes and toss.

Arrange the potatoes on an oiled baking sheet and bake about 35 minutes, turning every 15 minutes, until tender and well browned. Taste for seasoning.

Turn into a serving dish and serve immediately.

ADVANCE PREPARATION: This may be prepared 2 hours in advance and kept at room temperature. Reheat in a 350 degree Fahrenheit oven for 10 to 15 minutes. Serve with scrambled eggs, omelets, sautéed chicken or grilled veal chops.

Ingredient	Cal	Fat	Chol	Sod	Prot	Carb	Fiber
RED POTATOES	880	4	0	80	24	204	20
OIL	476	54	0	0	0	0	0
LEMON JUICE	22	0.3	0	2	1.2	8.7	0
OREGANO	1	0	0	1	0	0	0
THYME	0	0	0	0	0	0	0
PAPRIKA	2	0.1	0	0	0.1	0.3	0.1
BLACK PEPPER	1	0	0	0	0.1	0.4	0.1
Totals Per Serving:	230	9.7	0	14	4.2	35.6	3.4

POTATO CASSEROLE
6 servings (5 mcgs of vitamin K per serving)

1/2	cup	Onion, chopped
1/2	cup	Green pepper, chopped
2	tbsp	Olive oil, treated (See Dietary Tip # 10)
8	cups	Potatoes, peeled and cooked
1	can	Cream of Mushroom soup, lowfat
2	cups	Beans, green, cooked
6	oz	Cheddar cheese, shredded (about 1 1/2 cups)
1/2	tsp	Rosemary, fresh, minced
1/4	cup	Bread crumbs, dry, plain

Sauté onion and green pepper in olive oil.

Peel and slice (or dice) potatoes. Add to onion and green pepper mixture.

Mix this with the soup, green beans, cheddar cheese and rosemary.

Place in a 2-1/2 quart oiled baking dish.

Sprinkle bread crumbs on top of the casserole.

Bake in a preheated 350 degree Fahrenheit oven for 45 minutes to an hour, until all bubbly and potatoes are tender.

Ingredient	Cal	Fat	Chol	Sod	Prot	Carb	Fiber
ONION	32	0	0	0	0.8	6.8	1.2
GREEN PEPPER	32	0.4	0	0	1.2	7.2	2
OIL	238	27	0	0	0	0	0
POTATOES	960	0	0	64	25.6	224	19.2
CRM OF MSHRM SOUP	18	0.8	1	213	0.5	2.5	0.5
BEANS	144	0	0	32	16	32	32
CHEDDAR	660	54	180	1200	42	6	0
ROSEMARY	0	0	0	0	0	0	0
BREAD CRUMBS	106	1.4	0	232	3	19.2	1
Totals Per Serving:	**365**	**13.9**	**30**	**290**	**14.9**	**49.6**	**9.3**

VEGETABLES

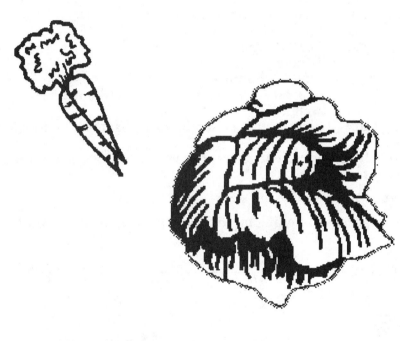

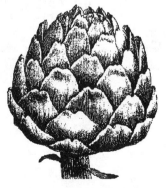

SMOTHERED GREENS
4 servings (VITAMIN K content = 400 mcg per cup)

3	oz	Bacon (2 or 3 slices)
3	cups	Water
1/2	tsp	Ground black pepper
2	tsp	Garlic cloves, minced
1/4	cup	Scallion, chopped
1	tsp	Ginger, dried, ground
1/4	cup	Onion, chopped
16	oz	Mustard greens, fresh, no stems (must be weighed)
16	oz	Turnip greens, fresh, no stems (must be weighed)

Add all the ingredients, except greens, to a large saucepan and bring to boil.

Cut greens into desired size.

Place greens in boiling mixture and cook 20 to 30 minutes.

Ingredient	Cal	Fat	Chol	Sod	Prot	Carb	Fiber
BACON	474	48	57	621	6	0	0
BLACK PEPPER	3	0.1	0	1	0.1	0.7	0.2
GARLIC	8	0	0	4	0.3	2	0
GREEN ONIONS	18	0	0	10	2	4	2
GINGER	16	0.3	0	2	0.4	3.4	0.3
ONION	16	0	0	0	0.4	3.4	0.6
MUSTARD GREENS	112	0	0	112	16	16	16
TURNIP GREENS	128	1.6	0	304	0	28.8	8
Totals Per Serving:	194	12.5	14	264	6.3	14.6	6.8

LIMA BEANS AND SPINACH
8 servings (VITAMIN K content = 260 mcg per cup)

4	cups	Lima beans, fresh
1	tbsp	Canola oil, treated (See Dietary Tip # 10)
1	cup	Onion, chopped
16	oz	Spinach leaves (no stems)
1	tbsp	Vinegar
1/4	tsp	Ground black pepper

Sauté onions in oil.

Boil the lima beans until tender. Drain.

Place the onions and spinach in the pot with the lima beans and cook until the spinach has wilted (approximately 2 minutes).

Add vinegar and pepper. Serve hot.

Ingredient	Cal	Fat	Chol	Sod	Prot	Carb	Fiber
LIMA BEANS	640	3.2	0	64	41.6	160	28.8
OIL	120	14	0	0	0	0	0
ONION	64	0	0	0	1.6	13.6	2.4
SPINACH LEAVES	64	0	0	256	8	11.2	3.2
VINEGAR	2	0	0	3	0	0	0
BLACK PEPPER	1	0	0	0	0.1	0.4	0.1
Totals Per Serving:	**111**	**2.2**	**0**	**40**	**6.4**	**23.1**	**4.3**

VEGETABLE STEW
12 servings (VITAMIN K content = 35 mcg per cup)

3	cups	Water
2	cups	Potatoes, peeled and diced
2	cups	Carrots, peeled and chopped
4	cups	Squash, zucchini, chopped
2	cups	Corn kernels, fresh or frozen
2	tsp	Garlic cloves, minced
1/2	cup	Green onions, chopped
1/4	cup	Green pepper, chopped
1	cup	Onion, chopped
1	cup	Tomato, chopped

Bring water to a boil.

Add carrots and potatoes. Cook for 10 minutes on low boil.

Add remaining ingredients except tomatoes and cook for 15 more minutes.

Add tomatoes and cook for 5 more minutes. Serve.

Ingredient	Cal	Fat	Chol	Sod	Prot	Carb	Fiber
POTATO	240	0	0	16	6.4	54.4	4.8
CARROTS	96	1.6	0	80	1.6	24	1.6
SQUASH	192	3.2	0	32	9.6	38.4	9.6
CORN KERNELS	384	4.8	0	64	14.4	86.4	14.4
GARLIC	8	0	0	4	0.3	2	0
GREEN ONIONS	36	0	0	20	4	8	4
GREEN PEPPER	16	0.2	0	0	0.6	3.6	1
ONION	64	0	0	0	1.6	13.6	2.4
TOMATO	40	0.8	0	16	1.6	8	2.4
Totals Per Serving:	**90**	**.9**	**0**	**19**	**3.3**	**19.9**	**3.4**

SUCCOTASH
6 servings (7 mcgs of vitamin K per serving)

1/4	cup	Ham, diced
1	lb	Lima beans, fresh or frozen
3	cups	Corn kernels, fresh or frozen
1/8	tsp	Ground black pepper
1/3	cup	Water
1/4	cup	Milk, skim

Brown the ham in a pan.

Add all ingredients except milk. Bring to a boil. Turn down heat to simmer. Cook for 20 to 25 minutes until the lima beans are tender.

Add milk and heat but do not boil.

Ingredient	Cal	Fat	Chol	Sod	Prot	Carb	Fiber
HAM	92	4.8	30	724	10.4	1.4	0
LIMA BEANS	512	3.2	0	32	30.4	91.2	16
CORN KERNELS	576	7.2	0	96	21.6	129.6	21.6
BLACK PEPPER	1	0	0	0	0	0.2	0.1
MILK, SKIM	22	0.2	2	32	2	3	0
Totals Per Serving:	**201**	**2.6**	**5**	**147**	**10.7**	**37.6**	**6.3**

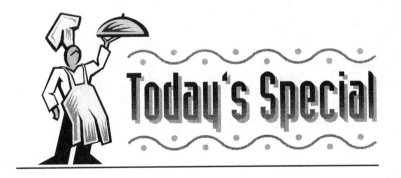

MAPLE WHIPPED BUTTERNUT SQUASH
7 to 8 servings (5 mcgs of vitamin K per serving)

2	lb	Butternut squash, peeled, quartered and seeded
1/2	cup	Butter, softened
1/4	cup	Maple syrup
1	tbsp	Sugar, light brown, firmly packed
1/4	tsp	Nutmeg, freshly grated
1/8	tsp	White pepper

Bring 1 1/2 inches of water to boil in a 5-quart sauce pot or Dutch oven.

Add squash and steam, covered, until tender, about 20 minutes. Drain, then return to pot and mash and stir over low heat about 5 minutes to evaporate some of the moisture.

Transfer to a large bowl and add butter, maple syrup, brown sugar and pepper. Beat with an electric mixer at medium speed, or with a potato masher, until smooth.

Sprinkle with nutmeg to serve.

Ingredient	Cal	Fat	Chol	Sod	Prot	Carb	Fiber
BUTTERNUT	416	0	0	32	0	96	0
BUTTER	800	92	280	720	0	0	0
MAPLE SYRUP	148	0	0	6	0	38	0
SUGAR, BROWN	48	0	0	0	0	12.5	0
NUTMEG	3	0.2	0	0	0	0.3	0.1
WHITE PEPPER	2	0	0	0	0.1	0.4	0.1
Totals Per Serving:	**177**	**11.5**	**35**	**95**	**0**	**18.4**	**0**

STUFFED ARTICHOKES
4 servings (13 mcgs of vitamin K per serving)

4	each	Artichokes, medium size
2	cups	Bread crumbs, dry, plain
4	oz	Parmesan cheese, grated (about 1 cup)
2	tsp	Garlic cloves, minced
1/4	tsp	Ground black pepper
1/4	cup	Olive oil, treated (See Dietary Tip # 10)

Cut off the artichoke stems very evenly so they stand up alone. Cut off the top fourth of the artichoke leaves. Spread the leaves so they resemble a rose and wash them. Turn the artichokes upside down to dry.

In a bowl, mix the remaining ingredients except for the olive oil.

Pour a little olive oil over the mixture to make a paste. (You may not need to use all the oil.)

Put some of the paste mixture in between every leaf and layer of the artichokes.

With a little water at the bottom of a large pot, steam the artichokes, covered, for approximately 1 hour. Add additional water as it evaporates.

Serve warm or at room temperature.

Ingredient	Cal	Fat	Chol	Sod	Prot	Carb	Fiber
ARTICHOKES	240	0.8	0	456	16.8	53.6	4
BREAD CRUMBS	848	11.2	0	1856	24	153.6	8
PARMESAN	444	30	96	1816	40.4	3.6	0
GARLIC	8	0	0	4	0.3	2	0
BLACK PEPPER	1	0	0	0	0.1	0.4	0.1
OIL	476	54	0	0	0	0	0
Totals Per Serving:	504	24	24	1033	20.4	53.3	3

BALSAMIC SQUASH PUREE
4 servings (4 mcgs of vitamin K per serving)

2	tbsp	Shallots, minced
1/4	cup	Butter
3	tbsp	Balsamic vinegar
2	cups	Butternut squash, roasted, pulp only
1/8	tsp	Nutmeg, freshly grated

Cook the shallots in a medium saucepan with 1 tablespoon of butter over medium heat until soft, about 3 to 5 minutes.

Add vinegar, increase heat to high, and cook until vinegar is reduced to syrup, another 3 to 5 minutes.

Add squash pulp and stir to combine. Reduce heat to low and cook until heated through, about 5 minutes.

Cut remaining butter into small cubes, add to squash, and beat in until fairly smooth.

Serve immediately, dusted with freshly grated nutmeg.

Ingredient	Cal	Fat	Chol	Sod	Prot	Carb	Fiber
SHALLOTS	14	0.1	0	2	0.7	3.4	0.2
BUTTER	400	46	140	360	0	0	0
VINEGAR	6	0	0	9	0	0	0
BUTTERNUT	208	0	0	16	0	48	0
NUTMEG	2	0.1	0	0	0	0.1	0.1
Totals Per Serving:	**158**	**11.6**	**35**	**97**	**0.2**	**12.9**	**0.1**

SUMMER SQUASH STIR-FRY

6 servings (5 mcgs of vitamin K per serving)

2	tbsp	Olive oil, treated (See Dietary Tip # 10)
1	tsp	Garlic cloves, minced
3/4	cup	Onion, sliced and separated into rings
1	lb	Zucchini, peeled, thinly sliced or julienne
1	lb	Squash, yellow summer squash, peeled, thinly sliced
8	each	Cherry tomatoes, cut in half or 2 tomatoes cut in 1/2 inch pieces
1/2	tsp	Ground black pepper
1	oz	Parmesan cheese, grated (about 1/4 cup)

Pour 2 tablespoons of oil around the top of a preheated wok, coating the sides. Heat at medium high (325 degrees Fahrenheit) for 1 minute.

Add garlic clove and onion, stir-fry 1 minute.

Add zucchini and yellow squash, stir-fry 3 minutes or until crisp-tender.

Add cherry tomatoes and pepper, stir-fry 1 minute or until thoroughly heated.

Transfer to a serving bowl. Sprinkle with cheese and serve immediately.

Ingredient	Cal	Fat	Chol	Sod	Prot	Carb	Fiber
OIL	238	27	0	0	0	0	0
GARLIC	4	0	0	2	0.2	1	0
ONION	66	0	0	6	1.8	14.4	30
SQUASH, ZUCCHINI	80	0	0	16	3.2	16	1.6
SQUASH, YELLOW	96	1.6	0	16	4.8	19.2	4.8
CHERRY TOMATOES	40	0.8	0	0	0.8	8.8	4.8
BLACK PEPPER	3	0.1	0	1	0.1	0.7	0.2
PARMESAN	111	7.5	24	454	10.1	0.9	0
Totals Per Serving:	**106**	**6.2**	**4**	**83**	**3.5**	**10.2**	**6.9**

STRING BEANS, SOUTHERN STYLE
4 servings (1 mcgs of vitamin K per serving)

1	lb	Green beans
1/2	cup	Water
3/4	cup	Onion, diced
1/3	cup	Ham, cut fine
1/8	tsp	Ground black pepper
1/8	tsp	Paprika

Wash the beans. Remove stem ends and cut slantwise into 1-inch lengths. Add water, onion, ham and seasonings. Bring to a boil.

Turn down heat to a simmer, cover pan and cook for 25 to 30 minutes until beans are tender and juices are reduced to one half.

Ingredient	Cal	Fat	Chol	Sod	Prot	Carb	Fiber
BEANS	144	0	0	32	16	32	32
ONION	48	0	0	0	1.2	10.2	1.8
HAM	123	6.4	40	965	13.9	1.9	0
BLACK PEPPER	1	0	0	0	0	0.2	0.1
PAPRIKA	1	0	0	0	0	0.2	0.1
Totals Per Serving:	79	1.6	10	249	7.8	11.1	8.5

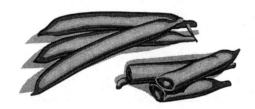

FRIED GARLIC GREEN BEANS
4 servings (9 mcgs of vitamin K per serving)

1	lb	Green beans, fresh or frozen
8	tsp	Garlic cloves, minced
1	tbsp	Olive oil, treated (See Dietary Tip # 10)
1/4	tsp	White pepper

If using fresh green beans, rinse and remove stem ends.

Steam the green beans until almost done. Try to time the steaming so that the green beans are ready at the same time as the garlic is ready in the next step.

Heat the olive oil in a skillet large enough to toss stuff about in without getting it all over the place. Add the garlic and sauté until it just begins to turn brown.

Add the green beans to the skillet along with the pepper and toss to coat with the oil and garlic.

Raise the heat a little and toss continuously until the green beans start to get brown and black in some spots. Then remove from the skillet into your serving dish. Serve hot.

Ingredient	Cal	Fat	Chol	Sod	Prot	Carb	Fiber
BEANS	144	0	0	32	16	32	32
GARLIC	32	0.1	0	16	1.2	8	0
OIL	119	13.5	0	0	0	0	0
WHITE PEPPER	4	0	0	0	0.1	0.8	0.3
Totals Per Serving:	75	3.4	0	12	4.3	10.2	8.1

BABY CARROTS GLAZED WITH BUTTER
8 servings (9 mcgs of vitamin K per serving)

| 2 | lb | Baby carrots, scraped (they usually come already scraped these days) |
| 3 | tbsp | Butter |

Place the carrots in a heavy saucepan and barely cover with water. Add the butter and cover.

Bring to a boil, reduce the heat, and cook 15 minutes or until still firm but easy to pierce with a fork.

Remove the cover and boil down until the liquid has evaporated and the carrots are coated with butter.

Watch them carefully or they will burn. Serve.

Ingredient	Cal	Fat	Chol	Sod	Prot	Carb	Fiber
BABY CARROTS	352	0	0	320	0	64	32
BUTTER	300	34.5	105	270	0	0	0
Totals Per Serving:	82	4.3	13	74	0	8	4

CAULIFLOWER PANCAKES
6 servings (4 mcgs of vitamin K per serving)

1 1/4	cups	Cauliflower, cut in small pieces
1/2	tbsp	All purpose flour
1	large	Egg
2	tsp	Grated onion (or 1 teaspoon powdered onion)
1/2	tsp	Baking powder
1/2	cup	Canola oil, treated (See DIETARY TIP # 10) for frying

Put everything in a blender, or food processor, and blend until there are no lumps.

Make small 2 inch pancakes. Fry in oil, turning once.

Good plain or with sour cream.

Ingredient	Cal	Fat	Chol	Sod	Prot	Carb	Fiber
CAULIFLOWER	30	0	0	10	3	6	1
FLOUR	12	0.1	0	0	0.4	2.8	0
EGG	75	5	213	63	6.3	0.6	0
GRATED ONION	4	0	0	0	0.1	0.8	1.7
BAKING POWDER	1	0	0	102	0	0.2	0
OIL	964	112	0	0	0	0	0
Totals Per Serving:	**181**	**19.5**	**36**	**29**	**1.6**	**1.7**	**0.4**

ZUCCHINI AND CHEDDAR BAKE
8 servings (4 mcgs of vitamin K per serving)

4	cups	Zucchini, peeled and coarsely grated
1/2	lb	Cheddar cheese, grated (about 2 cups)

Layer 1/3 zucchini, 1/3 cheese and pepper to taste. Repeat until you have used all the ingredients.

Bake at 350 degrees Fahrenheit for 40 minutes. Serve.

Ingredient	Cal	Fat	Chol	Sod	Prot	Carb	Fiber
ZUCCHINI	160	0	0	32	6.4	32	3.2
CHEDDAR	880	72	240	1600	56	8	0
Totals Per Serving:	**130**	**9**	**30**	**204**	**7.8**	**5**	**0.4**

CAULIFLOWER WITH TOMATOES
6 servings (12 mcgs of vitamin K per serving)

4	cups	fresh cauliflower in bite size pieces
1/2	cup	Water
1/2	tsp	Oregano leaves, fresh, minced
10	oz	Tomatoes, fresh, in wedges (about 2 medium tomatoes)
2	oz	Mozzarella cheese, shredded

Place cauliflower and water in a 2-quart dish, cover.

Microwave on HIGH for 5 to 8 minutes or until tender-crisp. Drain.

Stir in seasonings and tomatoes. Microwave uncovered, at HIGH 2 to 4 minutes, or until tomatoes are hot.

Sprinkle with Mozzarella cheese. Microwave 1 minute or until cheese melts. Serve.

Ingredient	Cal	Fat	Chol	Sod	Prot	Carb	Fiber
CAULIFLOWER	96	0	0	32	9.6	19.2	3.2
OREGANO	1	0	0	0	0	0	0
TOMATOES	60	1	0	30	2	13	4
MOZZARELLA	180	14	40	380	12	2	0
Totals Per Serving:	56	2.5	7	74	3.9	5.7	1.2

STUFFED PEPPERS
6 servings (37 mcgs of vitamin K per serving)

2 1/2	lb	Green peppers (6)
1	lb	Beef, lean, ground
1	cup	Rice, cooked
16	oz	Tomato sauce
1/4	tsp	Ground black pepper
1	tsp	Garlic cloves, minced
2	tbsp	Onion, chopped (not green onion or scallions)
1 1/2	quarts	Water

Cut a slice in the stem end of the peppers. Remove the seeds and thoroughly wash.

Bring the water to a boil, add peppers and cook for 5 minutes. Remove peppers and drain.

Preheat oven to 350 degrees Fahrenheit.

Cook the beef, garlic and onion in a skillet until the onion is tender. Drain off any fat.

Stir in the rice and half the tomato sauce. Heat.

Stuff each pepper and stand upright in a baking dish. Pour the rest of the tomato sauce over the peppers and bake, covered, for 45 minutes.

Uncover and bake 15 minutes. Serve.

Ingredient	Cal	Fat	Chol	Sod	Prot	Carb	Fiber
GREEN PEPPERS	320	4	0	0	12	72	20
BEEF GROUND	1056	80	320	304	80	0	0
RICE	392	11.2	0	8	26.4	104	0.8
TOMATO SAUCE	176	0	0	2640	8	35.2	0
BLACK PEPPER	1	0	0	0	0.1	0.4	0.1
GARLIC	4	0	0	2	0.2	1	0
ONION	9	0	0	5	1	1	0.5
Totals Per Serving:	**326**	**15.9**	**53**	**493**	**21.3**	**35.6**	**3.6**

ZUCCHINI CASSEROLE
4 servings (10 mcgs of vitamin K per serving)

1	lb	Zucchini, peeled and grated
1/3	cup	Onion, minced
4	oz	Cheddar cheese, sharp, grated (about 1 cup)
1	cup	Bread crumbs, dry, plain
2	large	Eggs, beaten
3	tbsp	Butter, melted
1/4	tsp	Ground black pepper
		HERB MIXTURE
1/4	cup	Celery leaves, chopped
1	tsp	Herbs, mixed fresh herbs, like thyme, sage and marjoram
1	tsp	Butter for pie plate

Drain the zucchini for 15 to 20 minutes. Combine the zucchini, onion, cheese, bread crumbs, eggs, butter and pepper.

For the herb mixture, chop the celery leaves together with the fresh herbs to freshen the flavor.

Stir herbs into the zucchini mixture.

Spoon the mixture into a buttered 9-inch pie plate. Bake at 350 degrees Fahrenheit for 40-45 minutes or until golden.

Let cool for about 10 minutes before serving.

Ingredient	Cal	Fat	Chol	Sod	Prot	Carb	Fiber
ZUCCHINI	80	0	0	16	3.2	16	1.6
ONION	21	0	0	0	0.5	4.5	0.8
CHEDDAR	440	36	120	800	28	4	0
BREAD CRUMBS	424	5.6	0	928	12	76.8	4
EGGS	150	11.2	426	126	12.6	1.2	0
BUTTER	300	34.5	105	270	0	0	0
BLACK PEPPER	1	0	0	0	0.1	0.4	0.1
CELERY LEAVES	4	0	0	26	0.2	1.2	0.2
HERBS	3	0	0	2	0.2	0.7	0.3
BUTTER	33	3.8	12	30	0	0	0
Totals Per Serving:	364	22.8	166	550	14.2	26.2	1.8

ZUCCHINI-TOMATO PIE

6 servings (7 mcgs of vitamin K per serving)

1	tbsp	Olive oil, treated (See Dietary Tip #10)
2	cups	Zucchini, peeled and chopped
1	cup	Tomato, chopped
1/2	cup	Onion, chopped
1/3	cup	Parmesan cheese, grated
1 1/2	cups	Milk, skim
3/4	cup	Bisquick , reduced fat
3	large	Eggs
1/4	tsp	Ground black pepper

Heat the oven to 400 degrees Fahrenheit.

Grease a 10 inch quiche dish or pie plate, 10 by 1 1/2 inches with the oil.

Sprinkle zucchini, tomato, onion and cheese into the dish.

Beat remaining ingredients until smooth, 15 seconds in blender on high or 1 minute with hand beater. Pour into dish.

Bake until knife inserted in center comes out clean, about 30 minutes.

Cool 5 minutes before serving.

Ingredient	Cal	Fat	Chol	Sod	Prot	Carb	Fiber
OLIVE OIL	119	13.5	0	0	0	0	0
ZUCCHINI	80	0	0	16	3.2	16	1.6
TOMATO	40	0.8	0	16	1.6	8	2.4
ONION	32	0	0	0	0.8	6.8	1.2
PARMESAN	109	7.5	21	453	10.1	1.1	0
MILK, SKIM	132	1.2	12	192	12	18	0
BISQUICK	336	6	0	1032	6.6	63	1.2
EGGS	225	16.8	639	189	18.9	1.8	0
SALT	0	0	0	1150	0	0	0
BLACK PEPPER	1	0	0	0	0.1	0.4	0.1
Totals Per Serving:	179	7.6	112	316	8.9	19.2	1.1

BASQUE PEPPER STEW
4 servings (28 mcgs of vitamin K per serving)

2	tbsp	Olive oil, treated (See Dietary Tip # 10)
1	cup	Onion, chopped
1	lb	Green peppers, cored, seeded, cut into 1/4 by 1/2 inch cubes.
2	tsp	Garlic cloves, minced
1 1/2	lb	Tomatoes, peeled, seeded and chopped (about 4 1/2 medium tomatoes)
1/8	tsp	Ground black pepper

Heat oil in a deep skillet over low heat.

Add onion and cook, stirring often, until soft but not brown, about 5 minutes.

Add green peppers and garlic and cook, stirring often, until peppers soften, about 7 minutes.

Add tomatoes and pepper.

Cook, uncovered, over medium heat, stirring often, until stew is thick, about 30 minutes.

Taste and adjust seasoning.

Ingredient	Cal	Fat	Chol	Sod	Prot	Carb	Fiber
OIL	238	27	0	0	0	0	0
ONION	64	0	0	0	1.6	13.6	2.4
GREEN PEPPERS	128	1.6	0	0	4.8	28.8	8
GARLIC	8	0	0	4	0.3	2	0
TOMATOES	144	2.4	0	72	4.8	31.2	9.6
BLACK PEPPER	1	0	0	0	0	0.2	0.1
Totals Per Serving:	146	7.8	0	19	2.9	18.9	5

BEST EVER BAKED BEANS
12 servings (4 mcgs of vitamin K per serving)

4 1/2	lb	Beans, baked, canned, with pork & tomato sauce
1/2	cup	Onion, chopped
1/2	cup	Celery, chopped
1/3	cup	Bell pepper, chopped
2	tbsp	Mustard
1/2	cup	Molasses
1	tsp	Worcestershire Sauce
4	drops	Tabasco sauce
1/2	cup	Barbecue sauce (See Recipe Index)
1/2	cup	Catsup
2	strips	Bacon, uncooked, and cut in half

Combine all ingredients, except bacon, in a large oven-proof container.

Lay bacon strips on top.

Place on a smoker barbecue grid and smoke-cook for 2 to 2 1/2 hours. (Or put them in your oven at 325 degrees Fahrenheit for 2 1/2 hours.)

Ingredient	Cal	Fat	Chol	Sod	Prot	Carb	Fiber
BEANS, BAKED	2016	0	144	9000	72	360	72
ONION	32	0	0	0	0.8	6.8	1.2
CELERY	8	0	0	52	0.4	2.4	0.4
BELL PEPPER	19	0	0	0	0.3	0.3	0.3
MUSTARD	20	1.2	0	360	1.8	2	0
MOLASSES	412	0	0	24	0	106.8	0
WORCESTERSHIRE	3	0	0	67	0	0.7	0
TABASCO SAUCE	20	0	0	0	0	0	0
BARBECUE SAUCE	144	.4	0	1440	1.6	32.8	0
CATSUP	116	0.4	0	1344	1.6	32	0
BACON	316	32	38	414	4	0	0
Totals Per Serving:	**259**	**2.8**	**15**	**1058**	**7.1**	**45.2**	**6.3**

F

ONION PANCAKES
6 servings (2 mcgs of vitamin K per serving)

1	lb	All purpose flour (4 cups sifted)

8	oz	Boiling water
1	cup	Cold water
1	lb	Onion, peeled and finely chopped
5	tbsp	Canola oil or olive oil, treated (See Dietary Tip # 10)
1/2	tsp	Salt

Sift the flour into a bowl. Pour in the boiling water, stirring all the time, to form a stiff dough. Add the cold water to the dough and when it is cool enough to handle, knead until smooth.

Cover the dough and leave to rest for about 30 minutes.

Roll the dough into a long sausage and cut into 10 pieces. Roll each piece into a ball, then flatten with the rolling pin into a small pancake about 3 to 4 inches in diameter.

Sprinkle each pancake with the chopped onion and salt. Fold the edges of the pancake into the middle and then roll out into a pancake again.

Heat 2 tablespoons of vegetable oil in a frying pan and put in the pancakes.

Fry in batches for 2 minutes on either side, or until golden brown, adding more oil as necessary.

Serve hot either by themselves or as an accompaniment to savory foods.

Ingredient	Cal	Fat	Chol	Sod	Prot	Carb	Fiber
FLOUR	1600	3.2	0	0	41.6	352	0
ONION	176	0	0	16	4.8	38.4	80
OIL	602	70	0	0	0	0	0
SALT	0	0	0	1150	0	0	0
Totals Per Serving:	396	12.2	0	194	7.7	65.1	13.3

LEMON VEGGIES

**4 servings (VITAMIN K content = 165 mcg per cup)
Be careful with serving this recipe! Make certain there are
approximately equal amounts of all vegetables! Also, you must
weigh the broccoli, not just measure the amount in a
measuring cup.)**

1	cup	Cauliflower, raw
8	oz	Broccoli, raw (about 1 cup)
1	cup	Carrots, peeled and thinly sliced
3	tbsp	Lemon juice
1	tbsp	Olive or Canola oil, treated (See Dietary Tip # 10)
1	tsp	Garlic cloves, minced

Steam vegetables until tender.

Mix the remaining ingredients in saucepan and cook over low heat for 3 minutes.

Pour sauce over vegetables in serving dish.

Ingredient	Cal	Fat	Chol	Sod	Prot	Carb	Fiber
CAULIFLOWER	24	0	0	8	2.4	4.8	0.8
BROCCOLI	64	0	0	16	11.2	22.4	4
CARROTS	48	0.8	0	40	0.8	12	0.8
LEMON JUICE	9	0	0	0	1.5	3	0
OIL	120	14	0	0	0	0	0
GARLIC	4	0	0	2	0.2	1	0
Totals Per Serving:	**67**	**3.9**	**0**	**29**	**2.8**	**8.2**	**2.2**

PINEAPPLE YAM BAKE
6 servings (5 mcgs of vitamin K per serving)

1 1/2	lb	Yams, peeled, sliced 1 inch thick, (About 3 medium yams.)
3/4	cup	Pineapple packed in juice, crushed, drained
4	tbsp	Maple syrup
2	each	Egg whites

Cook yams in boiling water for 25 to 35 minutes or until very soft and tender. Drain and mash thoroughly until consistency is smooth.

Preheat oven to 400 degrees Fahrenheit.

Mix the drained pineapple and 3 tablespoons of maple syrup into the mashed yams.

Spoon into a 9 inch round or 8 inch square non-stick baking pan.

Beat egg whites to soft peaks, add remaining 1 tablespoon syrup and beat until stiff. Spread with a spatula, using a swirling motion, on top of yam mixture.

Bake at 400 degrees Fahrenheit for 8 to 10 minutes, or until top is golden.

Ingredient	Cal	Fat	Chol	Sod	Prot	Carb	Fiber
YAMS	792	2.4	0	72	9.6	189.6	0
PINEAPPLE	108	0	0	12	0	27	1.2
MAPLE SYRUP	148	0	0	6	0	38	0
EGG WHITES	28	0	0	92	6	6	0
Totals Per Serving:	**179**	**0.4**	**0**	**30**	**2.6**	**43.4**	**0.2**

COOKIES

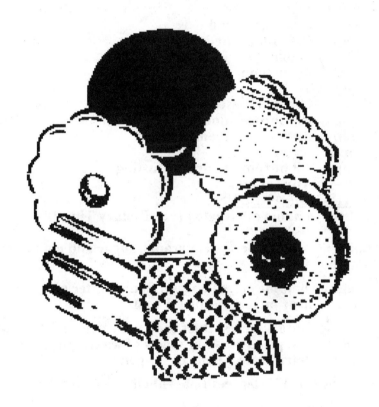

RUGALA
48 servings (1 mcg of VITAMIN K per serving)

<u>FILLING</u>

1	cup	Pecans, ground
1	cup	Raisins, packed
1/2	cup	Sugar
1	tsp	Cinnamon, ground

<u>DOUGH</u>

8	oz	Cream cheese, room temperature
2	cups	All purpose flour
1	cup	Butter, room temperature
2	tbsp	Sugar
1/4	cup	All purpose flour for dusting
12	oz	Apricot jam

<u>MISCELLANEOUS</u>

2	tbsp	Canola oil, treated (See Dietary Tip #10)

For filling: Combine pecans, currants, sugar and cinnamon in a mixing bowl.

For dough: Combine cream cheese, flour, butter and sugar in a food processor or mixer and blend well.

Divide dough into 4 pieces. Dust each with flour, shaking off excess. Roll each piece between sheets of waxed paper into 10 inch circles. Refrigerate 1 hour or longer.

Preheat oven to 375 degrees Fahrenheit.

Grease baking sheets with Canola oil.

Spread each circle of dough with apricot jam. Divide the filling among the circles of dough, spreading evenly.

Cut each circle into 12 pie shaped wedges. Roll up each wedge from bottom to point. Arrange on prepared sheets, point side down.

Bake until golden brown, about 16-17 minutes. Transfer at once to wire rack and let cool.

Store cookies in airtight container.

Tips: Be sure to work on just one circle at a time and keep the others refrigerated. Do not overdo the jam, cinnamon and pecan filling because they tend to overflow and will burn on your baking sheets.

Ingredient	Cal	Fat	Chol	Sod	Prot	Carb	Fiber
FILLING:							
PECANS	792	80	0	0	9.6	22.4	8
RAISINS	504	0.8	0	32	4	132	11.2
SUGAR	388	0	0	0	0	100	0
CINNAMON	6	1	0	1	0.1	1.7	0.6
DOUGH:							
CREAM CHEESE	792	79.2	240	680	16	8	0
FLOUR	800	3.2	0	0	22.4	176	0
BUTTER	1600	184	560	1440	0	0	0
SUGAR	97	0	0	0	0	25	0
DUSTING FLOUR	100	0.4	0	0	2.8	22	0
APRICOT JAM	1260	0	0	36	0	324	12
MISCELLANEOUS							
CANOLA OIL	241	28	0	0	0	0	0
Totals Per Serving:	137	7.8	17	46	1.1	16.9	0.7

PUMPKIN BARS WITH CREAM CHEESE FROSTING
50 servings (less than 1 mcg of VITAMIN K per serving)

2	cups	Sugar
8	oz	Pumpkin, canned w/out salt*
4	large	Eggs**
1/2	cup	Cottage cheese, lowfat
2	cups	Bisquick, reduced fat
1/2	cup	Raisins, packed
2	tbsp	Cinnamon
1	tbsp	Canola oil, treated (See Dietary Tip #10)
1	each	CREAM CHEESE FROSTING (See Recipe Index.)

*Papaya may be substituted for the pumpkin.

**Or 1 cup egg substitute. (This will change the nutrition values.)

Preheat oven to 350 degrees Fahrenheit. Grease a jelly roll pan, 15 1/2 by 10 1/2 by 1 inch size with the Canola oil.

Beat sugar, pumpkin, cottage cheese and eggs on medium speed in mixer for one minute.

Stir in Bisquick, cinnamon and raisins. Pour into prepared pan.

Bake until toothpick inserted in center comes out clean, about 25 to 30 minutes. Cool.

Frost and cut into 3 inch by 1 inch bars.

Ingredient	Cal	Fat	Chol	Sod	Prot	Carb	Fiber
PUMPKIN	80	0	0	8	0	16	8
SUGAR	1552	0	0	0	0	400	0
COTTAGE CHEESE	80	1.2	4	460	14	3.2	0
EGGS	300	22.4	852	252	25.2	2.4	0
CINNAMON	36	6	0	6	0.6	10	3.6
RAISINS	252	0.4	0	16	2	66	5.6
BISQUICK	896	16	0	2752	17.6	168	3.2
CREAM CHS FRSTING	1492	76.4	217	969	9.5	198.9	0
CANOLA OIL	120	14	0	0	0	0	0
Totals Per Serving:	96	2.7	21	89	1.4	17.3	0.4

CREAM CHEESE FROSTING

**Yields enough to frost two 9 inch layers or one sheet cake.
(VITAMIN K content = 9 mcg for the entire recipe)**

3	oz	Cream cheese, lowfat
1/3	cup	Butter
2	cups	Sugar, confectioners, sifted
1	tbsp	Milk, skim
1	tsp	Vanilla extract

Beat cream cheese, butter, milk and vanilla until creamy.

Stir in confectioners sugar and beat until smooth.

Ingredient	Cal	Fat	Chol	Sod	Prot	Carb	Fiber
CREAM CHEESE	180	15	30	480	9	6	0
BUTTER	533	61.3	187	480	0	0	0
SUGAR	768	0	0	0	0	192	0
MILK, SKIM	6	0.1	0	8	0.5	0.8	0
VANILLA EXTRACT	10	0	0	0	0	0.3	0
Totals Per Recipe:	**1497**	**76.4**	**217**	**968**	**9.5**	**199.1**	**0**

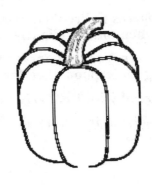

CHOCOLATE WALNUT SQUARES
24 servings (1 mcg of VITAMIN K per serving)

1 1/4	cups	All purpose flour, sifted
3/4	cup	Brown sugar, packed
1	each	Egg, large
3/4	tsp	Baking powder
1/4	cup	Coffee liqueur
1/2	tsp	Salt
1	cup	Chocolate chips, semi-sweet
1/2	cup	Butter, soft
1 1/2	oz	Walnuts, chopped (about 1/3 cup)
1	tbsp	Canola oil, treated (See Dietary Tip #10)
1	tbsp	Coffee liqueur for tops of bars
1	each	BROWN BUTTER ICING (See Recipe Index)

Resift flour with baking powder and salt.

Cream the butter, sugar and egg together.

Stir in the coffee liqueur, then the flour mixture, blending well.

Fold in the chocolate pieces and walnuts.

Grease a 7 by 11 by 1 1/2 inch baking pan with the Canola oil. Spread the mixture evenly in the baking pan

Bake in 350 degrees Fahrenheit oven, 30 minutes or until top springs back when touched lightly in the center.

Remove from oven, cool in pan, for 15 minutes. Then brush top with remaining tablespoon of coffee liqueur.

When cold, spread with BROWN BUTTER ICING.

When icing is set, cut into bars about 1 3/4 by 1 1/2 inches. Makes 2 dozen.

Ingredient	Cal	Fat	Chol	Sod	Prot	Carb	Fiber
FLOUR	500	2	0	0	14	110	0
BROWN SUGAR	618	0	0	0	0	160.2	0
EGG	75	5	213	63	6.3	0.6	0
BAKING POWDER	2	0	0	153	0	0.3	0
COFFEE LIQUEUR	40	0	0	2	0	40	0
SALT	0	0	0	1150	0	0	0
CHOCOLATE CHIPS	800	36	0	120	8	120	0
BUTTER	800	92	280	720	0	0	0
WALNUTS	273	26.4	0	4	6.2	7.8	2.1
CANOLA OIL	120	14	0	0	0	0	0
COFFEE LIQUEUR	3	0	0	0	0	0	0
BUTTER ICING	344	23.3	71	185	0.3	42.4	0
Totals Per Serving:	**149**	**8.3**	**24**	**100**	**1.4**	**20.1**	**0.1**

BROWN BUTTER ICING

1 recipe (VITAMIN K content = 2 mcg for the entire recipe)

2	tbsp	Butter
1	tbsp	Coffee liqueur
2	tsp	Milk*
1/3	cup	Sugar, confectioners, sifted

*OR light cream. (Adjust the nutrition values accordingly.)

Place 2 tablespoons butter in saucepan over low heat. Heat until lightly browned.

Remove from the heat and add 1 tablespoon coffee liqueur, 2 teaspoons milk or light cream, and 1/3 cup sifted powdered sugar. Beat smooth. (You may need to add a little more sugar to the icing if it is too thin.)

Use as directed in recipe.

Ingredient	Cal	Fat	Chol	Sod	Prot	Carb	Fiber
BUTTER	200	23	70	180	0	0	0
COFFEE LIQUEUR	10	0	0	0	0	10	0
MILK	6	0.3	1	5	0.3	0.4	0
SUGAR	128	0	0	0	0	32	0
Totals Per Recipe:	**344**	**23.3**	**71**	**185**	**0.3**	**42.4**	**0**

PEANUT BUTTER COOKIES
50 servings (1 mcg of VITAMIN K per serving)

1	tsp	Vanilla extract
1	cup	Sugar
1	cup	Brown sugar
1	cup	Butter
2	large	Eggs
1	cup	Peanut butter
3	cups	All purpose flour
1/8	tsp	Salt
2	tsp	Baking soda
1	tbsp	Canola oil, treated, (See Dietary Tip #10)

Cream together the shortening, vanilla and sugars. Add eggs.

Mix together the dry ingredients, add to the first mixture and mix well. It will be dry at first.

Form into small balls and place on cookie sheet greased with Canola oil. Press with a fork that has been dipped in sugar (to prevent sticking). Press to make a criss cross pattern. They will remain the same size in diameter, so what you see is what you get.

Bake at 375 degrees Fahrenheit for 10 minutes.

Ingredient	Cal	Fat	Chol	Sod	Prot	Carb	Fiber
VANILLA EXTRACT	10	0	0	0	0	0.3	0
SUGAR	776	0	0	0	0	200	0
BROWN SUGAR	824	0	0	0	0	213.6	0
BUTTER	1600	184	560	1440	0	0	0
EGGS	150	11.2	426	126	12.6	1.2	0
PEANUT BUTTER	1520	128	0	1240	72	48	0.8
FLOUR	1200	4.8	0	0	33.6	264	0
SALT	0	0	0	288	0	0	0
BAKING SODA	0	0	0	1642	0	0	0
CANOLA OIL	120	14	0	0	0	0	0
Totals Per Serving:	**124**	**6.8**	**20**	**95**	**2.4**	**14.5**	**0**

FUDGE BROWNIES
12 servings (VITAMIN K content = 3 mcg per serving)

1	tbsp	Canola oil, treated, (See Dietary Tip #10)
1/2	cup	Butter
2	oz	Unsweetened chocolate
1	cup	Sugar
2	large	Eggs
1	tbsp	Vanilla extract
3/4	cup	All purpose flour
1/2	cup	Walnuts, chopped
1	each	CHOCOLATE FROSTING (See Recipe Index)

Preheat oven to 350 degrees Fahrenheit. Grease an 8 by 8 inch baking pan with the Canola oil.

Melt butter and chocolate in a saucepan. Remove from heat and stir in the sugar. Add eggs and vanilla, beat lightly just until blended. Stir in flour and nuts.

Spread batter in pan. Bake 30 minutes. Cool. Ice with CHOCOLATE FROSTING (See Recipe Index for Frosting recipe.) and cut into bars.

Ingredient	Cal	Fat	Chol	Sod	Prot	Carb	Fiber
CANOLA OIL	120	14	0	0	0	0	0
BUTTER	800	92	280	720	0	0	0
CHOCOLATE	380	32	0	2	8	14	0
SUGAR	776	0	0	0	0	200	0
EGGS	150	11.2	426	126	12.6	1.2	0
VANILLA EXTRACT	30	0	0	0	0	0.9	0
FLOUR	300	1.2	0	0	8.4	66	0
WALNUTS	384	37.2	0	8	8.4	11.2	2.8
CHOC FROSTING	2630	66.7	107	304	10	505	0
Totals Per Serving:	**464**	**21.2**	**68**	**97**	**4**	**66.5**	**0.2**

CHOCOLATE FROSTING:

2 cups (VITAMIN K content = 3 mcg per recipe)

1	cup	Sugar
3	tbsp	Butter
2	oz	Unsweetened chocolate
1/4	cup	Milk, skim
3	cups	Confectioner's sugar, sifted

Melt butter, add chocolate and stir until chocolate melts.

Remove from heat and stir in sugar.

Add milk and put back on the burner. Cook, stirring constantly, until mixture is bubbly. Cool a little before using.

Use as directed in recipe.

Ingredient	Cal	Fat	Chol	Sod	Prot	Carb	Fiber
SUGAR	776	0	0	0	0	200	0
BUTTER	300	34.5	105	270	0	0	0
CHOCOLATE	380	32	0	2	8	14	0
MILK, SKIM	22	0.2	2	32	2	3	0
CONF SUGAR	1152	0	0	0	0	288	0
Totals Per Recipe:	**2630**	**66.7**	**107**	**304**	**10**	**505**	**0**

RAISIN-FILLED BARS

27 servings (2 mcgs of VITAMIN K per serving)

FILLING

2	cups	Raisins, packed
1 1/3	cups	Water
3	tbsp	Cornstarch
2	tbsp	Cold water
1	cup	Sugar
1	tsp	Vanilla extract
	COOKIE	
1	cup	Brown sugar, firmly packed
1 1/2	cups	Rolled oats
1	cup	Butter, melted
1 1/2	cups	All purpose flour
1	tsp	Baking soda
1/2	tsp	Salt
1	cup	Walnuts, chopped
1	tbsp	Canola oil, treated, (See Dietary Tip #10)

FILLING: Cook raisins in 1 1/3 cups water until tender. Dissolve cornstarch in 2 tablespoons cold water. Add sugar and cornstarch to raisins, stir until mix thickens. Remove from heat, add vanilla and set aside to cool.

COOKIE: Add brown sugar and oats to melted butter. Mix well. Sift together the flour, soda and salt. Add to the sugar and butter mixture. Stir in the nuts.

Oil a 9-inch square pan with the Canola oil. Pack half of mix into the bottom of the pan. Spread the raisin filling evenly on top. Top with the remaining crumb mixture.

Bake in a 350 degree Fahrenheit oven for 30 minutes. Remove from oven. Set pan on a rack to cool completely, then cut into 3 by 1 inch bars.

Ingredient	Cal	Fat	Chol	Sod	Prot	Carb	Fiber
CANOLA OIL	120	14	0	0	0	0	0
FILLING							
RAISINS	1008	1.6	0	64	8	264	22.4
CORNSTARCH	162	0	0	4	0	39	0
SUGAR	776	0	0	0	0	200	0
VANILLA EXTRACT	10	0	0	0	0	0.3	0
COOKIE							
BROWN SUGAR	824	0	0	0	0	213.6	0
ROLLED OATS	840	24	0	12	58.8	225.6	54
BUTTER	1600	184	560	1440	0	0	0
FLOUR	600	2.4	0	0	16.8	132	0
BAKING SODA	0	0	0	821	0	0	0
SALT	0	0	0	1150	0	0	0
WALNUTS	768	74.4	0	16	16.8	22.4	5.6
Totals Per Serving:	**248**	**11.1**	**21**	**130**	**3.7**	**40.6**	**3.1**

MEXICAN WEDDING COOKIES
36 servings (1 mcg of VITAMIN K per serving)

1	cup	Butter, softened
1	cup	Sugar, confectioners
2	cups	All purpose flour, sifted
1	cup	Walnuts, ground
1	tsp	Vanilla extract
1	tbsp	Canola oil, treated, (See Dietary Tip #10)

Combine all ingredients. Form into 1 1/2 inch balls.

Oil a cookie sheet with the Canola oil. Place balls on cookie sheet and bake at 350 degrees Fahrenheit for about 10-15 minutes or until set. These cookies will not spread.

Roll in powdered sugar while still warm.

Ingredient	Cal	Fat	Chol	Sod	Prot	Carb	Fiber
BUTTER	1600	184	560	1440	0	0	0
SUGAR	464	0	0	0	0	120	0
FLOUR	800	3.2	0	0	22.4	176	0
WALNUTS	488	48	0	0	16	8	4
VANILLA EXTRACT	10	0	0	0	0	0.3	0
CANOLA OIL	120	14	0	0	0	0	0
Totals Per Serving:	97	6.9	16	40	1.1	8.5	0.1

ALMOND BUTTER COOKIES
36 cookies (1 mcg of VITAMIN K per 3 cookies)

1	cup	Butter
1	tsp	Almond extract
1/4	tsp	Salt
2	cups	All purpose flour
1/2	cup	Sugar
1	tbsp	Canola oil, treated, (See Dietary Tip #10)

Oil a cookie sheet with the Canola oil.

Cream the butter and sugar with the almond extract. Add the salt and flour. Mix well. Chill the dough.

Form the dough into 1 inch balls and roll in sugar. Stamp each cookie with a cookie stamp, or the bottom of a glass, to flatten.

Bake at 350 degrees 12 to 15 minutes.

Ingredient	Cal	Fat	Chol	Sod	Prot	Carb	Fiber
BUTTER	1600	184	560	1440	0	0	0
ALMOND EXTRACT	5	0	0	1	0	0.2	0
SALT	0	0	0	575	0	0	0
FLOUR	800	3.2	0	0	22.4	176	0
SUGAR	388	0	0	0	0	100	0
CANOLA OIL	120	14	0	0	0	0	0
Totals Per Serving:	**78**	**5.2**	**16**	**56**	**0.6**	**7.7**	**0**

SOUR CREAM COOKIES
36 cookies (1 mcg of VITAMIN K per 3 cookies)

1/2	cup	Butter
1	large	Egg
1/2	cup	Sour cream, nonfat
2 1/2	cup	All purpose flour, sifted
1	cup	Sugar
1/2	tsp	Baking soda
1/2	tsp	Salt
1	tsp	Vanilla extract

Cream together the shortening and sugar.

Add the egg and beat well.

Add the sour cream.

Add the flour, soda and salt.

Blend all ingredients and drop onto an ungreased cookie sheet.

Dip the bottom of a small glass in water and then into sugar and press on top of dropped cookie dough, flattening the cookie a bit.

Bake 12 to 16 minutes at 335 degrees Fahrenheit.

Ingredient	Cal	Fat	Chol	Sod	Prot	Carb	Fiber
BUTTER	800	92	280	720	0	0	0
EGG	75	5	213	63	6.3	0.6	0
SOUR CREAM	60	0	0	60	12	4	0
FLOUR	1000	4	0	0	28	220	0
SUGAR	776	0	0	0	0	200	0
BAKING SODA	0	0	0	411	0	0	0
SALT	0	0	0	1150	0	0	0
VANILLA EXTRACT	10	0	0	0	0	0.3	0
Totals Per Serving:	76	2.8	14	67	1.3	11.8	0

CAKES

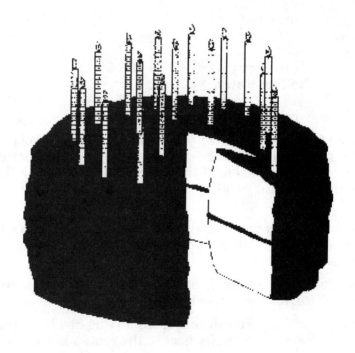

MARBLE CHEESECAKE

10 servings (1 mcg of VITAMIN K per serving. This recipe is also low in fat and calories.)

3	each	Graham crackers, crushed
15	oz	Ricotta cheese, nonfat
8	oz	Cream cheese, lowfat
1/4	cup	Sour cream, lowfat
1/2	cup	Sugar, plus
6	tbsp	Sugar
2	tbsp	All purpose flour
1 1/2	tsp	Vanilla extract
3	large	Egg whites
3	tbsp	Cocoa powder
1	tbsp	Coffee liqueur
1/8	tsp	Salt
1	tbsp	Butter for pan
		Boiling water

Preheat the oven to 350 degrees Fahrenheit.

Grease an 8-inch springform pan with butter (or Canola oil.) Sprinkle the graham cracker crumbs evenly over the bottom of the pan. Wrap the outside of the pan with heavy-duty foil. (If you do not have heavy-duty foil then just double up the regular foil.)

Combine ricotta, cream cheese, sour cream and 1/2 cup sugar in a food processor. Process until smooth, scraping sides occasionally.

Add the flour and vanilla. Process until just blended (about 15 seconds). Transfer the batter to a large bowl.

Beat the egg whites and salt in a clean mixing bowl on medium speed until foamy. Gradually beat in the remaining 6 tablespoons of sugar, 1 tablespoon at a time. Continue beating until the egg whites form soft peaks.

Carefully fold half the beaten whites into the cheese batter with a rubber spatula. Repeat with the remaining whites.

Transfer 1-1/2 cups of the batter to a medium bowl. Pour the remaining batter over the graham cracker crumbs in the springform pan.

Place the foil wrapped springform pan inside a larger baking pan.

Gently whisk the cocoa and liqueur into the reserved batter just until smooth.

Carefully spoon the cocoa mixture over the batter in the pan. Swirl a knife through to marbleize.

Place the pans, one inside the other, on the oven rack. Pour boiling water into the larger pan to reach 1 inch up the side of the springform pan.

Bake 45 minutes or until just set. Turn the oven off and let the cake stand in the oven for 1 hour with the oven door closed.

Remove the pan from the water bath. Remove foil; cool completely.

Cover and refrigerate overnight (or at least 4 to 5 hours). Remove sides of pan, cut and serve.

Ingredient	Cal	Fat	Chol	Sod	Prot	Carb	Fiber
GRAHAM CRACKERS	138	7.2	45	1086	15.6	2.1	0
RICOTTA CHEESE	750	52.5	150	675	52.5	15	0
CREAM CHEESE	480	40	80	1280	24	16	0
SOUR CREAM	80	4	10	70	4	8	0
SUGAR	388	0	0	0	0	100	0
SUGAR	291	0	0	0	0	75	0
FLOUR	50	0.2	0	0	1.4	11	0
VANILLA EXTRACT	15	0	0	0	0	.5	0
EGG WHITES	42	0	0	138	9	9	0
COCOA POWDER	30	1.5	0	9	3	8.4	0.6
COFFEE LIQUEUR	10	0	0	0	0	10	0
SALT	0	0	0	288	0	0	0
BUTTER FOR PAN	100	11.5	35	90	0	0	0
Totals Per Serving:	**237**	**11.7**	**32**	**364**	**11**	**25.5**	**0.1**

FRUIT COCKTAIL CAKE
8 servings (1 mcg of VITAMIN K per serving)

2	cups	All purpose flour
1 1/2	cups	Sugar
16	oz	Fruit cocktail, packed in juice
2	tsp	Baking soda
2	large	Eggs or 1/2 cup of an egg substitute
1/8	tsp	Salt

Mix all ingredients in a 9 x 13-inch pan.

Mix by hand.

Bake at 350 degrees Fahrenheit for about 40 minutes.

Ingredient	Cal	Fat	Chol	Sod	Prot	Carb	Fiber
FLOUR	800	3.2	0	0	22.4	176	0
SUGAR	1164	0	0	0	0	300	0
FRUIT COCKTAIL	208	0	0	16	1.6	52.8	3.2
BAKING SODA	0	0	0	1642	0	0	0
EGGS	150	11.2	426	126	12.6	1.2	0
SALT	0	0	0	288	0	0	0
Totals Per Serving:	**290**	**1.8**	**53**	**259**	**4.6**	**66.3**	**0.4**

CHEESECAKE
10 servings (2 mcgs of VITAMIN K per serving)

1	tbsp	Graham cracker crumbs
1	cup	Cottage cheese, lowfat
16	oz	Cream cheese, lowfat, softened*
2/3	cup	Sugar
2	tbsp	All purpose flour
2	tbsp	Milk, skim
1/4	cup	Almond extract
3	large	Eggs or 3/4 cup of an egg substitute**
1	tbsp	Butter for the pan

*Cream Cheese may be regular or nonfat.

**A liquid egg substitute such as EggBeaters can be used instead of whole eggs. Adjust the nutrition values accordingly.

Lightly grease the bottom of a 9-inch springform pan with the butter. Sprinkle with Graham cracker crumbs. Remove the excess crumbs and discard.

Put the cottage cheese in a blender container. Cover and process on high speed until smooth.

In a large mixing bowl of an electric mixer, combine the cottage cheese, cream cheese, sugar and flour. Mix at medium speed until well blended.

Add eggs, one at a time, mixing well after each addition.

Blend in milk and almond extract and pour into the pan.

Bake at 325 degrees Fahrenheit, 45 to 50 minutes or until center is almost set. (Center of cheesecake appears to be soft, but firms upon cooling.)

Cool. Loosen the cake from the rim of the pan and remove the rim. Chill and serve.

If you like, top with fresh slices of strawberries or blueberries. (Adding the fruit will add 1 to 2 mcgs of VITAMIN K per serving.)

Ingredient	Cal	Fat	Chol	Sod	Prot	Carb	Fiber
CRACKER CRUMBS	60	1.3	0	70	1	11	0.5
COTTAGE CHEESE	160	2.4	8	920	28	6.4	0
CREAM CHEESE	960	80	160	2560	48	32	0
SUGAR	517	0	0	0	0	133.3	0
FLOUR	50	0.2	0	0	1.4	11	0
MILK, SKIM	11	0.1	1	16	1	1.5	0
ALMOND EXTRACT	1	0	0	0	0	0	0
EGGS	225	16.8	639	189	18.9	1.8	0
BUTTER	100	10.1	81	376	9.8	19.7	0.1
Totals Per Serving:	208	11.2	84	385	9.8	19.7	0.1

PUMPKIN-RAISIN CAKE
12 servings (3 mcgs of VITAMIN K per serving)

1 2/3	cup	All purpose flour
2/3	cup	Sugar
1/4	cup	Milk, dry powdered skim
1	tsp	Baking soda
1/2	tsp	Baking powder
1/2	tsp	Salt
2	tsp	Pumpkin pie spice
1/2	cup	Raisins, packed
2	each	Egg whites
1	cup	Pumpkin, canned, no salt
1/3	cup	Corn syrup, light or dark
1/3	cup	Orange juice
1	tbsp	Butter for greasing pan

Butter a 9-inch square baking pan.

In a large bowl, combine the dry ingredients and the raisins.

In a medium bowl, combine the remaining ingredients.

Add to dry ingredients. Stir until smooth. Pour into prepared pan.

Bake in 350 degrees Fahrenheit oven 35 minutes or until toothpick inserted in center comes out clean.

Cool in pan on wire rack.

Ingredient	Cal	Fat	Chol	Sod	Prot	Carb	Fiber
FLOUR	667	2.7	0	0	18.7	146.7	0
SUGAR	517	0	0	0	0	133.3	0
MILK, DRY	192	2	12	300	19.2	28.8	0
BAKING SODA	0	0	0	821	0	0	0
BAKING POWDER	1	0	0	102	0	0.2	0
SALT	0	0	0	1150	0	0	0
PUMPKIN PIE SPICE	13	0.2	0	1	0.2	2.6	0.3
RAISINS	252	0.4	0	16	2	66	5.6
EGG WHITES	28	0	0	92	6	6	0
PUMPKIN	80	0	0	8	0	16	8
CORN SYRUP	320	0	0	187	0	80	0
ORANGE JUICE	45	0	0	0	0.5	8.5	0.3
BUTTER	100	11.5	35	90	0	0	0
Totals Per Serving:	**185**	**1.4**	**4**	**231**	**3.9**	**40.7**	**1.2**

GOLDEN FRUITCAKE
12 servings (4 mcg of VITAMIN K per serving)

1 1/4	cups	All purpose flour
1/2	tsp	Baking powder
1/2	tsp	Salt
2	cups	Candied fruits*
1	cup	Raisins, packed, golden
1	cup	Pecans
1/2	cup	Butter
1/2	cup	Sugar
3	large	Eggs
1/2	cup	Bourbon or cognac
1	tbsp	Butter

*I use one quarter pound each of candied cherries and small pieces of candied pineapple.

Line a well buttered 9 by 5 by 3 inch pan with wax paper.

Sift together the flour, baking powder and salt. Add the fruit and nuts.

Cream the butter and sugar. Beat in the eggs, 1 at a time.

Combine with the fruit and flour mix. Pour into pan.

Bake at 300 degrees Fahrenheit for 1 1/2 to 2 hours or until cake tester comes out clean.

Cool and anoint with bourbon or cognac. Wrap in foil to keep.

I usually make these 1 month ahead of when I want to serve them. This is the only fruitcake I ever make.

Ingredient	Cal	Fat	Chol	Sod	Prot	Carb	Fiber
ALL PURPOSE FLOUR	500	2	0	0	14	110	0
BAKING POWDER	1	0	0	102	0	0.2	0
SALT	0	0	0	1150	0	0	0
CANDIED FRUITS	1120	0	0	240	0	288	16
RAISINS	504	0.8	0	32	4	132	11.2
PECANS	792	80	0	0	9.6	22.4	8
BUTTER	800	92	280	720	0	0	0
SUGAR	388	0	0	0	0	100	0
EGGS	225	16.8	639	189	18.9	1.8	0
BOURBON	260	0	0	0	0	0	0
BUTTER	100	11.5	35	90	0	0	0
Totals Per Serving:	391	16.9	80	210	3.9	54.5	2.9

TANGERINE POUND CAKE
8 servings (Less than 1 mcg of VITAMIN K per serving)

1	tsp	Grated tangerine zest
1	cup	Whipped cream*
12	oz	Pound cake, nonfat
4	each	Tangerines
1/3	cup	Sugar
1	tbsp	Lemon juice

*Or your favorite whipped topping. Adjust nutrition values accordingly.

Stir the tangerine peel into the whipped cream and chill.

Pierce top and bottom of the cake with a fork. Place in a shallow baking pan. Heat in a 350 degree Fahrenheit oven for 10 minutes.

Peel 2 of the tangerines with a sharp knife, section and seed, reserving segments and juice separately. Squeeze juice from remaining tangerines to make 1/2 cup.

In a saucepan, combine the sugar, 1/2 cup tangerine juice and lemon juice. Boil 3 to 4 minutes until slightly thickened, stirring frequently.

Slowly spoon the hot syrup over the bottom, sides and top of the warm cake. Let stand 5 minutes.

To serve, slice cake and spoon topping over each piece. Garnish with reserved tangerine sections.

Ingredient	Cal	Fat	Chol	Sod	Prot	Carb	Fiber
TANGERINE ZEST	0	0	0	0	0.1	1.2	0
WHIPPED CREAM	416	44.8	168	48	2.4	3.2	0
POUND CAKE	960	0	0	1164	24	204	0
TANGERINES	140	0.8	0	8	2	32	0.8
SUGAR	259	0	0	0	0	66.7	0
LEMON JUICE	3	0	0	0	0.5	1	0
Totals Per Serving:	222	5.7	21	153	3.6	38.5	0.1

APPLE CAKE
10 servings (1 mcg of VITAMIN K per serving)

6	med	Apples, peeled, cored and sliced
5	tbsp	Sugar plus
2	cups	Sugar
5	tsp	Cinnamon
3	cups	All purpose flour
3	tsp	Baking powder
1/2	tsp	Salt
4	large	Eggs
1	cup	Canola oil, treated (See Dietary Tip # 10)
1/4	cup	Orange juice
1	tbsp	Vanilla extract
2	tbsp	Butter for pan

Combine the peeled apples and 5 tablespoons of the sugar. Add the cinnamon and mix well.

Sift flour, the rest of the sugar, baking powder and salt into a bowl.

Make a well in the center and pour in the oil, eggs, juice and vanilla. Beat with a spoon until blended.

Spoon 1/3 of the batter into a greased, 9 inch, angel food pan. Make a ring of 1/2 of the apple mix (drained). Spoon another 1/3 of the batter over apples, spread the remaining apples and top with the last 1/3 of the batter.

Bake in 375 degrees Fahrenheit oven for 1 hour or until done. Test with toothpick. Serve warm or cold.

Optional: Serve with whipped cream, whipped topping or ice cream.

Ingredient	Cal	Fat	Chol	Sod	Prot	Carb	Fiber
APPLES	438	0	0	0	0.6	114	14.4
SUGAR	242	0	0	0	0	62.5	0
SUGAR	1552	0	0	0	0	400	0
CINNAMON	30	5	0	5	0.5	8.3	3
FLOUR	1200	4.8	0	0	33.6	264	0
BAKING POWDER	6	0	0	612	0	1.4	0
SALT	0	0	0	1150	0	0	0
EGGS	300	22.4	852	252	25.2	2.4	0
OIL	1928	224	0	0	0	0	0
ORANGE JUICE	34	0	0	0	0.4	6.4	0.2
VANILLA EXTRACT	30	0	0	0	0	0.9	0
BUTTER	200	23	70	180	0	0	0
Totals Per Serving:	596	27.9	92	220	6	86	1.8

RASPBERRY WALNUT CAKE
8 servings (7 mcg of VITAMIN K per serving)

2 3/4	cup	All purpose flour
2 1/2	tsp	Baking powder
1/4	tsp	Salt
1/2	cup	Butter, (room temperature)
1 3/4	cup	Sugar
1	tsp	Vanilla extract
1/2	tsp	Black walnut flavoring
2	large	Eggs (room temperature)
1 1/4	cups	Milk, skim
1	cup	Walnuts, ground
5	tbsp	Raspberry jam or preserves PLUS
1	tsp	Raspberry jam or preserves (1/3 cup total raspberry jam)
1	each	CREAM CHEESE FROSTING (See Recipe Index)
1	tbsp	Butter for pans
2	tbs	All purpose flour for pans

Preheat oven to 350 degrees Fahrenheit. Grease and flour two cake pans.

Sift flour, baking powder and salt into bowl.

Using a mixer, cream butter with sugar in another bowl until light and fluffy. Blend in the vanilla and walnut flavoring. Beat in the eggs, 1 at a time.

Mix in the dry ingredients and milk alternately in 3 additions. Fold in 3/4 cup of walnuts. Pour batter into the pans.

Bake until golden brown and tester inserted in center comes out clean, 30 to 35 minutes.

Cool in pans on a rack for 10 minutes. Turn out onto rack and cool completely.

Heat the jam in a heavy small saucepan over low heat, stirring often.

Set 1 cake layer on a platter. Spread the top of the cake with half of the jam. Top with second layer. Spread with remaining jam.

Sprinkle with remaining walnuts. Spoon 2/3 cup frosting into pastry bag fitted with a star tip, set aside.

Ice sides of cake with remaining frosting. Pipe rosettes of frosting around the edge of the cake. Refrigerate until frosting is set. (Can do one day ahead.)

Let stand 1 hour before serving.

Ingredient	Cal	Fat	Chol	Sod	Prot	Carb	Fiber
FLOUR	1100	4.4	0	0	30.8	242	0
BAKING POWDER	5	0	0	510	0	1.1	0
SALT	0	0	0	575	0	0	0
BUTTER	800	92	280	720	0	0	0
SUGAR	1358	0	0	0	0	350	0
VANILLA EXTRACT	10	0	0	0	0	0.3	0
WALNUT FLAVOR	5	0	0	0	0	0	0
EGGS	150	11.2	426	126	12.6	1.2	0
MILK, SKIM	110	1	10	160	10	15	0
WALNUTS	488	48	0	0	16	8	4
RASPBERRY JAM	270	0	0	38	0	60	0
RASPBERRY JAM	18	0	0	3	0	4	0
FROSTING	1492	76.4	217	969	9.5	198.9	0
BUTTER	100	11.5	35	90	0	0	0
FLOUR	50	.2	0	0	1.4	11	0
Totals Per Serving	**596**	**24.5**	**97**	**319**	**8**	**89.2**	**0.4**

CHOCOLATE PUDDING CAKE
6 servings (4 mcgs of VITAMIN K per serving)

CAKE

1	cup	All purpose flour
2	tsp	Baking powder
1/2	tsp	Salt
3/4	cup	Sugar
2	tbsp	Cocoa powder
1/2	cup	Milk, skim
1	tsp	Vanilla extract
2	tbsp	BLENDER MAYONNAISE #2 (See Recipe Index)
3/4	cup	Walnuts, chopped

TOPPING

3/4	cup	Brown sugar
1/4	cup	Cocoa powder
1 3/4	cup	Hot water

Sift dry ingredients together.

Add milk, vanilla and mayonnaise. Mix until smooth. Add nuts. Pour into a 9 inch cake pan.

Mix brown sugar and cocoa. Sprinkle over the batter in the pan. Pour hot water over the top of the batter.

Bake at 350 degrees Fahrenheit for 40 to 45 minutes.

Note: You can substitute pecans for the walnuts.

Ingredient	Cal	Fat	Chol	Sod	Prot	Carb	Fiber
CAKE							
FLOUR	400	1.6	0	0	11.2	88	0
BAKING POWDER	4	0	0	408	0	0.9	0
SALT	0	0	0	1150	0	0	0
SUGAR	582	0	0	0	0	150	0
COCOA POWDER	20	1	0	6	2	5.6	0.4
MILK, SKIM	44	0.4	4	64	4	6	0
VANILLA EXTRACT	10	0	0	0	0	0.3	0
MAYONNAISE	153	16.8	21	75	0.6	0.3	0
WALNUTS	576	55.8	0	12	12.6	16.8	4.2
TOPPING							
BROWN SUGAR	618	0	0	0	0	162	0
COCOA POWDER	40	2	0	12	4	11.2	0.8
Totals Per Serving:	408	12.9	4	288	5.7	73.2	0.9

ANGEL FOOD CAKE
8 servings (Less than 1 mcg of VITAMIN K per serving)

1	cup	Cake flour, sifted
1 1/4	cups	Sugar, granulated, sifted
1	cup	Egg whites at room temperature
1/4	tsp	Salt
1	tsp	Cream of tartar
3/4	tsp	Vanilla extract
1/4	tsp	Almond extract

Sift flour once, measure, add 1/4 cup sugar, and sift together four times.

Beat the egg whites and salt with a rotary egg beater or flat wire whisk. When foamy, add the cream of tartar and continue beating until the eggs are stiff enough to hold up in peaks, but not dry. Add the remaining 1 cup sugar, 2 tablespoons at a time, beating with the rotary egg beater or whisk after each addition until sugar is just blended. Fold in the flavorings.

Sift about 1/4 cup of the flour mixture over the egg whites and fold in lightly. Repeat this step until all flour is used.

Turn into an ungreased angel food pan. Cut gently through batter with knife to remove air bubbles.

Bake in a slow oven (325 degrees Fahrenheit) 45 to 50 minutes. Remove from oven and invert pan 1 hour, or until cold.

Ingredient	Cal	Fat	Chol	Sod	Prot	Carb	Fiber
CAKE FLOUR	400	1.6	0	0	10.4	88	0
SUGAR	970	0	0	0	0	250	0
EGG WHITES	112	0	0	368	24	24	0
SALT	0	0	0	575	0	0	0
CREAM OF TARTAR	8	0	0	0	0	0.3	0
VANILLA EXTRACT	8	0	0	0	0	0.2	0
ALMOND EXTRACT	1	0	0	0	0	0	0
Totals Per Serving:	187	0.2	0	118	4.3	45.3	0

APPLE COFFEE CAKE
9 servings (1 mcg of VITAMIN K per serving)

2	cups	All purpose flour
1 1/4	cups	Sugar
1 1/2	tsp	Cinnamon, ground
1 1/4	tsp	Baking soda
1/2	tsp	Salt
1/4	tsp	Cloves, ground
1/4	tsp	Nutmeg, ground
2	large	Eggs, beaten
1	tsp	Vanilla extract
1/2	cup	Applesauce, unsweetened (replaces 1/2 cup oil)
1/3	cup	Apple juice
2	cups	Apples, peeled, cored and chopped
1/4	cup	Brown sugar, packed
1/4	cup	Walnuts, chopped
1	tbsp	Butter for pan

Sift together the flour, sugar, cinnamon, baking soda, salt, cloves, and nutmeg into mixing bowl. Stir to blend.

Add the eggs, vanilla, applesauce and apple juice. Stir just until blended. Fold in the peeled apples.

Spoon the batter into a buttered 8-inch square baking pan.

Combine the brown sugar and walnuts. Sprinkle evenly over top of batter.

Bake at 350 degrees Fahrenheit 40 to 45 minutes or until a toothpick inserted in the center of the cake comes out clean.

Ingredient	Cal	Fat	Chol	Sod	Prot	Carb	Fiber
FLOUR	800	3.2	0	0	22.4	176	0
SUGAR	970	0	0	0	0	250	0
CINNAMON	9	1.5	0	2	0.2	2.5	0.9
BAKING SODA	0	0	0	1026	0	0	0
SALT	0	0	0	1150	0	0	0
CLOVES	2	0.1	0	1	0	0.3	0.2
NUTMEG	3	0.2	0	0	0	0.3	0.1
EGGS	150	11.2	426	126	12.6	1.2	0
VANILLA EXTRACT	10	0	0	0	0	0.3	0
APPLESAUCE	48	0	0	4	0.8	0	0
APPLE JUICE	40	0	0	5	0	8.8	0
APPLES	256	0	0	0	1.6	64	16
BROWN SUGAR	206	0	0	0	0	53.4	0
WALNUTS	192	18.6	0	4	4.2	5.6	1.4
BUTTER FOR PAN	100	11.5	35	90	0	0	0
Totals Per Serving:	**310**	**5.1**	**51**	**268**	**4.6**	**62.5**	**2.1**

FUZZY NAVEL CHEESECAKE
12 servings (2 mcgs of VITAMIN K per serving)

COOKIE CRUST

3/4	cup	All purpose flour
2 1/2	tbsp	Sugar
1	large	Egg, beaten lightly
1/4	cup	Butter, softened
1/2	tsp	Vanilla extract
1	tbsp	Butter for the pan

FILLING

24	oz	Cream cheese, lowfat
3/4	cup	Sugar
1/4	cup	Sour cream, lowfat
5	tsp	Cornstarch
3	large	Eggs
1	each	Egg yolk
1/2	cup	Orange juice concentrate, thawed
1/4	cup	Peach Schnapps
2	tsp	Lemon juice
1 1/4	tsp	Vanilla extract

ORANGE MARMALADE GLAZE

2/3	cup	Orange marmalade
3	tbsp	Peach schnapps
1 1/2	tbsp	Cornstarch
1 1/2	tbsp	Orange juice concentrate, thawed
2	tsp	Lemon juice

CRUST: In a medium bowl, stir together the flour and sugar. Add the egg, butter and vanilla. Beat with an electric mixer until well combined. With greased fingers press dough evenly on to the bottom of greased 9 inch springform pan.

Bake at 350 degrees Fahrenheit for 12-15 minutes or until lightly browned. Remove from oven and set aside.

FILLING: In a large bowl combine the cream cheese, sugar, sour cream and cornstarch. Beat with an electric mixer until smooth.

Add eggs and yolk, one at a time, beating well after each addition. Beat in orange juice, schnapps, lemon juice and vanilla. Pour mixture over the crust.

Bake at 350 degrees Fahrenheit for 15 minutes. Lower the oven temperature to 200 degrees Fahrenheit and bake for an additional hour and 10 minutes or until center no longer looks shiny or wet. Remove the cake from the oven and run a knife around the edge of the pan. Chill uncovered, overnight.

GLAZE: In a small saucepan combine all ingredients. Cook and stir until thickened and bubbly. Cook and stir 2 minutes more. Pour over cheesecake. Chill until serving time.

Ingredient	Cal	Fat	Chol	Sod	Prot	Carb	Fiber
COOKIE CRUST							
FLOUR	300	1.2	0	0	8.4	66	0
SUGAR	121	0	0	0	0	31.3	0
EGG, BEATEN	75	5.6	213	63	6.3	0.6	0
BUTTER	400	46	140	360	0	0	0
VANILLA EXTRACT	5	0	0	0	0	0.2	0
BUTTER	100	11.5	35	90	0	0	0
FILLING							
CREAM CHEESE	1440	120	240	3840	72	48	0
SUGAR	582	0	0	0	0	150	0
SOUR CREAM	80	4	10	70	4	8	0
CORNSTARCH	90	0	0	3	0	21.7	0
EGGS	225	16.8	639	189	18.9	1.8	0
EGG YOLK	101	8.8	363	12	4.8	0.5	0
ORANGE JUICE	248	0.8	0	0	4.8	61.6	12.4
PEACH SCHNAPPS	250	0	0	4	0	28	0
LEMON JUICE	2	0	0	0	0.3	0.7	0
VANILLA EXTRACT	13	0	0	0	0	0.4	0
ORANGE MARMALADE GLAZE							
MARMALADE	576	0	0	0	0	128	0
PEACH SCHNAPPS	188	0	0	3	0	21	0
CORNSTARCH	81	0	0	2	0	19.5	0
ORANGE JUICE	46	0.2	0	0	0.9	11.6	2.3
LEMON JUICE	2	0	0	0	0.3	0.7	0
Totals Per Serving:	**410**	**17.9**	**137**	**386**	**10.1**	**49.9**	**1.3**

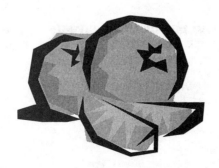

CARROT/ZUCCHINI/APRICOT/PINEAPPLE CAKE
24 servings (3 mcgs of VITAMIN K per serving)

2	large	Eggs
2	each	Egg whites
2	cups	All purpose flour
2	cups	Sugar
2	tsp	Baking powder
1 1/2	tsp	Baking soda
1	tsp	Salt
2	tsp	Cinnamon, ground
1 1/2	cups	APRICOTS, PUREED (See Recipe Index)*
2	cups	Carrots, peeled and grated
8	oz	Pineapple packed in juice, crushed, drained, and the juice reserved
1	cup	Raisins, packed
1/2	cup	Walnuts, chopped
8	oz	Sugar, confectioners
1	tbsp	Butter for the pan

*Pureed figs or peeled, grated Zucchini may be used in place of the apricots.

Preheat oven to 350 degrees Fahrenheit. Use the 1 tablespoon butter for greasing the pan.

Lightly beat together the eggs and egg whites in a bowl.

Sift together the flour, sugar, baking powder, baking soda, salt and cinnamon into a mixing bowl. Stir to blend.

Add pureed apricots, beaten eggs, carrots, pineapple, raisins and nuts until blended. Turn into the buttered 13 by 9 inch baking pan.

Bake at 350 degrees Fahrenheit 35 to 40 minutes or until cake tests done in center.

While cake cools, blend powdered sugar and 2 tablespoons reserved pineapple juice until smooth and of spreading consistency. Drizzle over cake while it is still hot.

Most people think of carrot cake as a healthy cake. What they forget is that most carrot cakes are made with oil. In the oil version of this recipe there is 1-1/2 cups. But replace the oil with pureed apricots and you reduce the percentage of calories from fat from an extremely high 50% to just 4%.

Though they are traditionally added to carrot cake, you may want to omit the walnuts, which are high in fat. However, walnuts are so good for you in so many other ways that I always leave them in.

Note: You can substitute pecans for the walnuts.

Ingredient	Cal	Fat	Chol	Sod	Prot	Carb	Fiber
EGGS	150	11.2	426	126	12.6	1.2	0
EGG WHITES	28	0	0	92	6	6	0
FLOUR	800	3.2	0	0	22.4	176	0
SUGAR	1552	0	0	0	0	400	0
BAKING POWDER	4	0	0	408	0	0.9	0
BAKING SODA	0	0	0	1232	0	0	0
SALT	0	0	0	2300	0	0	0
CINNAMON	12	2	0	2	0.2	3.3	1.2
APRICOTS	629	1.6	0	33	9.6	160.2	22.4
CARROTS	96	1.6	0	80	1.6	24	1.6
PINEAPPLE	144	0	0	16	0	36	1.6
RAISINS	504	0.8	0	32	4	132	11.2
WALNUTS	384	37.2	0	8	8.4	11.2	2.8
SUGAR	464	0	0	0	0	120	0
BUTTER	100	11.5	35	90	0	0	0
Totals Per Serving:	**203**	**2.9**	**19**	**184**	**2.7**	**44.6**	**1.7**

PUREED APRICOTS
1 1/2 cups (5 mcgs of VITAMIN K for the entire recipe)

2	cups	apricots, dried
3/4	cup	Boiling water
2	tsp	Vanilla extract

Pour the boiling water over the apricots and let sit for 1/2 hour.

Puree the apricots, water and vanilla in a blender or food processor. Makes 1-1/2 cups.

You can use dried figs in place of the apricots. Figs will double the calories.

Ingredient	Cal	Fat	Chol	Sod	Prot	Carb	Fiber
APRICOTS, DRIED	624	1.6	0	32	9.6	160	22.4
VANILLA EXTRACT	10	0	0	0	0	0.3	0
Totals Per Recipe:	634	1.6	0	33	9.6	160.3	22.4

CRANBERRY SWIRL CHEESECAKE
12 servings (2 mcgs of VITAMIN K per serving)

12	oz	Fresh cranberries
1 1/3	cups	Sugar
2	tbsp	Sugar
2	lb	Cream cheese, lowfat, at room temperature, cut in pieces
2	tsp	Vanilla extract
4	large	Eggs, at room temperature
2	cups	Sour cream, lowfat, at room temperature
1	tbsp	Butter
2	tbsp	All purpose flour

In a medium non-reactive saucepan, combine the cranberries and 3/4 cup water. Bring to a boil over moderate heat and boil, stirring occasionally, until the cranberries burst and the mixture reduces to 1-1/4 cups, about 12 minutes. Remove from the heat and stir in 1/3 cup of the sugar until dissolved. Strain the mixture through a coarse sieve and let the puree cool completely.

Preheat the oven to 275 degrees Fahrenheit. Butter and flour a 9-by-2-3/4 inch springform pan.

In a large bowl, using an electric mixer, beat the cream cheese with the remaining 1 cup plus 2 tablespoons sugar and the vanilla at low speed until smooth. Beat in the eggs one at a time, beating until just blended. Stir in the sour cream.

Spoon half of the cream cheese mixture into the prepared pan. Drop 8 or 9 rounded teaspoons of the cranberry puree randomly over the top. Spoon half of the remaining cheesecake mixture evenly over the first layer and dot with half of the remaining puree. Repeat with the remaining cheesecake mixture and puree. (Do not drop puree in the center of the pan in more than 1 layer.) With a blunt knife, cut through the batter in a swirling motion to distribute the cranberry puree.

Place the pan on a baking sheet and bake in the lower part of the oven for 1 hour. Turn the oven off and leave the cheesecake in for 1 hour longer. Transfer the cake to a rack and let cool to room temperature.

Cover and refrigerate overnight before serving.

Ingredient	Cal	Fat	Chol	Sod	Prot	Carb	Fiber
CRANBERRIES	72	0.2	0	12	0.6	18	6
SUGAR	1035	0	0	0	0	266.7	0
SUGAR	97	0	0	0	0	25	0
CREAM CHEESE	1920	160	320	5120	96	64	0
VANILLA EXTRACT	20	0	0	0	0	0.6	0
EGGS	300	22.4	852	252	25.2	2.4	0
SOUR CREAM	640	32	80	560	32	64	0
BUTTER	100	11.5	35	90	0	0	0
FLOUR	50	0.2	0	0	1.4	11	0
Totals Per Serving:	**353**	**18.8**	**107**	**503**	**13**	**37.6**	**0.5**

HUNGARIAN COFFEE CAKE
8 servings (3 mcgs of VITAMIN K per serving)

2	cups	Brown sugar
1	cup	Butter
3	cups	All purpose flour
2	large	Eggs, beaten
1	cup	Buttermilk
1/2	tsp	Salt
1	tsp	Baking soda
1	tbsp	Butter for the pan

Using a pastry blender, cut the butter into the flour and brown sugar, until crumbly. Remove 1 cup of this mixture to a small bowl and add 1/8 teaspoon cinnamon and 3 tablespoons white sugar. Set aside for topping.

Beat the eggs. Add the buttermilk, baking soda and salt and mix well.

Add remaining flour mixture and beat well with an electric mixer. Turn into two greased 9 inch round pans or one 9x13 inch pan. Top with crumb mixture and if desired, sprinkle with powdered sugar.

Bake at 350 degrees Fahrenheit for 25 to 30 minutes or until done (use toothpick to test).

OPTIONS:

BERRIES: Sprinkle 2 cups of blueberries or raspberries with 1/2 cup sugar and lightly toss. Arrange the berries on top of the cake, then sprinkle with the crumb mixture. Bake longer (45-50 minutes.) and watch closely at the end. Make sure you bake this longer because of the fruit. (Adds 14 mcgs of VITAMIN K to each cake.)

PEACHES: Peel, pit and thinly slice peaches (about 2 cups), toss with 1/2 cup sugar. Arrange peach slices overlapping on top of cakes, top with crumb mixture. Bake until done (takes longer than regular cake also). (Adds 8 mcgs of VITAMIN K to each cake.)

APPLES: Same as above. Be sure to peel, and slice apples very thin. (Negligible affect on the VITAMIN K content.)

Ingredient	Cal	Fat	Chol	Sod	Prot	Carb	Fiber
BROWN SUGAR	1648	0	0	0	0	427.2	0
BUTTER	1600	184	560	1440	0	0	0
FLOUR	1200	4.8	0	0	33.6	264	0
EGGS	150	11.2	426	126	12.6	1.2	0
BUTTERMILK	88	1.6	8	240	7.2	11.2	0
SALT	0	0	0	1150	0	0	0
BAKING SODA	0	0	0	821	0	0	0
BUTTER	100	11.5	35	90	0	0	0
Totals Per Serving:	**598**	**26.6**	**129**	**483**	**6.7**	**88**	**0**

RAINBOW CAKES

8 servings (Less than 1 mcg of VITAMIN K per serving)

2	layers	Cake, yellow (See Recipe Index)
3	ounces	Lemon or lime gelatin*
3	ounces	Orange gelatin*
2	cups	Water, boiling
8	ounces	Whipped cream

*Use sugar free gelatin to reduce calories.

Place cake layers top side up, in 2 clean layer pans, prick each cake with utility fork at 1/2 inch intervals.

Dissolve each flavor of gelatin separately in one cup of boiling water. Carefully pour one flavor of the gelatin over one cake layer and the other flavor over the second layer. Chill 4 hours or more.

Dip one cake pan in warm water for 10 seconds. Unmold, and place on serving plate. Top with 1 cup of whipped cream. Place second layer on top, finish frosting with the remaining whipped cream. Chill.

Ingredient	Cal	Fat	Chol	Sod	Prot	Carb	Fiber
CAKE	3312	146.5	493	3248	45.4	472.6	0
LEMON GELATIN	320	0	0	500	4	76	0
ORANGE GELATIN	320	0	0	300	8	76	4
WHIPPED CREAM	832	89.6	336	96	4.8	6.4	0
Totals Per Serving:	**478**	**23.6**	**83**	**414**	**6.2**	**63.1**	**04**

GLAZED BLUEBERRY SHORTCAKE
8 servings (1 mcg of VITAMIN K per serving)

1/2	cup	Sugar
2	tsp	Cornstarch
1/8	tsp	Salt
1/2	cup	Water
2	pints	Blueberries, thawed if frozen
1	tsp	Grated lime zest
1	tbsp	Lime juice
1	each	BISCUIT SHORTCAKE (See Recipe Index)
1	cup	Whipping cream*

*Or 2 cups of your favorite whipped topping. (Adjust the nutrition values accordingly.)

In a saucepan mix the sugar, cornstarch, salt and water. Add 1 pint blueberries and bring to boil. Simmer uncovered, stirring until clear and thickened, about 3 or 4 minutes. Remove from heat, stir in lime peel and juice. Cool. Stir in remaining 1 pint of blueberries.

Assemble just before serving. Slice the BISCUIT SHORTCAKE in half horizontally.

Whip the cream with 1 tablespoon sugar until soft peaks form. Spread half the blueberry mixture on the bottom half of the shortcake and then spread half of whipped cream on top of the blueberries. Top with other half of the shortcake, remaining blueberry mix and remaining whipped cream.

Ingredient	Cal	Fat	Chol	Sod	Prot	Carb	Fiber
SUGAR	388	0	0	0	0	100	0
CORNSTARCH	36	0	0	1	0	8.7	0
SALT	0	0	0	288	0	0	0
BLUEBERRIES	448	3.2	0	64	6.4	112	19.2
LIME ZEST	0	0	0	0	0.1	1.2	0
LIME JUICE	4	0	0	0	0.1	1.4	0
BISCUIT SHORTCAKE	1837	101.3	498	2396	7.1	62.5	3
WHIPPING CREAM	824	88	328	88	4.8	6.4	0
Totals Per Serving:	**442**	**24.1**	**103**	**355**	**2.3**	**36.5**	**2.8**

YELLOW CAKE
8 servings (3 mcg of VITAMIN K per serving)

2 1/4	cup	Cake Flour
3	tsp	Baking Powder
1	tsp	Salt
1 1/4	cups	Sugar
1/2	cup	Canola Oil, Treated (see Dietary Tip # 10)
1	cup	Milk
2	large	Eggs
2	tsp	Vanilla Extract
1	tbsp	Butter for the pan
2	tbsp	All purpose flour

Preheat the oven to 350 degrees Fahrenheit.

Butter and lightly flour two 8-onch round cake pans.

Mix the flour, baking powder, salt and sugar in a bowl. Stir in the oil and milk, and beat for 2 minutes. Add the eggs and vanilla and beat for another 2 minutes.

Pour into the, buttered and floured, pans and bake for 25 to 30 minutes, or until a toothpick inserted in the center comes out clean. Cool in the pans for 5 minutes before turning out onto cake racks.

Frost with your favorite frosting.

Ingredient	Cal	Fat	Chol	Sod	Prot	Carb	Fiber
CAKE FLOUR	900	3.6	0	0	23.4	198	0
BAKING POWDER	6	0	0	612	0	1.4	0
SALT	0	0	0	2300	0	0	0
SUGAR	970	0	0	0	0	250	0
CANOLA OIL	964	112	0	0	0	0	0
MILK	152	8	32	120	8	10.4	0
EGGS	150	11.2	426	126	12.6	1.2	0
VANILLA EXTRACT	20	0	0	0	0	0.6	0
BUTTER	100	11.5	35	90	0	0	0
FLOUR	50	0.2	0	0	1.4	11	0
Totals Per Serving:	**331**	**14.7**	**49**	**325**	**4.5**	**47.3**	**0**

CHOCOLATE HAZELNUT TORTE
6 servings (9 mcgs of VITAMIN K per serving)

1	tbsp	Butter for cake pan
1	tbsp	All purpose flour for cake pan
1 1/2	cups	Hazelnuts,(Filberts) toasted and skinned
1	cup	Sugar, granulated
6	oz	Bittersweet chocolate, finely chopped (6 squares)
4	oz	Butter, at room temperature (1 stick)
5	large	Eggs, separated, at room temperature
1/4	tsp	Salt
2	tbsp	Liqueur, Frangelico*
2	tbsp	Sugar, confectioners to dust cake

*Or 1 teaspoon of Vanilla extract instead of the liqueur.

Place the oven rack in the center of the oven. Preheat to 350 degrees Fahrenheit. Butter and flour a 9 inch cake pan. Line the bottom of the pan with parchment or wax paper. Butter the paper.

In a food processor or blender, pulse the hazelnuts with 3 tablespoons of sugar until they are finely ground, about 1 minute. Do not over-process or the nuts will turn into hazelnut butter.

Melt together the chocolate, butter and remaining sugar, stirring frequently. Beat the egg yolks (1 at a time) into the chocolate mixture, blending well after each addition. Blend in the liqueur or vanilla. Blend in the nut mixture.

Whip egg whites with salt until they hold firm, but not stiff peaks, about 10 minutes. Gently fold the whites into the chocolate mixture.

Pour the batter into the prepared pan. Bake 35 minutes, until the cake feels firm in the center when pressed lightly. Remove from the oven and cool the cake in the pan on a rack for 20 minutes. Place a cardboard round or a plate over the pan and invert. Remove the pan and peel off the parchment. Let cool completely. Can be made a day ahead.

When cool, wrap completely in plastic wrap and store at room temperature.

Dust with confectioners sugar just before serving.

(Large strawberries arranged around the cake, on the platter, make a great presentation.)

Ingredient	Cal	Fat	Chol	Sod	Prot	Carb	Fiber
BUTTER FOR PAN	100	11.5	35	90	0	0	0
FLOUR	25	0.1	0	0	0.7	5.5	0
HAZELNUTS	1092	108	0	0	24	27.6	12
SUGAR	776	0	0	0	0	200	0
CHOCOLATE	900	54	24	120	6	120	0
BUTTER	800	92	280	720	0	0	0
EGGS	375	28	1065	315	31.5	3	0
SALT	0	0	0	575	0	0	0
FRANGELICO	20	0	0	1	0	10	0
SUGAR	58	0	0	0	0	15	0
Totals Per Serving:	**415**	**29.4**	**140**	**182**	**6.2**	**38.1**	**1.2**

DARK RUM GLAZE
1 cup (9 mcgs of VITAMIN K per cup)

1/4	lb	Butter
1/4	cup	Water
1	cup	Sugar
1/2	cup	Dark rum

Melt the butter and stir all the ingredients except the rum over a low flame for 5 minutes. Keep stirring and wiping the sides of the pan.

Add rum and use as a glaze to dress up a store bought (fat free of course) pound cake.

Ingredient	Cal	Fat	Chol	Sod	Prot	Carb	Fiber
BUTTER	800	92	280	720	0	0	0
SUGAR	776	0	0	0	0	200	0
DARK RUM	296	0	0	0	0	0	0
Totals Per Recipe:	**1872**	**92**	**280**	**720**	**0**	**200**	**0**

SEVEN MINUTE FROSTING
1 recipe (Less than 1 mcg of VITAMIN K per recipe)

2	each	Egg whites, unbeaten
1 1/2	cups	Sugar
5	tbsp	Water
1 1/2	tbsp	Corn syrup
1	tsp	Vanilla extract
		Boiling water

Combine the egg whites, sugar, water, and corn syrup in the top of a double boiler. Beat with hand mixer or rotary egg beater until thoroughly mixed. Place over rapidly boiling water, beating constantly with mixer or rotary egg beater, and cook 7 minutes, or until frosting will stand in peaks.

Remove from boiling water; add vanilla and beat until thick enough to spread.

Makes enough frosting to cover tops and sides of two 9" layers or generously cover the top and sides of an 8 x 8 x 2" cake, or about 2 dozen cup cakes, or top and sides of a small angel food cake.

To cover top and sides of 3 10" layers, prepare this single recipe twice.

Variations:

TINTED SEVEN MINUTE FROSTING: Use this recipe and add red, green or yellow coloring to hot frosting to give a delicate tint. Remove from boiling water, add vanilla and beat until thick enough to spread.

MINT FROSTING: Use this recipe, using green coloring and 1/4 teaspoon peppermint extract in place of the vanilla. Add coloring gradually to the hot frosting to give a delicate tint. Remove from boiling water, add flavoring and beat until thick enough to spread.

Ingredient	Cal	Fat	Chol	Sod	Prot	Carb	Fiber
EGG WHITES	28	0	0	92	6	6	0
SUGAR	1164	0	0	0	0	300	0
CORN SYRUP	90	0	0	52	0	22.5	0
VANILLA EXTRACT	10	0	0	0	0	0.3	0
Total Per Recipe:	**1292**	**0**	**0**	**144**	**6**	**328.8**	**0**

SEVEN MINUTE COFFEE FROSTING
1 recipe (Less than 1 mcgs of VITAMIN K per recipe)

1	tbsp	Espresso instant coffee powder
1/4	cup	Hot water
3	each	Egg whites
1 1/2	cups	Sugar, light brown, packed
1	tsp	Cream of tartar
1	tsp	Vanilla extract

Dissolve the coffee in hot water. Combine the egg whites, brown sugar, coffee mixture and cream of tartar in the top of a double boiler. Beat with a mixer until frosting forms stiff peaks, 5 to 7 minutes. Remove from the heat. Beat in the vanilla. Makes about 5 cups, enough to frost a 2 layer cake or 1 angel food cake.

Ingredient	Cal	Fat	Chol	Sod	Prot	Carb	Fiber
ESPRESSO POWDER	34	0.1	0	5	1.8	5.9	0
EGG WHITES	42	0	0	138	9	9	0
SUGAR, BROWN	1152	0	0	0	0	288	0
CREAM OF TARTAR	8	0	0	0	0	0.3	0
VANILLA EXTRACT	10	0	0	0	0	0.3	0
Total Per Recipe:	**1246**	**0.1**	**0**	**143**	**10.8**	**303.5**	**0**

BISCUIT SHORTCAKE

6 servings (3 mcgs of VITAMIN K per serving without the
fruit. If you use a pound of strawberries add 2 mcgs of
VITAMIN K per serving. For a pound of blueberries add 5
mcgs per serving. For a pound of peaches add 3 mcgs per
serving. For a pound of sweet pitted cherries add 1.5 mcgs per
serving.)

2	cups	All purpose flour
1/2	cup	Butter
2	tbsp	Sugar
1	large	Egg, beaten
3	tsp	Baking powder
2/3	cup	Milk, skim
1/2	tsp	Salt
1	lb	Strawberries or other fruit
2	cups	Whipped cream*

*You can substitute any other whipped topping of your choice,
just remember to change the nutrition values.

In a large bowl, sift together the flour, sugar, baking powder
and salt.

Cut in the butter until the mixture resembles coarse crumbs.

Combine the egg and milk and add it all at once to the dry
ingredients, stirring just enough to moisten.

Spread the dough in a greased 8 by 1 1/2 inch round layer pan,
slightly building up the edges.

Bake at 450 degrees Fahrenheit oven for 15 to 18 minutes or
until golden. Remove from the pan and cool on a rack for 3
minutes. With a serrated knife, split the biscuit horizontally
into 2 layers. Lift the top off carefully.

Spoon fruit, then whipped cream between layers and then over the top. Garnish and cut in 6 wedges.

Ingredient	Cal	Fat	Chol	Sod	Prot	Carb	Fiber
FLOUR	800	3.2	0	0	22.4	176	0
BUTTER	800	92	280	720	0	0	0
SUGAR	97	0	0	0	0	25	0
EGG, BEATEN	75	5.6	213	63	6.3	0.6	0
BAKING POWDER	6	0	0	612	0	1.4	0
MILK, SKIM	59	0.5	5	85	5.3	8	0
SALT	0	0	0	1150	0	0	0
STRAWBERRIES	112	1.6	0	0	1.6	24	1.6
WHIPPED CREAM	832	89.6	336	96	4.8	6.4	0
Totals Per Serving:	**464**	**32.1**	**139**	**454**	**6.7**	**40.2**	**0.3**

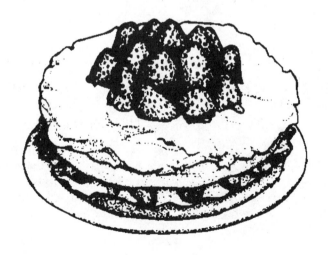

DESSERTS

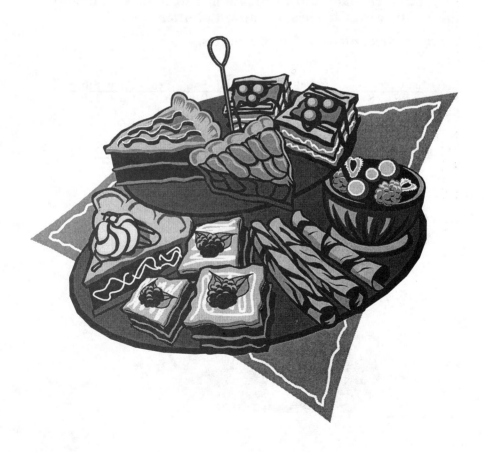

BAKED PEARS IN WINE
2 servings (1 mcg of VITAMIN K per serving)

2	each	Whole pears, firm
1/3	cup	Orange marmalade or apricot jam
1/4	cup	Vermouth, white
2	tbsp	Butter

Preheat oven to 350 degrees Fahrenheit.

Peel, quarter and core pears. Cut into 1/2 inch strips. Arrange in two serving dishes.

Mix the marmalade and vermouth in a small bowl and pour this mixture over the pears. Top with butter.

Place in oven and cook for 20 minutes.

Ingredient	Cal	Fat	Chol	Sod	Prot	Carb	Fiber
WHOLE PEARS	34	0.2	0	0	0.2	8.6	1.4
MARMALADE	48	0	0	3	1.1	8	2.7
VERMOUTH	66	0	0	0	0	1.6	0
BUTTER	200	23	70	180	0	0	0
Totals Per Serving:	174	11.6	35	92	0.6	9.1	2

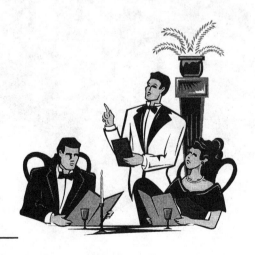

KIWI FRUIT ICE

4 servings (22 mcg of VITAMIN K per serving)

1	cup	Water
1/2	cup	Sugar
1/2	cup	Corn syrup, light
1 1/2	cups	Kiwi fruit, pared
5	tbsp	Lemon juice
1/4	tsp	Lemon peel, grated

Combine water, sugar and corn syrup in saucepan. Cook and stir 2 minutes or until sugar is dissolved.

Puree kiwi in food processor or blender to equal 3/4 cup puree. Add lemon juice, peel and sugar mixture.

Pour into shallow metal pan and freeze for approximately 1 hour or until the mixture is firm, but not solid.

When chilled, spoon into a chilled bowl and beat with an electric mixer until the mix is light and fluffy. Return it to the freezer for approximately 2 hours or until firm enough to scoop.

Ingredient	Cal	Fat	Chol	Sod	Prot	Carb	Fiber
SUGAR	388	0	0	0	0	100	0
CORN SYRUP	480	0	0	280	0	120	0
KIWI FRUIT	204	1.2	0	12	3.6	50.4	12
LEMON JUICE	15	0	0	0	2.5	5	0
LEMON PEEL	1	0	0	0	0	0.2	0.1
Totals Per Serving:	**181**	**0.2**	**0**	**49**	**1**	**45.9**	**2**

FRUITY BREAD PUDDING
6 servings (7 mcg of VITAMIN K per serving)

10	oz	Bread cubes, a little dried out (about 10 slices)
3	large	Eggs, beaten
2	cups	Sugar
1/2	cup	Butter
1	cup	Raisins
1	cup	Pecans, pieces
1	cup	Fruit cocktail, packed in juice, undrained
12	oz	Milk, evaporated skim
1	cup	Water
2	tbsp	Vanilla butternut flavoring
1	tbsp	Butter for the pan

Put everything in a large bowl and mix it. Turn the mixture into a greased 9 by 13-inch pan and bake in a 400 degree Fahrenheit oven for 1 hour and 20 minutes.

Serve warm or cold.

Ingredient	Cal	Fat	Chol	Sod	Prot	Carb	Fiber
BREAD CUBES	760	10	0	1530	23	140	7
EGGS, BEATEN	225	16.8	639	189	18.9	1.8	0
SUGAR	1552	0	0	0	0	400	0
BUTTER	800	92	280	720	0	0	0
RAISINS	504	0.8	0	32	4	132	11.2
PECANS, PIECES	792	80	0	0	9.6	22.4	8
FRUIT COCKTAIL	104	0	0	8	0.8	26.4	1.6
MILK, EVAP SKIM	300	1.2	12	444	28.8	20.4	0
VANILLA BUTTERNUT	30	0	0	3	0	1	0
BUTTER	100	11.5	35	90	0	0	0
Totals Per Serving:	**431**	**17.7**	**81**	**251**	**7.1**	**62**	**2.3**

FRUIT COCKTAIL TORTE
9 servings (2 mcg of VITAMIN K per serving)

1	cup	All purpose flour
3/4	cup	Sugar
1	large	Egg
1	tsp	Baking soda
1/4	tsp	Salt
16	oz	Fruit cocktail, packed in juice, drained
1/2	cup	Brown sugar
1/2	cup	Walnuts, chopped

If you mix this with a fork, the fruit stays whole. If you mix with a beater, the fruit gets chopped. Either way is great.

Mix all ingredients except brown sugar and nuts. Place in an ungreased 8-inch square pan. Spread top with brown sugar and nuts.

Bake at 300 degrees Fahrenheit for 1 hour. Cool, cut and serve.

Optional: Garnish with whipped cream, whipped topping or ice cream. (Do not forget to add the additional counts to the nutrition totals.)

Ingredient	Cal	Fat	Chol	Sod	Prot	Carb	Fiber
FLOUR	400	1.6	0	0	11.2	88	0
SUGAR	582	0	0	0	0	150	0
EGG	75	5	213	63	6.3	0.6	0
BAKING SODA	0	0	0	821	0	0	0
SALT	0	0	0	575	0	0	0
FRUIT COCKTAIL	208	0	0	16	1.6	52.8	3.2
BROWN SUGAR	412	0	0	0	0	106.8	0
WALNUTS	384	37.2	0	8	8.4	11.2	2.8
Totals Per Serving:	**229**	**4.9**	**24**	**165**	**3.1**	**45.5**	**0.7**

STRAWBERRIES NAPOLEAN
8 servings (3 mcgs of VITAMIN K per serving)

PASTRY

2	cups	All purpose flour, sifted
1/2	tsp	Salt
1/3	cup	Butter
1/3	cup	Shortening (Nothing else will do as well)*
5	tbsp	Ice water, approximately

CREAMY STRAWBERRY FILLING

1	pint	Strawberries (or one 10 ounce package frozen)
1/2	cup	Sugar
5	tbsp	All purpose flour
2	cups	Milk, skim
2	tbsp	Butter
2	each	Egg yolks
1/2	cup	Whipping cream
1/2	tsp	Almond extract
1/2	cup	Walnuts, chopped

*This is one of those recipes you make when it's a special treat and you throw dietary rules to the winds. It's not heart healthy but it tastes great!

Set oven at 425 degrees Fahrenheit.

Sift flour, then work in the butter and shortening. When the mixture resembles cornmeal, sprinkle the water into it, stirring gently but quickly until the dough holds together, no more.

Roll out one quarter of the dough on a lightly floured baking sheet to form a thin rectangle 8 by 4 inches. Prick surface several times with a fork.

Bake 15 to 20 minutes covered with a sheet of brown paper (to keep edges from getting too brown). Remove from baking sheet and bake the remaining three pieces of dough the same way.

Cut the berries into quarters. (When using frozen berries, thaw and drain well.)

Mix the sugar, flour and salt in a saucepan. Stir in the milk and butter. Cook over medium heat, stirring constantly until mix is as thick as a thick custard.

Beat egg yolks slightly, then stir a little of the hot sauce into the egg yolks and then add the remaining sauce. Return it all to the saucepan and cook 2 minutes longer. Chill.

Whip the cream stiff and then fold the cream gently into the custard along with the almond extract and the berries.

Spread this filling between the 4 layers of pastry, making a stack.

To Ice: Beat 2 cups confectioners sugar with 2 tablespoons water and 1/8 teaspoon almond extract. Spread over the top of the stack and let it drizzle down the sides.

Sprinkle with 1/2 cup chopped nuts.

Ingredient	Cal	Fat	Chol	Sod	Prot	Carb	Fiber
PASTRY							
FLOUR	800	3.2	0	0	22.4	176	0
SALT	0	0	0	1150	0	0	0
BUTTER	533	61.3	187	480	0	0	0
SHORTENING	613	68.3	0	0	0	0	0
CREAMY STRAWBERRY FILLING							
STRAWBERRIES	112	1.6	0	0	1.6	24	1.6
SUGAR	388	0	0	0	0	100	0
FLOUR	125	0.5	0	0	3.5	27.5	0
MILK, SKIM	176	1.6	16	256	16	24	0
BUTTER	200	23	70	180	0	0	0
EGG YOLKS	202	17.6	726	24	9.6	1	0
WHIPPING CREAM	412	44	164	44	2.4	3.2	0
ALMOND EXTRACT	3	0	0	0	0	0.1	0
WALNUTS	384	37.2	0	8	8.4	11.2	2.8
Totals Per Serving:	**494**	**32.3**	**145**	**268**	**8**	**45.9**	**0.6**

CREME TOPPING

6 servings (Less than 1 mcg of VITAMIN K per serving)

1	cup	Cottage cheese, lowfat
2	tbsp	Milk, skim
2	tsp	Vanilla extract
3	tbsp	Sugar
1/4	tsp	Lemon extract

In a blender container, combine all ingredients. Blend until smooth. Chill.

Can be used as a dip for fruit or on top of pies, fruit desserts or cakes.

For a variation try coconut, almond or orange extract in place of the lemon.

Ingredient	Cal	Fat	Chol	Sod	Prot	Carb	Fiber
COTTAGE CHEESE	160	2.4	8	920	28	6.4	0
MILK, SKIM	11	0.1	1	16	1	1.5	0
VANILLA EXTRACT	20	0	0	0	0	.6	0
SUGAR	146	0	0	0	0	37.5	0
LEMON EXTRACT	5	0	0	0	0	0	0
Totals Per Serving:	57	0.4	2	156	4.8	7.7	0

FUDGE SAUCE

8 servings (Less than 1 mcg of VITAMIN K per serving)

3/4	cup	Sugar
1/4	cup	Cocoa powder plus
1	tbsp	Cocoa powder
4	tsp	Cornstarch
2/3	cup	Milk, evaporated skim
1	tsp	Vanilla extract

Mix the sugar, all the cocoa powder and cornstarch together. Add the milk. Stir and cook until bubbly. Continue cooking for about two minutes. Add Vanilla.

Stir and serve.

Ingredient	Cal	Fat	Chol	Sod	Prot	Carb	Fiber
SUGAR	582	0	0	0	0	150	0
COCOA POWDER	40	2	0	12	4	11.2	0.8
COCOA POWDER	10	0.5	0	3	1	2.8	0.2
CORNSTARCH	72	0	0	2	0	17.3	0
MILK, EVAP SKIM	133	0.5	5	197	12.8	9.1	0
VANILLA EXTRACT	10	0	0	0	0	0.3	0
Totals Per Serving:	**106**	**0.4**	**1**	**27**	**2.2**	**23.8**	**0.2**

WHIPPED CREAM

2 cups - 8 servings (VITAMIN K content = less than 1 mcg per cup)

1   cup   Whipping cream

Whip the cream until soft peaks form, add 1 tablespoon sugar or sugar substitute, if desired. Continue whipping until the cream is stiff. Cover and refrigerate.

When ready to serve, whisk the cream lightly.

Ingredient	Cal	Fat	Chol	Sod	Prot	Carb	Fiber
WHIPPING CREAM	824	88	328	88	4.8	6.4	0
Totals Per Serving:	**103**	**11**	**41**	**11**	**.6**	**.8**	**0**

VANILLA SAUCE
6 servings (Less than 1 mcg of VITAMIN K per serving)

1 1/2	tbsp	Butter
1 1/2	tbsp	All purpose flour or cornstarch
1	cup	Boiling water
1/8	tsp	Salt
2	tbsp	Sugar
1	tsp	Vanilla extract

Melt the butter in a saucepan, stir in the flour or cornstarch and blend well.

Stir in the boiling water, salt and sugar, mixing constantly.

Cook over low heat, stirring constantly, until the mixture thickens. Remove from heat and add the vanilla.

Serve warm or cold. Serve on cake or apple pie

Ingredient	Cal	Fat	Chol	Sod	Prot	Carb	Fiber
BUTTER	150	17.3	52	135	0	0	0
FLOUR	38	0.2	0	0	1.1	8.3	0
SALT	0	0	0	288	0	0	0
SUGAR	97	0	0	0	0	25	0
VANILLA EXTRACT	10	0	0	0	0	0.3	0
Totals Per Serving:	49	2.9	9	71	0.2	5.6	0

TART APRICOT SAUCE
6 servings (Less than 1 mcg of VITAMIN K per serving)

8	oz	Apricots, dried
1 1/2	cups	Water
2	tbsp	Sugar
2	tbsp	Lemon juice, fresh
2	inch	Piece of vanilla bean

Combine the apricots, water, vanilla bean and sugar in a 4 cup glass measure. Cover tightly with plastic wrap. Cook in a 650 to 700 watt microwave at 100% for 7 minutes. Prick plastic to release steam.

Remove from microwave oven and uncover carefully. Drain apricots, reserving juice, and remove vanilla bean.

Scrape the apricots into a blender. Add the lemon juice and puree until smooth.

Add as much of the reserved cooking liquid as you wish to get the texture that you like.

You can use glazed apricots for a sweeter sauce. I like it sweeter myself. It is yummy over ice cream, cakes, etc.

Ingredient	Cal	Fat	Chol	Sod	Prot	Carb	Fiber
APRICOTS, DRIED	536	0	0	24	8	144	24
SUGAR	97	0	0	0	0	25	0
LEMON JUICE	22	0.3	0	2	1.2	8.7	0
VANILLA BEAN	0	0	0	0	0	0	0
Totals Per Serving:	109	0.1	0	4	1.5	29.6	4

PEACH MELBA TRIFLE
12 servings (3 mcgs of VITAMIN K per serving)

14	oz	Sweetened condensed milk, nonfat
1 1/2	cups	Water
1	pkg	Vanilla instant pudding mix
2	cups	Whipping cream, whipped*
5	tbsp	Orange juice
1	each	ANGELFOOD CAKE (See Recipe Index)
4	cups	Peaches, fresh, peeled, sliced
1/4	cup	Raspberry preserves, warmed
2	oz	Almonds, slivered, toasted
2	tbsp	Raspberry preserves, warmed

*Or 4 cups of your favorite whipped topping. (Adjust the nutrition values accordingly.)

In a large bowl, combine the sweetened condensed milk and the water. Mix well.

Add the pudding mix and beat until well blended. Chill for 5 minutes.

Fold in the whipped cream and 1 tablespoon of the orange juice.

Tear the cake into small pieces. Place half the cake pieces in a 2 quart bowl. Sprinkle with 2 tablespoons orange juice. Top with half the peach slices, the preserves and 1/2 of the pudding mixture. Repeat layering with remaining cake, orange juice, peaches and pudding.

Chill. Garnish with almonds and additional preserves.

Ingredient	Cal	Fat	Chol	Sod	Prot	Carb	Fiber
SWTND COND MILK	1120	30.8	14	420	28	182	0
PUDDING MIX	360	0	0	1300	0	92	0
WHIPPING CREAM	1648	176	656	176	9.6	12.8	0
ORANGE JUICE	42	0	0	0	0.5	8	0.3
ANGELFOOD CAKE	1499	1.6	0	943	34.4	362.6	0
PEACHES	288	0	0	0	6.4	76.8	12.8
RASPBERRY JAM	216	0	0	30	0	48	0
ALMONDS	122	3.2	260	88	16.6	2.2	0
RASPBERRY JAM	108	0	0	15	0	24	0
Totals Per Serving:	450	17.6	78	248	8	67.4	1.1

CHOCOLATE BREAD PUDDING
6 servings (Less than 1 mcg of VITAMIN K per serving)

1	tbsp	Butter for pan
8	oz	Bread cubes, (about 8 slices)
2/3	cup	Sugar
2	tbsp	Cocoa powder (2 heaping tablespoons)
2	cups	Milk, skim
2	large	Eggs, beaten
1	tsp	Vanilla extract

Put the bread cubes into a greased 2 quart casserole dish. It should be about 2/3 full.

Mix the sugar and cocoa and toss lightly with bread. Add the well beaten eggs and vanilla to the milk. Pour this mixture over the bread and it should just cover the pieces.

Bake at 350 degrees Fahrenheit for about 45 minutes. Serve warm.

Optional: Serve with milk or with a lump of butter melting into the warm pudding or with whipped cream or whipped topping. (Do not forget to add these counts to the nutrition values.)

Ingredient	Cal	Fat	Chol	Sod	Prot	Carb	Fiber
BUTTER	100	11.5	35	90	0	0	0
BREAD CUBES	608	8	0	1224	18.4	112	5.6
SUGAR	517	0	0	0	0	133.3	0
COCOA POWDER	20	1	0	6	2	5.6	0.4
MILK, SKIM	176	1.6	16	256	16	24	0
EGGS	150	11.2	426	126	12.6	1.2	0
VANILLA EXTRACT	10	0	0	0	0	0.3	0
Totals Per Serving:	**264**	**5.6**	**80**	**284**	**8.2**	**46.1**	**1**

PEPPERED STRAWBERRIES
4 servings (2 mcgs of VITAMIN K per serving)

1	lb	Strawberries
1	tsp	Black pepper, coarsely ground
4	tbsp	Sugar
1	tbsp	Pernod
1	tbsp	Grand Marnier
4	tbsp	Heavy cream
2	small	Cantaloupes (or 1 large cut into 4 quarters.)

Wash, dry and hull the strawberries. Sprinkle with pepper. Add sugar and toss gently. Add Pernod and Grand Marnier and toss gently.

Peel the cantaloupe, halves and scoop out the seeds. Cut partially down through the center of each half. Fan out the slices and top with the strawberry mixture.

Ingredient	Cal	Fat	Chol	Sod	Prot	Carb	Fiber
STRAWBERRIES	112	1.6	0	0	1.6	24	1.6
BLACK PEPPER	5	0.1	0	1	0.2	1.4	0.3
SUGAR	194	0	0	0	0	50	0
PERNOD	58	0.1	0	2	0	8.2	0
GRAND MARNIER	58	0	0	2	0	8.2	0
HEAVY CREAM	206	22	82	22	1.2	1.6	0
CANTALOUPES	372	0.2	0	6	0.4	4.8	0.6
Totals Per Serving:	251	6	21	8	0.9	24.5	0.6

PIES

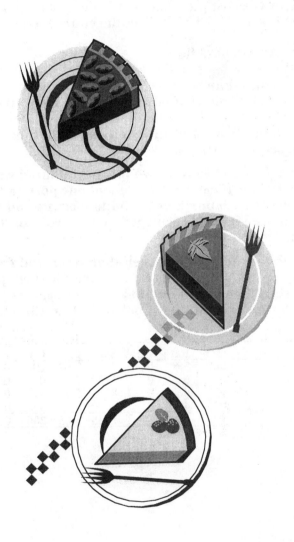

PIE CRUST

One 8 inch two crust pie shell or two single 8 inch pie shells (12 mcgs VITAMIN K in the entire recipe)

2 1/4	cup	All purpose flour
1/2	tsp	Salt
2/3	cup	Milk, skim
3 1/2	tbsp	Canola oil, treated (See Dietary Tip # 10)

Combine all ingredients and stir gently until thoroughly mixed. Divide into 2 equal portions.

Roll out each portion between two pieces of floured wax paper. Use one portion for the bottom crust and one portion for the top crust. Or use both portions for bottom crusts and freeze one until you need it. This recipe will make two, 8 or 9 inch pie shells. Use as directed in recipe.

If your recipe calls for just one shell than wrap and freeze the other. If the dessert recipe calls for a baked pie shell, prick all around the shell with a fork and bake at 375 degrees Fahrenheit for 8 to 12 minutes. Cool and use as directed.

Ingredient	Cal	Fat	Chol	Sod	Prot	Carb	Fiber
FLOUR	900	3.6	0	0	25.2	198	0
SALT	0	0	0	1150	0	0	0
MILK, SKIM	59	0.5	5	85	5.3	8	0
OIL	422	49	0	0	0	0	0
Totals Per Recipe:	1381	53.1	5	1235	30.5	206	0

SWEET POTATO PIE
8 Servings (Less then 4 mcg VITAMIN K per serving)

3	cups	Sweet potatoes, peeled, cooked and mashed
3	large	Eggs, beaten
1/4	cup	Sugar, granulated white
1/4	cup	Brown sugar
1/2	tsp	Salt
1/4	cup	Milk, evaporated skim
1	tsp	Vanilla extract
1/4	tsp	Nutmeg, ground
1	each	PIE CRUST, single crust (See Recipe Index.)

Preheat the oven to 350 degrees Fahrenheit.

Mix all the ingredients except the pie crust in a mixer, on medium speed, for 2 minutes. Pour the filling into the unbaked pie crust and bake for one hour.

Crust will be golden brown.

Ingredient	Cal	Fat	Chol	Sod	Prot	Carb	Fiber
SWEET POTATOES	480	0	0	24	7.2	156	9.6
EGGS	225	16.8	639	189	18.9	1.8	0
SUGAR, WHITE	194	0	0	0	0	50	0
BROWN SUGAR	206	0	0	0	0	53.4	0
SALT	0	0	0	1150	0	0	0
MILK, EVAP SKIM	50	0.2	2	74	4.8	3.4	0
VANILLA EXTRACT	10	0	0	0	0	0.3	0
NUTMEG	3	0.2	0	0	0	0.3	0.1
PIE CRUST	699	15.3	105	501	0	26.6	2.7
Totals Per Serving:	**233**	**4.1**	**93**	**99**	**3.9**	**36.5**	**1.6**

PUMPKIN PIE
8 servings (5 mcgs of VITAMIN K per serving)

1/3	cup	Brown sugar
1/2	tsp	Cinnamon, ground
1/4	tsp	Nutmeg, ground
1/4	tsp	Salt
1	large	Egg, beaten
3	tsp	Vanilla extract
1	cup	Pumpkin, canned, no salt
2/3	cup	Milk, evaporated skim
1	each	PIE CRUST, single crust (See Recipe Index)

Preheat the oven to 325 degrees Fahrenheit.

Mix all the ingredients except the pie crust, in a mixer, on medium speed, for 2 minutes. Pour the filling into the unbaked pie crust and bake for 50 minutes or until a small fork stuck in the middle of the pie comes out clean.

Ingredient	Cal	Fat	Chol	Sod	Prot	Carb	Fiber
BROWN SUGAR	275	0	0	0	0	71.2	0
CINNAMON	3	0.5	0	1	0.1	0.8	0.3
NUTMEG	3	0.2	0	0	0	0.3	0.1
SALT	0	0	0	575	0	0	0
EGG, BEATEN	75	5.6	213	63	6.3	0.6	0
VANILLA EXTRACT	30	0	0	0	0	.9	0
PUMPKIN	80	0	0	8	0	16	8
MILK, EVAP SKIM	133	0.5	5	197	12.8	9.1	0
PIE CRUST	699	15.3	105	501	0	26.6	2.7
Totals Per Serving:	162	2.8	40	168	2.4	15.7	1.4

FUDGE PECAN PIE
8 servings (8 mcgs of VITAMIN K per serving)

1/3	cup	Butter
1/4	cup	Cocoa powder plus
1	tbsp	Cocoa powder
2/3	cup	Sugar
1/4	tsp	Salt
3	large	Eggs, beaten slightly
3/4	cup	Corn syrup, light
1	cup	Pecans, chopped
4	oz	Pecan halves
1	cup	Whipped cream*
1	each	PIE CRUST, single crust, 8 inch, Unbaked (See Recipe Index)

*Or your favorite topping. (Adjust the nutrition values accordingly.)

Preheat the oven to 375 degrees Fahrenheit.

Melt the butter over low heat. Add all the cocoa and stir until smooth. Remove from heat and cool slightly.

Stir in sugar, salt, eggs and corn syrup. Blend thoroughly.

Stir in chopped nuts. Pour into the unbaked pie shell. Place pecan halves over top.

Bake for 40 minutes. Cool.

Let stand 8 hours before serving. Garnish with sweetened whipped cream.

Ingredient	Cal	Fat	Chol	Sod	Prot	Carb	Fiber
BUTTER	533	61.3	187	480	0	0	0
COCOA POWDER	40	2	0	12	4	11.2	0.8
COCOA POWDER	10	0.5	0	3	1	2.8	0.2
SUGAR	517	0	0	0	0	133.3	0
SALT	0	0	0	575	0	0	0
EGGS	225	16.8	639	189	18.9	1.8	0
CORN SYRUP, LIGHT	720	0	0	420	0	180	0
PECANS	792	80	0	0	9.6	22.4	8
PECAN HALVES	360	36	0	0	4	10	3.6
WHIPPED CREAM	416	44.8	168	48	2.4	3.2	0
PIE CRUST	699	15.3	105	501	0	26.6	2.7
Totals Per Serving:	**539**	**32.1**	**137**	**279**	**5**	**48.9**	**1.9**

CREAM RAISIN PIE
8 servings (less than 1 mcg of VITAMIN K per serving)

1	cup	Sour cream, lowfat
1	cup	Sugar
1	cup	Raisins, packed
1	large	Egg
1	each	PIE CRUST, single crust, 8 inch (See Recipe Index)

Mix the first 4 ingredients thoroughly and pour into the unbaked pie shell.

Bake at 275 degrees Fahrenheit for 90 minutes, until the filling is golden brown.

Ingredient	Cal	Fat	Chol	Sod	Prot	Carb	Fiber
SOUR CREAM	320	16	40	280	16	32	0
SUGAR	776	0	0	0	0	200	0
RAISINS	504	0.8	0	32	4	132	11.2
EGG	75	5	213	63	6.3	0.6	0
PIE CRUST	699	15.3	105	501	0	26.6	2.7
Totals Per Serving:	297	4.6	45	110	3.3	48.9	1.7

BANANA CREAM PIE
8 servings (Less than 1 mcg of VITAMIN K per serving)

1	each	PIE CRUST, single crust, baked (See Recipe Index)
1	pkg	Vanilla instant pudding mix
1	cup	Milk, skim
1	cup	Sour cream, lowfat
3	each	Bananas, whole

Bake the pie crust as instructed. Cool.

Make the pudding using the milk and sour cream.

Slice the bananas into the pie crust. Cover with the pudding. Chill.

Optional: Decorate with bananas or whipped cream just before serving.

Ingredient	Cal	Fat	Chol	Sod	Prot	Carb	Fiber
PIE CRUST	699	15.3	105	501	0	26.6	2.7
PUDDING MIX	360	0	0	1300	0	92	0
MILK, SKIM	88	0.8	8	128	8	12	0
SOUR CREAM	320	16	40	280	16	32	0
BANANAS	360	3	0	0	3	84	9
Totals Per Serving:	228	4.4	19	276	3.4	30.8	1.5

QUICK & EASY APPLE PIE
8 servings (less than 3 mcgs of VITAMIN K per serving)

1/2	cup	All purpose flour
3/4	cup	Sugar*
1/8	tsp	Salt
2	tsp	Baking powder
1 1/2	cups	Apples, peeled, cored and diced
1/2	cup	Walnuts, chopped
1	large	Egg, beaten
1	tsp	Vanilla extract
2	tsp	Canola oil, treated (See Dietary Tip #10)

*You can also try half brown and half white sugar. (The change in nutrition values is negligible.)

Mix together the flour, sugar, salt and baking powder. Add to the peeled apples and nuts.

Beat the egg and vanilla together. Mix everything together. Oil a 9 inch pie plate with Canola oil. Spread the mixture onto the oiled pie plate.

Bake at 25 minutes at 350 degrees Fahrenheit.

Optional: Serve warm with vanilla ice cream, whipped cream or whipped topping.

Ingredient	Cal	Fat	Chol	Sod	Prot	Carb	Fiber
FLOUR	200	0.8	0	0	5.6	44	0
SUGAR	654	0	0	0	0	169.2	0
SALT	0	0	0	288	0	0	0
BAKING POWDER	4	0	0	408	0	0.9	0
APPLES	192	0	0	0	1.2	48	12
WALNUTS	384	37.2	0	8	8.4	11.2	2.8
EGG	75	5.6	213	63	6.3	0.6	0
VANILLA EXTRACT	10	0	0	0	0	0.3	0
CANOLA OIL	80	9.3	0	0	0	0	0
Totals Per Serving:	200	6.6	27	96	2.7	34.3	1.9

APPLE CRUMB PIE
8 servings (3 mcgs of VITAMIN K per serving)

3	lg	Cooking apples, peeled, cored, and thinly sliced
1	each	Pie Crust, Single Crust, unbaked
1	tsp	Ground cinnamon
1	cup	Sugar, divided*
3/4	cup	All purpose flour
1/3	cup	Butter

*You can use brown or white sugar. (The change in nutrition values is negligible.)

Arrange the apple slices evenly in the pastry shell. Combine the cinnamon and 1/2 cup sugar. Stir well, and sprinkle the mixture over the apples.

Combine the flour and the remaining sugar. Stir well.

Cut the butter into the flour mixture with a pastry blender until it resembles course meal.

Sprinkle the mixture over the apples. Bake at 400 degrees Fahrenheit for 40 to 50 minutes.

Ingredient	Cal	Fat	Chol	Sod	Prot	Carb	Fiber
APPLES	219	1.2	0	0	0.6	57	7.2
PIE CRUST	699	15.3	105	501	0	26.6	2.7
CINNAMON	6	0.1	0	1	0.1	1.8	1.2
SUGAR	776	0	0	0	0	200	0
FLOUR	300	1.2	0	0	8.4	66	0
BUTTER	533	61.3	187	480	0	0	0
Totals Per Serving:	317	9.9	37	123	1.1	43.9	1.4

SALADS, DRESSINGS & SAUCES

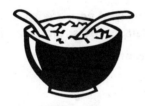

LETTUCE SALAD

1 serving. (Select the ingredients for your salad from the list below. Measure them carefully. Add the number of mcgs (for each of the ingredients selected) together. This will give you the total number of mcgs of vitamin K.)

1	oz	Iceberg lettuce contains 9 mcgs of vitamin K. (See DIETARY TIP # 17)
1	oz	Tomato contains 6 mcgs of vitamin K
1	oz	Carrot contains 5 mcgs of vitamin K.
1	oz	Cucumber, peeled and sliced, contains 2 mcgs of vitamin K. (Cucumbers must be peeled!)
1	oz	Onion contains 2 mcgs of vitamin K. (Do not use spring onions!)
1	oz	Green peppers contains 17 mcgs of vitamin K.

Toss ingredients together and serve with your choice of salad dressings. (See Recipe Index for salad dressings.)

Do not forget to add the number of mcgs, of vitamin K, in the salad dressing as well.

Ingredient	Cal	Fat	Chol	Sod	Prot	Carb	Fiber
ICEBERG LETTUCE	3	0	0	2	0.2	0.4	0.1
TOMATO	6	0	0	3	0	1	0
CARROT	6	0.1	0	5	0.1	1.5	0.1
CUCUMBER	3	0	0	1	0.1	0.3	0.1
ONION	11	0	0	1	0.3	2.4	5
GREEN PEPPERS	8	0.1	0	0	0.3	1.8	0.5
Totals Per Serving:	37	0.2	0	12	1	7.4	5.8

ELBOW MACARONI WITH GRAPES
4 servings (less than 8 mcgs of VITAMIN K per serving)

1/2	lb	Elbow macaroni
1	cup	Green grapes, seedless,
1/4	cup	Celery, sliced
1/4	tsp	Salt
1/2	cup	BLENDER MAYONNAISE #2 (See Recipe Index)
1/2	cup	Sour cream, nonfat

Whip the mayonnaise and sour cream together, add it to everything else. Serve.

Ingredient	Cal	Fat	Chol	Sod	Prot	Carb	Fiber
ELBOW MACARONI	840	4	0	0	28	168	0
GREEN GRAPES	160	1.6	0	8	1.6	40	1.6
CELERY	4	0	0	26	0.2	1.2	0.2
SALT	0	0	0	575	0	0	0
MAYONNAISE	612	67.2	84	300	2.4	1.2	0
SOUR CREAM	60	0	0	60	12	4	0
Totals Per Serving:	**419**	**18.2**	**21**	**242**	**11.1**	**53.6**	**0.5**

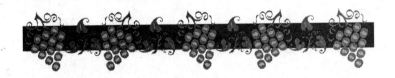

TOMATO AND CABBAGE SALAD

10 servings (VITAMIN K content = 30 mcg per 1/2 cup. Be careful with this recipe! Make certain it is well mixed and each serving contains proportionate amounts of vegetables. Also, you must weigh both types of cabbage.)

4	oz	Red cabbage, chopped and carefully weighed (about 1 cup)
2	oz	Cabbage, chopped and carefully weighed (about 1/2 cup)
2 1/2	cups	Tomatoes, diced
1	cup	Radishes, sliced
1	tsp	Cilantro, fresh, chopped
1/2	tsp	Salt
2	tsp	Olive or Canola oil, treated (See Dietary Tip # 10)
2	tbsp	Vinegar or lemon juice
1	tsp	Ground black pepper

Mix all the ingredients in a large bowl.

Ingredient	Cal	Fat	Chol	Sod	Prot	Carb	Fiber
RED CABBAGE	8	0	0	8	0.4	2	0.8
CABBAGE	4	0	0	4	0.2	1	0.4
TOMATOES	100	2	0	40	4	20	6
RADISHES	16	0	0	32	0.8	4	1.6
CILANTRO	1	0	0	0	0.1	0.1	0
SALT	0	0	0	1150	0	0	0
OIL	80	9.3	0	0	0	0	0
VINEGAR	22	0.3	0	2	1.2	8.7	0
BLACK PEPPER	5	0.1	0	1	0.2	1.4	0.4
Totals Per Serving:	**24**	**1.2**	**0**	**124**	**0.7**	**3.7**	**0.9**

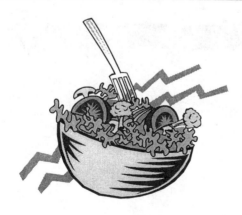

PIZZA STYLE TOMATO SALAD
8 servings (10 mcgs of VITAMIN K per serving)

3	lb	Tomatoes, fresh, thick sliced (about 6 large tomatoes)
1 1/2	oz	Pepperoni, thin sliced and diced
5	each	Black olives, large, canned, sliced
1/2	cup	Bell pepper, green, diced
1/3	cup	Onions, red, sliced thin
1	tbsp	Basil, fresh, minced
4	tbsp	ITALIAN HERB DRESSING (See Recipe Index)
4	oz	Mozzarella cheese, shredded (about 1 cup)*

*Nonfat Mozzarella cheese my be substituted.

Arrange tomatoes on a large heat proof platter, slightly overlapping the tomatoes. Sprinkle with pepperoni, olives, green pepper, onions and basil.

Drizzle with dressing, top with cheese.

Just before serving, place under broiler until cheese is barely melted.

Ingredient	Cal	Fat	Chol	Sod	Prot	Carb	Fiber
TOMATOES	288	4.8	0	144	9.6	62.4	19.2
PEPPERONI	45	0.9	0	9	1.8	12.6	2.7
BLACK OLIVES	25	2.5	0	190	0	1.5	0.5
BELL PEPPER	28	0	0	0	0.4	0.4	0.4
ONIONS	29	0	0	3	0.8	6.4	13.3
BASIL	0	0	0	0	0.1	0.1	0.1
ITALIAN DRESSING	324	36.2	0	346	0	0.2	0
MOZZARELLA	360	28	80	760	24	4	0
Totals Per Serving:	137	9.1	10	239	4.6	11	4.5

CUMIN FLAVORED CARROT SALAD
4 servings (3 mcgs of VITAMIN K per serving)

1/2	lb	Carrots, peeled, ends trimmed
1	cup	Chicken broth
2	tbsp	White wine vinegar
1 1/2	tbsp	Water
1	tsp	Garlic cloves, pressed
1/4	tsp	Oregano leaves, fresh, minced
1/4	tsp	Cumin, ground
1/4	tsp	Paprika

Place the carrots in a saucepan with a mixture of water and chicken broth to barely cover.

Bring to a boil, cover and simmer for about 10 minutes until just done but still slightly crisp. Cool and cut into 1/4 inch slices.

In a small bowl, mix together the remaining ingredients. Fold gently into the carrots. Marinate for several hours or overnight.

Ingredient	Cal	Fat	Chol	Sod	Prot	Carb	Fiber
CARROTS	48	0.8	0	40	0.8	12	0.8
CHICKEN BROTH	32	0	0	1320	1.6	5.6	0
VINEGAR	4	0	0	6	0	0	0
GARLIC	4	0	0	2	0.2	1	0
OREGANO	0	0	0	0	0	0	0
CUMIN	2	0	0	1	0.1	0.2	0.1
PAPRIKA	2	0.1	0	0	0.1	0.3	0.1
Totals Per Serving:	23	0.2	0	342	0.7	4.8	0.2

ITALIAN MARINATED TOMATOES
2 servings (14 mcgs of VITAMIN K per serving)

1	lb	Tomatoes, fresh, ripe (about 2 large tomatoes)
3	tsp	Garlic cloves, minced
1	tsp	Balsamic vinegar*
1/8	tsp	Salt
1/4	tsp	Ground black pepper

*Or use your favorite vinegar.

Slice tomatoes into thick slices and arrange them on a plate in one layer.

Sprinkle the garlic over the tomatoes. Make sure you get some on each slice!

Sprinkle the teaspoon of vinegar evenly over tomatoes. (If you like, 3 finely chopped fresh basil leaves can be sprinkled on the tomatoes at this point. This will add an additional 40mcg of VITAMIN K to the entire dish, or an additional 20mcg per serving.)

Let stand at least an hour at room temperature. Just before serving add the salt and pepper.

These are good by themselves, on bread, or in a salad.

Ingredient	Cal	Fat	Chol	Sod	Prot	Carb	Fiber
TOMATOES	96	1.6	0	48	3.2	20.8	6.4
GARLIC	12	0.1	0	6	0.5	3	0
VINEGAR	1	0	0	1	0	0	0
SALT	0	0	0	288	0	0	0
BLACK PEPPER	1	0	0	0	0.1	0.4	0.1
Totals Per Serving:	55	0.8	0	172	1.9	12.1	3.3

PINEAPPLE COLESLAW
8 servings (85 mcgs of VITAMIN K per serving)

DRESSING

1/2	cup	Sour cream, lowfat
1/2	cup	BLENDER MAYONNAISE #2 (See Recipe Index)
2	tsp	Sugar
1	tbsp	Onion, finely chopped
1	tsp	Lemon juice

SALAD

2	cups	Cabbage, green, shredded
1	cup	Apple, peeled, cored and chopped
1	cup	Carrots, peeled and shredded
3/4	cup	Pineapple tidbits packed in juice, drained

In a small bowl combine all the dressing ingredients and blend well.

In a large bowl combine all the salad ingredients and toss lightly. Pour dressing over salad. Mix well.

Cover and refrigerate to blend flavors.

Ingredient	Cal	Fat	Chol	Sod	Prot	Carb	Fiber
DRESSING							
SOUR CREAM	160	8	20	140	8	16	0
MAYONNAISE	612	67.2	84	300	2.4	1.2	0
SUGAR	32	0	0	0	0	8.3	0
ONION	6	0	0	0	0.2	1.2	2.5
LEMON JUICE	1	0	0	0	0.2	0.3	0
SALAD							
CABBAGE	32	0	0	32	1.6	8	3.2
APPLE	128	0	0	0	0.8	32	8
CARROTS	48	8.8	0	40	0.8	12	0.8
PINEAPPLE	102	0.6	0	12	0	27	1.2
Totals Per Serving:	**140**	**10.6**	**13**	**66**	**1.7**	**13.3**	**2**

GREEN BEANS CAESAR
8 servings (10 mcgs of VITAMIN K per serving)

1	lb	Green beans, cooked and chilled
1	tsp	Dijon mustard
1	tbsp	Lemon juice
1/2	tsp	Worcestershire Sauce
4	each	Anchovies (*or Anchovy paste)
1/2	cup	Olive oil, treated (See Dietary Tip # 10)
1	tsp	Garlic clove, minced
1	tsp	Black pepper, fresh ground
1/2	cup	Parmesan cheese, grated
1		Egg, raw or coddled**
1	cup	Croutons, plain

*If you use anchovies you need four. If you use the paste it takes more to get the same flavor.

**You can substitute sour cream for the egg if you do not want to eat raw egg. (Adjust the nutrition values accordingly.)

Put the mustard, pepper, lemon juice, anchovies (or paste), garlic, Worcestershire Sauce and 1/3 cup of oil into blender. Puree ingredients.

Taste at this point and adjust seasonings if necessary. Add remaining olive oil, Parmesan cheese and egg (or sour cream) to blender. Puree until well blended.

Toss with green beans until dressing is evenly distributed throughout the beans. Add croutons. Toss again.

Serve. You can vary the amount of any of the ingredients to suit your taste.

Ingredient	Cal	Fat	Chol	Sod	Prot	Carb	Fiber
BEANS	144	0	0	32	16	32	32
DIJON MUSTARD	5	0	0	120	0	0.2	0
LEMON JUICE	3	0	0	0	0.5	1	0
WORCESTERSHIRE	2	0	0	33	0	0.3	0
ANCHOVIES	32	1.6	0	588	4.8	0	0
OIL	952	108	0	0	0	0	0
GARLIC CLOVE	4	0	0	2	0.2	1	0
BLACK PEPPER	5	0.1	0	1	0.2	1.4	0.3
PARMESAN	164	11.2	32	680	15.2	1.6	0
EGG	75	5	213	63	6.3	0.6	0
CROUTONS	120	2.4	0	208	4	22.4	1.6
Totals Per Serving:	**188**	**16**	**31**	**216**	**5.9**	**7.6**	**4.2**

CUCUMBER "NOODLES" WITH TOMATO SALSA
6 servings (11 mcgs of VITAMIN K per serving)

2	lb	Cucumbers, seedless, peeled (about 2 large cucumbers)
1	tbsp	Salt

FOR THE SALSA

1	lb	Plum tomatoes, peeled, seeded, and chopped
1/4	cup	Onion, minced
1	tsp	Garlic, peeled and minced
1	each	Jalapeno pepper, seeded and minced, (pickled is fine)
1	tbsp	White-wine vinegar
1/4	tsp	Sugar

With a sharp knife cut the peeled cucumbers lengthwise into 1/8 inch thick "noodles" about 1/2 inch wide. In a bowl toss with salt and let stand for 10 minutes.

Make the salsa while cucumber noodles are standing. Stir together the salsa ingredients.

Drain the cucumbers in a colander and rinse off the salt under cold water. Pat dry on paper towels.

Just before serving toss the salsa and 'noodles' to combine.

Ingredient	Cal	Fat	Chol	Sod	Prot	Carb	Fiber
CUCUMBERS	96	0	0	32	3.2	9.6	3.2
SALT	0	0	0	1150	0	0	0
SALSA							
PLUM TOMATOES	96	0	0	48	3.2	20.8	6.4
ONION	16	0	0	0	0.4	3.4	0.6
GARLIC	4	0	0	2	0.2	1	0
JALAPENO PEPPER	9	0	0	0	0	2	1
VINEGAR	2	0	0	3	0	0	0
SUGAR	4	0	0	0	0	1	0
Totals Per Serving:	**38**	**0**	**0**	**206**	**1.2**	**6.4**	**1.9**

TOMATO AND CUCUMBER SALAD
10 servings (24 mcgs of VITAMIN K per serving)

2	tbsp	Ginger root, fresh, peeled and minced
2	tbsp	Garlic, peeled and chopped
1/3	cup	Balsamic vinegar
1	cup	Olive oil, treated (See Dietary Tip # 10)
20	oz	Cucumber, peeled seeded, thinly sliced (about 2 medium cucumbers)
4	cups	Plum tomatoes, quartered (approximately 15 tomatoes)
1/4	cup	Scallions, thinly sliced
3	each	Basil leaves, in thin strips

In a food processor, place the ginger and garlic, and puree them together. With the processor running, slowly add the balsamic vinegar and olive oil. Set the vinaigrette aside.

In a medium large bowl place the peeled cucumbers, Roma tomatoes, scallion, and basil leaves. Mix the ingredients together.

Add the vinaigrette and toss it in.

Serve the salad at room temperature.

Ingredient	Cal	Fat	Chol	Sod	Prot	Carb	Fiber
GINGER ROOT	20	0.2	0	4	0.5	4.3	0.3
GARLIC	24	0.1	0	12	.9	6	0
VINEGAR	11	0	0	16	0	0	0
OIL	1904	216	0	0	0	0	0
CUCUMBER	60	0	0	20	2	6	2
PLUM TOMATOES	192	0	0	96	6.4	41.6	12.8
SCALLIONS	8	0.2	0	4	0.4	1.6	0.4
BASIL	3	0	0	0	0.3	0.6	0.3
Totals Per Serving:	222	21.7	0	15	1.1	6	1.6

HOLLANDAISE SAUCE
4 servings (3 mcgs of VITAMIN K per serving)

3	each	Egg yolks
2	tbsp	Boiling water
1/2	lb	Butter, melted, hot
1	tbsp	Lemon juice
		Dash of cayenne pepper

Put the egg yolks in an electric blender or food processor. If using the blender, turn to low speed.

Slowly add the boiling water, and then add the butter very s l o w l y. Add the lemon juice and cayenne.

Makes about 1 1/4 cups.

Ingredient	Cal	Fat	Chol	Sod	Prot	Carb	Fiber
EGG YOLKS	303	26.4	1089	36	14.4	1.5	0
BUTTER	1600	184	560	1440	0	0	0
LEMON JUICE	3	0	0	0	0.5	1	0
CAYENNE PEPPER	0	0	0	0	0	0	0
Totals Per Serving:	**477**	**52.6**	**412**	**369**	**3.7**	**0.6**	**0**

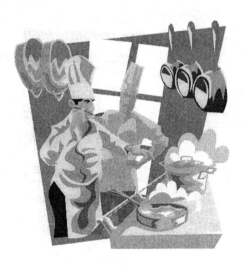

EASY BEARNAISE SAUCE
4 servings (3 mcgs of VITAMIN K per serving)

1	tbsp	Shallots, minced
2	tbsp	Vinegar
1/2	tsp	Tarragon, fresh minced
3	each	Egg yolks
2	tbsp	Boiling water
1/2	lb	Butter, melted, hot
		Dash of cayenne pepper

Cook the minced shallots with 2 tablespoons vinegar and 1/2 teaspoon fresh tarragon until reduced to 1 tablespoon.

Put the egg yolks in the electric blender or food processor. If using the blender, turn to low speed.

Slowly add the boiling water, and then add the hot melted butter very s l o w l y. Add the vinegar mix and cayenne.

Makes about 1 1/4 cups.

Ingredient	Cal	Fat	Chol	Sod	Prot	Carb	Fiber
SHALLOT	7	0.1	0	1	0.4	1.7	0.1
VINEGAR	4	0	0	6	0	0	0
TARRAGON	0	0	0	0	0	0	0
EGG YOLKS	303	26.4	1089	36	14.4	1.5	0
BUTTER	1600	184	560	1440	0	0	0
CAYENNE PEPPER	0	0	0	0	0	0	0
Totals Per Serving:	479	52.6	412	371	3.7	0.8	0

BEARNAISE SAUCE
8 servings or 2 cups (20 mcgs of VITAMIN K per serving)

1/4	cup	Apple cider or tarragon vinegar
1/4	cup	Onion, chopped
1/4	cup	Dry white wine*
1	tbsp	Parsley, fresh, minced
1	tbsp	Chives, fresh, minced
3	each	Egg yolks
1/2	cup	Butter
3/4	cup	BLENDER MAYONNAISE #2 (See Recipe Index)

*Water may be substituted.

Simmer vinegar and onion until liquid evaporates. Stir in the water or wine, parsley and chives and set aside.

Beat the egg yolks until very thick and lemon colored.

Melt the butter. Beat the melted butter into the egg yolks, a small amount at a time. Turn the butter mixture into a heavy saucepan. Cook over very low heat, stirring constantly, until it is thick.

Remove from heat and stir in the wine mixture.

Fold in the mayonnaise.

For meat, fish, seafood, vegetables or meat fondues.

Ingredient	Cal	Fat	Chol	Sod	Prot	Carb	Fiber
APPLE CIDER	146	0.8	0	2	0.6	38	2.2
ONION	16	0	0	0	0.4	3.4	0.6
WHITE WINE	44	0	0	2	0	1.4	0
PARSLEY	2	0.1	0	2	0.1	0.3	0
CHIVES	4	0	0	0	0.5	0.5	0.5
EGG YOLKS	303	26.4	1089	36	14.4	1.5	0
BUTTER	800	92	280	720	0	0	0
MAYONNAISE	918	100.8	126	450	3.6	1.8	0
Totals Per Serving:	**279**	**27.5**	**187**	**152**	**2.5**	**5.9**	**0.4**

HAND-MADE MAYONNAISE

20 servings, 1 1/4 cups (20 mcgs of VITAMIN K for the entire recipe or 1 mcg per serving)

1	each	Egg yolk
1/4	tsp	Salt
1/2	tsp	Dijon mustard*
1	tbsp	Lemon juice or white wine vinegar
1	cup	Canola or Olive oil, or combination, treated (See Dietary Tip # 10)
		Hot water

*Or more to taste.

Quickly bring the egg to room temperature by setting it in a bowl of hot water for 2 or 3 minutes, or until the egg no longer feels chilled when held in your hand. Then separate the yolk and discard the white (or freeze it for later use.)

Combine the egg yolk, salt, mustard and lemon juice or vinegar in a bowl. Set the bowl on a folded towel to keep it from moving around. Briskly whisk the ingredients together until they are thoroughly blended, then begin adding the oil, drop by drop at first, then in gradually increasing amounts.

When the oil is completely incorporated, taste the mayonnaise and add more salt or lemon juice or vinegar if desired.

A very thick mayonnaise can be thinned by stirring in a spoonful or two of hot water until you get the consistency you want.

Ingredient	Cal	Fat	Chol	Sod	Prot	Carb	Fiber
EGG YOLK	101	8.8	363	12	4.8	0.5	0
SALT	0	0	0	575	0	0	0
DIJON MUSTARD	3	0	0	60	0	0.1	0
LEMON JUICE	11	0.2	0	1	0.6	4.4	0
OIL	1904	216	0	0	0	0	0
Totals Per Serving:	**101**	**11.2**	**18**	**32**	**0.3**	**0.2**	**0**

BLENDER MAYONNAISE #1

24 servings, 1 1/2 cups (20 mcgs of VITAMIN K per recipe or .8 mcg per serving)

1	each	Egg
2	tbsp	Lemon juice
1	tsp	Mustard, powdered
1/4	tsp	Salt
1/4	tsp	White pepper
1	cup	Canola or Olive oil, or combination, treated (See Dietary Tip # 10)
		Hot water

Combine the egg, lemon juice, mustard, salt and white pepper in a blender or food processor.

Cover and blend at low speed until mixed. Remove center cap. Increase speed to high.

Add oil in a thin, s-l-o-w, steady stream. Blend until all the oil is added and the mayonnaise is smooth and creamy.

If necessary, turn the motor off and stir occasionally. Replace the cover before turning the motor back on.

A very thick mayonnaise can be thinned by stirring in a spoonful or two of hot water until you get the consistency you want.

Keep mayonnaise refrigerated and use within 7 to 10 days.

Ingredient	Cal	Fat	Chol	Sod	Prot	Carb	Fiber
EGG	75	5	213	63	6.3	0.6	0
LEMON JUICE	6	0	0	0	1	2	0
MUSTARD	19	0	0	0	0	0	0
SALT	0	0	0	575	0	0	0
WHITE PEPPER	4	0	0	0	0.1	0.8	0.3
OIL	1904	216	0	0	0	0	0
Totals Per Serving:	**100**	**11.1**	**11**	**32**	**0.4**	**0.2**	**0**

BLENDER MAYONNAISE #2

40 servings, 2 1/2 cups (28 mcgs of VITAMIN K per recipe or .7 mcg per serving)

2	large	Eggs
1	tsp	Mustard, powdered
4	tbsp	Apple cider vinegar
1/4	tsp	Salt
1 1/2	cups	Canola or Olive oil, or combination, treated (See Dietary Tip # 10)
		Hot water

Blend eggs, vinegar, mustard and salt in the blender.

Add oil very s-l-o-w-l-y (steady flow) while blender continues to run. You may need to stir toward the end of adding the oil. (Make sure you turn the blender off to stir.)

A very thick mayonnaise can be thinned by stirring in a spoonful or two of hot water until you get the consistency you want. Makes 2 1/2 cups.

Ingredient	Cal	Fat	Chol	Sod	Prot	Carb	Fiber
EGGS	150	11.2	426	126	12.6	1.2	0
MUSTARD	19	0	0	0	0	0	0
VINEGAR	8	0	0	0	0	4	0
SALT	0	0	0	575	0	0	0
OIL	2880	326.4	0	0	0	0	0
Totals Per Serving:	76	8.4	11	18	0.3	0.1	0

TOFU MAYONNAISE

1 1/4 cups or 20 tablespoons (10 mcgs of VITAMIN K per recipe .5 mcg per tablespoon)

8	oz	Tofu, raw, firm, mashed
1	tsp	Garlic cloves, minced
1	tsp	Dijon mustard
2	tsp	Apple cider vinegar
1/4	tsp	Salt
1/4	cup	Canola or Olive oil, or combination, treated (See Dietary Tip # 10)
		Hot water

Place all ingredients but the oil in a blender, or food processor using the steel blade. Process until smooth and creamy, continue to process as you s-l-o-w-l-y drizzle in the oil.

A very thick mayonnaise can be thinned by stirring in a spoonful or two of hot water until you get the consistency you want.

Makes about 1 1/4 cups. Keeps 1 week in the refrigerator.

Ingredient	Cal	Fat	Chol	Sod	Prot	Carb	Fiber
TOFU	216	16	0	24	24	8	0
GARLIC	4	0	0	2	0.2	1	0
DIJON MUSTARD	5	0	0	120	0	0.2	0
VINEGAR	1	0	0	0	0	0.7	0
SALT	0	0	0	575	0	0	0
OIL	476	54	0	0	0	0	0
Totals Per Serving:	**35**	**3.5**	**0**	**36**	**1.2**	**0.5**	**0**

CAJUN MAYONNAISE
40 tablespoons, 2 1/2 cups (.8 mcg of VITAMIN K per tablespoon)

2	each	Egg yolks
1/4	tsp	Salt
1	tsp	Garlic clove, minced
1/4	cup	Onion, chopped fine
4	drops	Tabasco sauce
1 1/2	tbsp	Lemon juice (about 1/2 of a lemon)
2	cups	Canola or Olive oil, or combination, treated (See Dietary Tip # 10)

Place all the ingredients except the oil in a blender (with the center of the lid removed) or a food processor fitted with a steel blade and blend or process for 2 minutes. (If you are using a food processor you should scrape down the sides after 1 minute.)

Pour the oil in a very thin stream, s-l-o-w-l-y, through the top or down the feed tube until it has all been incorporated. Blend or process for 30 seconds more.

Makes about 2 1/4 cups.

Ingredient	Cal	Fat	Chol	Sod	Prot	Carb	Fiber
EGG YOLKS	202	17.6	726	24	9.6	1	0
SALT	0	0	0	575	0	0	0
GARLIC CLOVE	4	0	0	2	0.2	1	0
ONION	22	0	0	2	0.6	4.8	10
TABASCO SAUCE	20	0	0	0	0	0	0
LEMON JUICE	16	0.2	0	2	0.9	6.5	0
OIL	3808	432	0	0	0	0	0
Totals Per Serving:	**102**	**11.2**	**18**	**15**	**0.3**	**0.3**	**0.3**

VINEGAR & ONION SALAD DRESSING
1 1/2 cups (12 mcgs of VITAMIN K per recipe)

4	oz	Onion, peeled (about 1/2 cup)
1/2	cup	Olive oil, treated (See Dietary Tip # 10)
1/2	cup	Apple cider vinegar
1/4	cup	Wine vinegar
3	tsp	Garlic cloves

Peel the garlic.

Put everything in the blender. Process on high for 1 to 2 minutes until pureed.

Serve over the LETTUCE SALAD. (See Recipe Index.)

Ingredient	Cal	Fat	Chol	Sod	Prot	Carb	Fiber
ONION	44	0	0	4	1.2	9.6	20
OIL	952	108	0	0	0	0	0
VINEGAR	16	0	0	0	0	8	0
WINE VINEGAR	8	0	0	12	0	0	0
GARLIC	12	0.1	0	6	0.5	3	0
Totals Per Recipe:	1032	108.1	0	22	1.7	20.6	20

SALSA
8 servings, 4 cups (VITAMIN K content = 11 mcg per cup)

3	cups	Tomatoes, diced
1/2	cup	Onion, minced
1	tsp	Garlic clove, minced
1/4	cup	Jalapeno pepper, chopped
1	tsp	Cilantro, fresh, chopped
2	tbsp	Juice from one lime
1/8	tsp	Oregano leaves, fresh, minced
1/8	tsp	Salt
1/4	tsp	Ground black pepper

Mix all ingredients in a bowl.

May be served immediately (for best flavor) or after refrigeration.

Ingredient	Cal	Fat	Chol	Sod	Prot	Carb	Fiber
TOMATOES	120	2.4	0	48	4.8	24	7.2
ONION	32	0	0	0	0.8	6.8	1.2
GARLIC CLOVE	4	0	0	2	0.2	1	0
JALAPENO PEPPER	18	0	0	0	0	4	2
CILANTRO	1	0	0	0	0.1	0.1	0
JUICE FROM LIME	7	0	0	1	0.1	2.5	0.1
OREGANO	0	0	0	0	0	0	0
SALT	0	0	0	288	0	0	0
BLACK PEPPER	1	0	0	0	0.1	0.4	0.1
Totals Per Serving:	**23**	**0.3**	**0**	**42**	**0.8**	**4.9**	**1.3**

BASIC VINAIGRETTE
8 servings (1 mcg of VITAMIN K per serving)

1	tbsp	Vinegar or lemon juice
8	tbsp	Olive oil, treated (See Dietary Tip # 10)
1/8	tsp	Salt
1	tsp	Dijon mustard
1/2	tsp	Ground black pepper

Place all ingredients in a jar and shake thoroughly. Add more lemon juice or vinegar to taste.

Serve over LETTUCE SALAD. (See Recipe Index) You can add crushed garlic or Bleu cheese for a different flavor.

Ingredient	Cal	Fat	Chol	Sod	Prot	Carb	Fiber
VINEGAR	11	0.2	0	1	0.6	4.4	0
OIL	952	108	0	0	0	0	0
SALT	0	0	0	288	0	0	0
DIJON MUSTARD	5	0	0	120	0	0.2	0
BLACK PEPPER	3	0.1	0	1	0.1	0.7	0.2
Totals Per Serving:	**121**	**13.5**	**0**	**51**	**0.1**	**0.7**	**0**

BALSAMIC VINAIGRETTE DRESSING
8 servings (VITAMIN K content = 1.5 mcg per serving)

1	tsp	Yogurt, plain, lowfat
1	tsp	Dijon mustard
1/4	cup	Balsamic vinegar
1/8	tsp	White pepper
1/3	cup	Olive oil, treated (See Dietary Tip # 10)

Whip together all but oil. Add oil s l o w l y, while whipping.

Ingredient	Cal	Fat	Chol	Sod	Prot	Carb	Fiber
YOGURT	3	0.1	0	4	0.3	0.3	0
DIJON MUSTARD	5	0	0	120	0	0.2	0
VINEGAR	8	0	0	12	0	0	0
WHITE PEPPER	2	0	0	0	0.1	0.4	0.1
OIL	635	72	0	0	0	0	0
Totals Per Serving:	82	9	0	17	0	0.1	0

ITALIAN HERB DRESSING
8 servings (VITAMIN K content = 7 mcg per serving or 56 mcg per cup)

2/3	cup	Olive oil, treated (See Dietary Tip # 10)
1/8	tsp	Salt
1/2	tsp	Oregano leaves, fresh, minced
1/2	cup	Wine or white vinegar
1/2	tsp	Basil, fresh, minced
1/4	tsp	Crushed dried red pepper
1	clove	Garlic, crushed

Combine all ingredients in a jar. Cover and shake well.

Chill to blend flavors.

Remove garlic. Shake again before serving. Makes 1 cup.

Ingredient	Cal	Fat	Chol	Sod	Prot	Carb	Fiber
OIL	1269	144	0	0	0	0	0
SALT	0	0	0	288	0	0	0
OREGANO	1	0	0	0	0	0	0
WINE VINEGAR	16	0	0	24	0	0	0
BASIL	0	0	0	0	0	0	0
DRIED RED PEPPER	2	0.1	0	0	0	0	0
Totals Per Serving:	161	18	0	39	0	0	0

GREEK SALAD DRESSING
3/4 cup = 8 servings (VITAMIN K content = 56 mcg for the entire recipe or 7 mcg per serving)

1/2	cup	Vinegar, white
1/4	cup	Olive oil, treated (See Dietary Tip # 10) and
1/4	cup	Canola oil, treated (See Dietary Tip # 10)
1	tsp	Oregano leaves, fresh, minced
1	tsp	Garlic cloves, minced

Simply combine and use. Can be refrigerated for several days.

Ingredient	Cal	Fat	Chol	Sod	Prot	Carb	Fiber
VINEGAR, WHITE	16	0	0	24	0	0	0
OIL	480	54.4	0	0	0	0	0
OIL	482	56	0	0	0	0	0
OREGANO	1	0	0	1	0	0	0
GARLIC	4	0	0	2	0.2	1	0
Totals Per Serving:	123	13.8	0	3	0	0.1	0

HONEY MUSTARD SALAD DRESSING
4 servings (1 mcg of VITAMIN K per serving)

2	tbsp	Dijon mustard
2	tbsp	Honey
2	tbsp	BLENDER MAYONNAISE #2 (See Recipe Index)
1/4	cup	Sour cream, lowfat

Whisk honey and mustard together. Add the last 2 ingredients.

At this point you should taste and add more of whatever you think it needs.

May be used as a salad dressing or as a dipping sauce.

Ingredient	Cal	Fat	Chol	Sod	Prot	Carb	Fiber
DIJON MUSTARD	30	0	0	720	0	1	0
HONEY	87	0	0	1	0.1	23.5	0
MAYONNAISE	153	16.8	21	75	0.6	0.3	0
SOUR CREAM	80	4	10	70	4	8	0
Totals Per Serving:	88	5.2	8	217	1.2	8.2	0

WHITE SAUCE
5 servings, 1 1/4 cups (VITAMIN K content = 3 mcg per cup)

2   tbsp   Butter
2   tbsp   All purpose flour
1/4   tsp   Ground black pepper
1 1/4 cups   Milk, skim, heated

Melt the butter in a sauce pan. Blend in the flour and cook, stirring constantly until thick and starting to bubble. Do not let it brown. Should take about 2 minutes.

Add the hot milk and continue to stir as the sauce thickens. Bring to a boil. Add pepper.

Lower heat and cook, stirring constantly, for 2 to 3 minutes more. Remove from heat. Use as directed.

Ingredient	Cal	Fat	Chol	Sod	Prot	Carb	Fiber
BUTTER	200	23	70	180	0	0	0
FLOUR	50	0.2	0	0	1.4	11	0
BLACK PEPPER	1	0	0	0	0.1	0.4	0.1
MILK, SKIM	110	1	10	160	10	15	0
Totals Per Serving:	72	4.8	16	68	2.3	5.3	0

CHEDDAR CHEESE SAUCE
6 servings (VITAMIN K content = 4 mcg per cup)
Make the WHITE SAUCE and stir in 1/2 cup grated cheddar cheese during the last 2 minutes of cooking time.

Makes about 1 1/2 cups.

Ingredient	Cal	Fat	Chol	Sod	Prot	Carb	Fiber
BUTTER	200	23	70	180	0	0	0
FLOUR	50	0.2	0	0	1.4	11	0
BLACK PEPPER	1	0	0	0	0.1	0.4	0.1
MILK, SKIM, HEATED	110	1	10	160	10	15	0
CHEDDAR	220	18	60	400	14	2	0
Totals Per Serving:	97	7	23	123	4.2	4.7	0

MUSHROOM CREAM SAUCE

7 servings, 1 3/4 cups (VITAMIN K content = 3 mcg per cup)
Make the White Sauce and stir in 1 cup sliced mushrooms
during the last 2 minutes of cooking time.

Ingredient	Cal	Fat	Chol	Sod	Prot	Carb	Fiber
BUTTER	200	23	70	180	0	0	0
FLOUR	50	0.2	0	0	1.4	11	0
BLACK PEPPER	1	0	0	0	0.1	0.4	0.1
MILK, SKIM, HEATED	110	1	10	160	10	15	0
MUSHROOMS	56	0	0	8	4.8	10.4	3.2
Totals Per Serving:	**60**	**3.5**	**11**	**50**	**2.3**	**5.3**	**0.5**

SAVORY WHITE SAUCE

5 servings, 1 1/4 cups (VITAMIN K content = 2 mcg per cup)

2	tbsp	Butter
3	tbsp	All purpose flour
1	cup	Chicken broth, hot
1/4	tsp	Ground black pepper

Melt the butter in a sauce pan. Blend in the flour and cook,
stirring constantly until thick and starting to bubble. Do not let
it brown. Should take about 2 minutes.

Add the hot chicken broth and continue to stir as the sauce
thickens. Bring to a boil. Add pepper. Lower heat and cook,
stirring constantly, for 2 to 3 minutes more.

Remove from heat.

Ingredient	Cal	Fat	Chol	Sod	Prot	Carb	Fiber
BUTTER	200	23	70	180	0	0	0
FLOUR	75	0.3	0	0	2.1	16.5	0
CHICKEN BROTH	32	0	0	1320	1.6	5.6	0
BLACK PEPPER	1	0	0	0	0.1	0.4	0.1
Totals Per Serving:	**62**	**4.7**	**14**	**300**	**0.7**	**4.5**	**0**

SEASONED SALT
120 shakes, 1/2 cup (VITAMIN K content = 3 mcg per shake)

1/4	cup	Kosher salt
1/2	tsp	Garlic powder
2	tbsp	Dried Chives
1/4	tsp	Paprika
2	tsp	Black Pepper
1/4	tsp	Ground Thyme
1/2	tsp	Ground Sage
1/4	tsp	Crushed dried red pepper or less according to how hot you like it.
2	tbsp	Parsley
2	tsp	Onion Flakes

Blend all the above ingredients until well blended. A coffee grinder works very well.

Ingredient	Cal	Fat	Chol	Sod	Prot	Carb	Fiber
KOSHER SALT	0	0	0	22560	0	0	0
GARLIC POWDER	5	0	0	1	0.3	1	0.1
CHIVES	9	0	0	1	1	1	1
PAPRIKA	2	0.1	0	0	0.1	0.3	0.1
BLACK PEPPER	10	0.2	0	2	0.4	2.8	0.6
GROUND THYME	1	0	0	0	0	0.2	0.1
GROUND SAGE	1	0.1	0	0	0	0.2	0.1
DRIED RED PEPPER	2	0.1	0	0	0	0	0
PARSLEY FLAKES	8	0.2	0	12	0.6	1.4	0.2
ONION FLAKES	31	0	0	2	0.8	7.9	0.3
Totals Per Serving:	**1**	**0**	**0**	**188**	**0**	**0.1**	**0**

BARBEQUE SAUCE

6 servings, 1 1/2 cups(VITAMIN K content = 1.5 mcg per serving)

1/4	cup	Onion, minced
1	tsp	Garlic cloves, minced
2	tbsp	Butter
1	cup	Catsup
1/4	cup	Brown sugar, firmly packed
1/4	cup	Lemon juice
1	tbsp	Worcestershire sauce
1	tsp	Mustard
1/8	tsp	Hot Sauce

In a small saucepan, cook the onion and garlic in butter until tender.

Add the remaining ingredients and bring to a boil. Reduce heat; simmer uncovered 15 to 20 minutes.

Use as basting sauce for pork, chicken or beef.

MICROWAVE Directions: In a one quart glass measure, microwave butter on full power (high) 30 to 45 seconds or until melted. Add onion and garlic. Microwave on full power (high) 1 1/2 to 2 minutes, or until tender. Add remaining ingredients; cover with waxed paper. Microwave on full power (high) 3 to 5 minutes or until mixture boils. Microwave on 2/3 power (medium-high) 4 to 5 minutes to blend flavors.

Ingredient	Cal	Fat	Chol	Sod	Prot	Carb	Fiber
ONION	16	0	0	0	0.4	3.4	0.6
GARLIC	4	0	0	2	0.2	1	0
BUTTER	200	23	70	180	0	0	0
CATSUP	232	0.8	0	2688	3.2	64.6	3.2
BROWN SUGAR	206	0	0	0	0	53.4	0
LEMON JUICE	12	0	0	0	2	4	0
WORCESTERSHIRE	10	0	0	200	0	2	0
MUSTARD	3	0.2	0	60	0.3	0.5	0
HOT SAUCE	0	0	0	14	0	0	0
Totals Per Serving:	**114**	**4**	**12**	**524**	**1**	**21**	**0.6**

SAVORY BARBECUE SAUCE
6 servings, 1 1/2 cups(VITAMIN K content = 1.5 mcg per serving)

1/2	cup	Celery, minced
3	tbsp	Onion, minced
2	tbsp	Butter
1	cup	Catsup
1/4	cup	Lemon juice
2	tbsp	Vinegar
2	tbsp	Sugar
1	tbsp	Worcestershire sauce
1	tsp	Mustard, powdered
1/8	tsp	Black pepper, fresh ground

Cook the celery and onion in butter until tender but not brown.

Stir in all remaining ingredients. Simmer for 12 minutes.

Yield: About 1 1/2 cups.

Ingredient	Cal	Fat	Chol	Sod	Prot	Carb	Fiber
CELERY	8	0	0	52	0.4	2.4	0.4
ONION	12	0	0	0	0.3	2.6	0.5
BUTTER	200	23	70	180	0	0	0
CATSUP	232	0.8	0	2688	3.2	64.6	3.2
LEMON JUICE	12	0	0	0	2	4	0
VINEGAR	4	0	0	6	0	0	0
SUGAR	97	0	0	0	0	25	0
WORCESTERSHIRE	10	0	0	200	0	2	0
MUSTARD	19	0	0	0	0	0	0
BLACK PEPPER	1	0	0	0	0	0.2	0
Totals Per Serving	**99**	**4**	**12**	**521**	**1**	**16.3**	**0.7**

CURTIDO SALVADORENO
10 to 12 servings (VITAMIN K content = 165 mcg per cup)

1 1/2	lb	Cabbage, shredded (about 4 cups)
1	cup	Carrots, peeled and shredded
1/2	tsp	Red pepper
1	tsp	Olive oil, treated (See Dietary Tip # 10)
1	tsp	Brown sugar
1/2	cup	Water
1/4	cup	Vinegar
1/4	tsp	Salt
1/2	tsp	Oregano leaves, fresh, minced
1/2	cup	Onion, chopped

Blanch cabbage in boiling water for one minute. Place cabbage in a container and add the remainder of the ingredients. (Use a fresh 1/2 cup of water.) Refrigerate.

Note: When preparing this recipe, it is essential that the cabbage is actually weighed and 24 ounce used. Also, be aware that this recipe contains a high amount of VITAMIN K and should be consumed accordingly.

Ingredient	Cal	Fat	Chol	Sod	Prot	Carb	Fiber
CABBAGE	48	0	0	48	2.4	12	4.8
CARROTS	48	8.8	0	40	0.8	12	0.8
RED PEPPER	3	0.2	0	0	0.1	0.5	0.2
OIL	40	4.5	0	0	0	0	0
BROWN SUGAR	17	0	0	0	0	4.5	0
VINEGAR	8	0	0	12	0	0	0
SALT	0	0	0	575	0	0	0
OREGANO	1	0	0	0	0	0	0
ONION	32	0	0	0	0.8	6.8	1.2
Totals Per Serving:	**20**	**1.3**	**0**	**68**	**0.4**	**3.6**	**0.7**

BEVERAGES

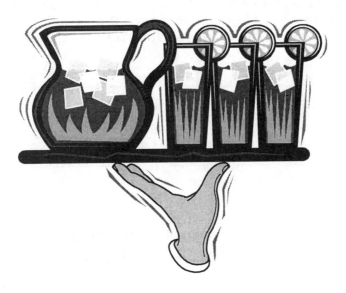

SUMMER FRUIT BLEND
3 servings (VITAMIN K content = 2 mcg per cup)

1	cup	Yogurt, plain, nonfat
1/2	cup	Strawberries
1	cup	Pineapple packed in juice, crushed, undrained
1	each	Banana, whole
1	tsp	Vanilla extract
4	each	Ice cubes

Puree all the ingredients in a blender to desired smoothness. If you like it sweeter, add sugar or sugar substitute. (You will need to recalculate the nutrition values if you use sugar.)

Ingredient	Cal	Fat	Chol	Sod	Prot	Carb	Fiber
YOGURT	120	0	0	200	12	0	0
STRAWBERRIES	28	0.4	0	0	0.4	6	0.4
PINEAPPLE	144	0	0	16	0	36	1.6
BANANA	120	1	0	0	1	28	3
VANILLA EXTRACT	10	0	0	0	0	0.3	0
Totals Per Serving:	141	0.5	0	72	4.5	23.4	1.7

ORANGE JULIUS TYPE DRINK
4 servings (VITAMIN K content = less than 1 mcg per cup)

1/2	cup	Sugar
1	cup	Milk, skim
1 1/2	cups	Orange juice
1	cup	Cold water
1	cup	Finely crushed ice

Add all these ingredients in a 48oz blender, adjust quantities for individual taste. Blend on highest speed for around 5 to 10 seconds and pour.

To achieve a closer taste to the real thing use carbonated water, but regular tap water will do.

You can also substitute strawberries or pineapple for the orange juice or mix the flavors.

Ingredient	Cal	Fat	Chol	Sod	Prot	Carb	Fiber
SUGAR	388	0	0	0	0	100	0
MILK, SKIM	88	0.8	8	128	8	12	0
ORANGE JUICE	204	0	0	0	2.4	38.4	1.2
Totals Per Serving:	**170**	**0.2**	**2**	**32**	**2.6**	**37.6**	**0.3**

FRUIT SMOOTHIE
4 servings (VITAMIN K content = 2 mcg per serving)

8	oz	Fruit cocktail, packed in juice, chilled
1	cup	Milk, skim
1/4	cup	Milk, dry powdered skim
1/2	tsp	Vanilla extract
1/2	cup	Ice cubes
1/8	tsp	Cinnamon, ground

In a blender container, combine the undrained fruit cocktail and remaining ingredients. Cover and blend until combined. Add ice cubes, cover and blend until smooth.

Sprinkle with additional cinnamon (for garnish) if desired. Serve immediately.

Ingredient	Cal	Fat	Chol	Sod	Prot	Carb	Fiber
FRUIT COCKTAIL	104	0	0	8	0.8	26.4	1.6
MILK, SKIM	88	0.8	8	128	8	12	0
MILK, DRIED SKIM	192	2	12	300	19.2	28.8	0
VANILLA EXTRACT	5	0	0	0	0	0.2	0
CINNAMON	1	0.1	0	0	0	0.2	0.1
Totals Per Serving:	**98**	**0.7**	**5**	**109**	**7**	**16.9**	**0.4**

CIDER SNAP

2 servings (VITAMIN K content is less than 1 mcg per cup)

2	cups	Apple cider or apple juice
4	tsp	Red Cinnamon Candies
2	oz	Apple slices (4 slices)

In a 4-cup measure, combine apple cider and cinnamon candies. Micro cook, uncovered, on 100% power for 4 to 5 minutes or until the candies dissolve and the cider is steaming hot, stirring once.

Serve in mugs. Garnish with apple slices if desired.

Ingredient	Cal	Fat	Chol	Sod	Prot	Carb	Fiber
APPLE	224	0	0	0	0	52.8	0
CINNAMON CANDIES	73	0	0	10	0	18	0
APPLE SLICES	32	0	0	0	0.2	8	2
Totals Per Serving:	165	0	0	5	.1	39.4	1

HOT BUTTERED RUM

2 servings (VITAMIN K content = less than 1 mcg per serving)

2	tbsp	Brown Sugar
4	tsp	Butter, softened
	pinch	Cinnamon, ground
	pinch	Nutmeg, ground
1 1/2	cups	Warm Water
1/2	cup	Rum*
		Lemon Slices (Optional)

*You can always substitute rum flavoring to taste.

In a 2-cup measure, stir together the brown sugar, butter, cinnamon, and nutmeg. Stir in the warm water.

Micro-cook, uncovered, on 100% power for 3 to 4 minutes or until steaming hot. Stir in the rum.

Serve in mugs. Garnish with lemon slices, if desired.

Ingredient	Cal	Fat	Chol	Sod	Prot	Carb	Fiber
BROWN SUGAR	103	0	0	0	0	26.7	0
BUTTER, SOFTENED	133	15.3	47	120	0	0	0
CINNAMON	0	0	0	0	0	0	0
NUTMEG	0	0	0	0	0	0	0
RUM	256	0	0	0	0	0	0
LEMON SLICES	0	0	0	0	0	0	0
Totals Per Serving:	246	7.7	24	60	0	13.4	0

MULLED CIDER

8 (8 ounce) servings (VITAMIN K content is less than 1 mcg per serving)

2	quarts	Apple cider
3/4	cup	Lemon juice
1	cup	Sugar, light brown, packed
8	each	Cloves
8	each	Cinnamon sticks

In a large saucepan, combine all the ingredients. Bring to a boil, reduce heat and simmer uncovered for 10 minutes. Remove spices.

Serve hot or cold. Makes two quarts.

Note: Some folks have been known to add rum on cold winter days.

Ingredient	Cal	Fat	Chol	Sod	Prot	Carb	Fiber
APPLE CIDER	896	0	0	0	0	211.2	0
LEMON JUICE	36	0	0	0	6	12	0
SUGAR, BROWN	768	0	0	0	0	192	0
CLOVES	0	0	0	0	0	0	0
CINNAMON STICKS	0	0	0	0	0	0	0
Totals Per Serving:	213	0	0	0	.8	51.9	0

BLONDE SANGRIA
6 servings (VITAMIN K content is less than 1 mcg per serving)

1	quart	Dry white wine
3	tsp	Lemon juice
1	cup	Pineapple juice
1/3	cup	Orange juice
1	tsp	Lime juice
1/4	cup	Sugar
		Ice cubes
7	oz	Bottle club soda, sodium free

Mix all ingredients together. Garnish with lemon and lime slices.

Ingredient	Cal	Fat	Chol	Sod	Prot	Carb	Fiber
DRY WHITE WINE	704	0	0	32	0	22.4	0
LEMON JUICE	3	0	0	0	0.5	1	0
PINEAPPLE JUICE	128	0	0	0	0.8	34.4	0
ORANGE JUICE	45	0	0	0	0.5	8.5	0.3
LIME JUICE	1	0	0	0	0	0.5	0
SUGAR	194	0	0	0	0	50	0
Totals Per Serving:	**90**	**0**	**0**	**3**	**0.2**	**9.7**	**0**

STRAWBERRY SHAKE
2 servings (VITAMIN K content = 1 mcg per serving)

1/2	cup	Strawberries
2	tbsp	Honey
1	cup	Milk, skim, cold
1	cup	Yogurt, plain, lowfat
2	each	Strawberries, whole berries

Puree 1/2 cup of the strawberries and all the honey in a blender or food processor.

Add the milk and yogurt. Blend until smooth.

Pour into glasses, garnish each with a whole strawberry.
Makes about 2 cups.

Ingredient	Cal	Fat	Chol	Sod	Prot	Carb	Fiber
STRAWBERRIES	28	0.4	0	0	0.4	6	0.4
HONEY	87	0	0	1	0.1	23.5	0
MILK, SKIM, COLD	88	0.8	8	128	8	12	0
YOGURT	128	4	16	200	16	16	0
STRAWBERRIES	14	0.2	0	0	0.2	3	0.2
Totals Per Serving:	**173**	**2.7**	**12**	**165**	**12.4**	**30.3**	**0.3**

PUNCH

20 (4 ounce) servings (VITAMIN K content = less than 1 mcg per serving)

2	quart	Grape juice, white
1	quart	Club soda, no sodium
56	oz	Seven (7)-Up

Mix ingredients. Serve well chilled.

Ingredient	Cal	Fat	Chol	Sod	Prot	Carb	Fiber
GRAPE JUICE	1280	0	0	64	0	320	0
CLUB SODA	0	0	0	0	0	0	0
SEVEN (7) UP	840	0	0	112	0	140	0
Totals Per Serving:	**106**	**0**	**0**	**9**	**0**	**23**	**0**

RED SANGRIA
12 (6 ounce) servings (VITAMIN K content = less than 1 mcg per serving)

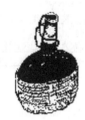

25	oz	Wine, red
1/4	cup	Brandy or Cognac
1/4	cup	Triple Sec or Cointreau
1	cup	Orange juice
1	cup	Apple cider*
1/4	cup	Lemon juice**
1	quart	Club soda, no sodium
		Oranges and/or lemons, sliced
1/4	cup	Sugar (or less)
12	each	Strawberries

*OR pineapple juice.

**OR use 3 ounces of lemonade concentrate. (Adjust the nutrition values accordingly.)

Mix all ingredients together except for the club soda.

Refrigerate until chilled.

Just before serving, stir in the club soda. Garnish with fruit, if desired.

Ingredient	Cal	Fat	Chol	Sod	Prot	Carb	Fiber
WINE, RED	550	0	0	25	0	0	0
BRANDY	120	2.4	0	4	9	36	5
TRIPLE SEC	40	0	0	2	0	4	0
ORANGE JUICE	136	0	0	0	1.6	25.6	0.8
APPLE CIDER	112	0	0	0	0	26.4	0
LEMON JUICE	44	0.6	0	4	2.4	17.4	0
ORANGES	0	0	0	0	0	0	0
SUGAR	194	0	0	0	0	50	0
STRAWBERRIES	84	1.2	0	0	1.2	18	1.2
Totals Per Serving:	**107**	**0.4**	**0**	**3**	**1.2**	**14.8**	**0.6**

VITAMIN K TABLE

Vitamin K Table

Food item	Vitamin K micrograms per ounce
Abalone, mixed species, raw	6.440
Algae, green 1 average	1.120
Algae, purple 1 average	387.800
Almond extract	trace
Almond oil	1.960
Amaranth leaf, raw	319.200
American, processed cheese	0.448
Apple (no peel)	0.092
Apple juice	0.028
Apple juice, canned or bottled	0.028
Apple peel, green	16.800
Apple peel, red	5.600
Apple pie, fresh/frozen, commercial	3.080
Apple sauce, bottled	0.168
Apple sauce, canned	0.140
Apple with peel	1.260
Apple without skin, raw	0.112
Apple, red, raw	0.504
Apricot, raw	0.924
Apricots, canned water pack with skin	1.400
Artichoke, raw	3.920
Asatsuki, leaf	53.200
Ashitaba, leaf	165.200
Asparagus, fresh/frozen, boiled	22.400
Avocado, peeled	11.200
Bagel, plain	0.112
Baking powder	trace
Banana raw	0.140
Barley flour	0.280
Basella raw leaf	44.800
Bean, raw pod	13.160
Beans, Navy, dry	0.560
Beans, snap raw	13.160
Beef chuck roast, baked	0.196

Beef, hamburger (20% fat)	0.60
Beef ground regular raw	0.140
Beef lean	1.890
Beef, veal cutlet, pan-cooked	1.848
Beefsteak, loin, pan-cooked	0.504
Beer	trace
Beets	2.268
Bell tree dahlia, cooked leaf	310.800
Bell tree dahlia, raw leaf	176.400
Blueberries, canned heavy syrup pack	1.680
Blueberry (canned)	1.792
Blueberry muffin, commercial	7.000
Bologna, sliced	0.084
Bran flakes	0.560
Bread, assorted types	0.840
Bread, cracked wheat	0.980
Bread, rye	0.840
Bread, white	0.850
Bread, white	0.532
Bread, whole wheat	0.952
Bream, white	0.945
Bresaola	2.025
Broccoli, cooked	75.600
Broccoli. Raw	57.400
Brown gravy, homemade	0.084
Brownies, commercial	3.920
Brussels sprouts, fresh/frozen, boiled	80.920
Brussels sprouts, raw	49.560
Brussels sprouts, top leaf	122.640
Buckwheat flour, whole groats cooked	1.960
Butter, regular (salted)	1.960
Butterfly bream, raw	0.056
Buttermilk curd, cow	1.418
Cabbage, fresh, boiled	27.440
Cabbage, red raw	12.320
Cabbage, Sauerkraut solids and liquids, canned	7.000
Cabbage, sauerkraut, canned	3.640
Cabbage, turnip, raw	0.560
Cabbage. Raw	40.600
Cake doughnuts with icing, any flavor	2.744

Cake, chocolate (snack cake) with chocolate icing	1.596
Cake, chocolate with chocolate icing, commercial	3.640
Cake, yellow with white icing	2.380
Cantaloupe raw	0.280
Caramel candy	0.476
Carrots	2.835
Carrot, cooked	5.040
Casein	0.008
Cauliflower, fresh/frozen, boiled	5.600
Cauliflower, raw	1.400
Celery, raw	8.960
Cereal, crisped rice	trace
Cereal, fruit-flavored, sweetened	0.056
Cereal, granola	0.504
Certosino cheese	1.890
Chayote leaf, cooked	75.600
Chayote leaf, raw	56.000
Cheese, bel paese	1.418
Cheese, cheddar	0.840
Cheese, cream	0.812
Cheese, fontina	1.418
Cheese, mozzarella	1.063
Cheese, parmesan	1.418
Cheese, Pecorino, raw	1.42
Cheese, provolone	1.418
Cheese, swiss	0.784
Cherries, sweet raw	0.420
Chicken (whole)	1.289
Chicken breast, roasted	trace
Chicken breasts(poached, 3% fat)	0.003
Chicken meat , raw	0.028
Chicken noodle soup, canned, condensed	0.028
Chicken nuggets, fast food	0.420
Chicken, fried (breast, leg, and thigh), fast food	0.364
Chicken, light meat	1.890
Chingentsuai, raw green	33.600
Chive. Raw	53.200

Chocolate milkshake, fast food	0.056
Chocolate pudding, from instant mix	0.112
Chocolate syrup dessert topping	0.056
Chrysanthemum, garland raw	98.000
Clam	0.056
Clam chowder, New England, canned, condensed	0.084
Coffee	2.800
Coffee, decaffeinated, from instant	0.006
Coffee, Freshly brewed	trace
Coffee, Freshly brewed decaffeinated	trace
Coffee, from ground beans	trace
Coffee, Maxwell House instant	trace
Coffee, Sanka instant	trace
Cola, carbonated beverage	0.006
Cola, Coca-Cola (regular)	trace
Cola, Coca-Cola, diet	trace
Cola, diet	trace
Cola, low-calorie carbonated beverage	trace
Cola, regular	0.001
Cola, Shasta diet	trace
Coleslaw, fast food	15.960
Collards, fresh/frozen, boiled	123.200
Cookies, chocolate chip, commercial	2.800
Coriander, cooked leaf	422.800
Coriander. Raw leaf	86.800
Corn chips	2.044
Corn flakes	0.011
Corn meal flour, yellow	1.063
Corn sweet. Raw	0.140
Corn, cream style, canned	0.008
Corn, fresh/frozen, boiled	0.084
Cottage cheese, 4% milk fat	0.112
Cowpeas, common raw	1.400
Crackers, butter-type	3.668
Crackers, graham	14.840
Crackers, saltine	1.008
Cranberry juice, cocktail	0.001
Cranberry sauce, canned sweetened	0.280
Cream substitute, frozen	1.596
Cream, half and half	0.364

Cream, sour cultured	0.280
Cucumber skin, raw	100.800
Cucumber, peeled raw	0.560
Cucumber, whole raw	5.320
Eel, mixed species raw	0.006
Egg noodles, boiled	0.025
Egg, cheese, and ham on English muffin, fast food	1.036
Eggplant, fresh, boiled	0.812
Eggplant. Raw	0.140
Eggs	0.56
Eggs fried	1.932
Eggs white, raw	0.003
Eggs yolk, raw	0.56
Emmenthal	1.418
Endive raw	64.680
English muffin, plain, toasted	0.084
Fish sandwich on bun, fast food	4.760
Fish sticks, frozen, heated	1.904
Fish, tuna	2.835
Fish, Tuna, bluefin raw	0.008
Fish, Tuna, canned in oil	3.240
Fish, tuna, canned in oil, drained	6.720
Flat fish	4.819
Flour, Wheat, all-purpose	0.168
Flour, white	0.140
Flour, White-rice	0.011
Flour, whole-wheat	0.308
Frankfurter on bun, fast food	1.232
Frankfurters, beef, boiled	0.504
French salad dressing, regular commercial	14.280
Frozen meal-salisbury steak with gravy	0.644
Frozen meal-turkey with gravy	1.484
Fruit cocktail, canned in heavy syrup	0.728
Fruit cocktail, canned water pack	0.224
Fruit drink, canned	0.006
Fruit drink, from powder	trace
Fruit spread, assorted flavors	0.140
Garlic powder	0.196
Gelatin dessert, any flavor	0.006

Ginger ale, diet	trace
Ginger ale, regular	trace
Grape juice	0.056
Grape juice, canned or bottled	0.056
Grape juice, from frozen concentrate	0.112
Grapefruit juice	0.006
Grapefruit juice, canned	0.056
Grapefruit juice, from frozen concentrate	0.014
Grapefruit, fresh	0.006
Grapes, European type (adherent skin) raw	0.840
Grapes, red/green, seedless, raw	2.324
Green pepper, raw	0.700
Grits, corn regular, cooked	trace
Haddock, pan-cooked	1.456
Ham luncheon meat, sliced	trace
Ham, thin slice, raw	2.062
Honey	0.006
Horse meat	1.890
Italian salad dressing, low calorie, commercial	0.812
JELLO gelatin	trace
Jelly, any flavor	3.360
Kaiwaredaikon. Raw leaf	22.400
Kale raw leaf	228.760
Kellogg's bran flakes	0.504
Kidney beans, dry	5.320
Kidney beans, dry, boiled	2.352
Kiwi fruit	7.000
Komatsuna raw leaf	78.400
Lamb	1.607
Lamb chop, pan-cooked	1.288
Leek, raw	3.920
Lemon extract	trace
Lemon peel, raw	0.056
Lemon, fresh	0.056
Lemonade, from frozen concentrate	0.017
Lentils, dry	6.160
Lettuce leaf, raw	58.800
Lettuce, iceburg raw	8.680
Lettuce, raw heading and bib	34.160

Lettuce, red. Leaf	58.800
Lima beans, dry	1.680
Lima beans, immature, frozen, boiled	1.428
Liver, beef, fried	0.756
Macaroni and cheese, from box mix	1.484
Macaroni, boiled	0.014
Mackerel., Atlantic, raw	1.400
Malabar gourd leaf, raw	6.160
Margarine regular, hard stick, mainly soybean oil	14.280
Margarine, stick, regular	9.240
Martini	trace
Mayonnaise, regular, bottled	22.68
Milk chocolate candy bar, plain	0.112
Milk evaporated canned	0.448
Milk skim	0.003
Milk whole	0.284
Milk, chocolate fluid	0.056
Milk, chocolate. 2 % fat	0.112
Milk, low-fat (2% fat), fluid	0.056
Milk, skim fluid	0.003
Milk, whole (3.3%)	0.084
Milk. Dried whole	0.560
Millet, uncooked	0.252
Mint leaf, cooked	240.800
Mint leaf, raw	64.400
Miso, dry	3.080
Mituba, raw leaf & stalk	103.600
Mixed vegetables, frozen, boiled	5.320
Mullet	1.050
Mushroom	1.814
Mushroom soup, canned, condensed	0.560
Mustard greens, raw	47.600
Mustard, yellow	0.616
Nightshade leaf, cooked	196.000
Nightshade leaf, raw	173.600
Nuts, mixed, no peanuts, dry roasted	3.640
Noodles, egg, boiled	0.025
Oat ring cereal	0.224
Oatmeal	0.756
Oatmeal cereal mix, Quaker	70.000

Oatmeal instant, dry plain	0.840
Oatmeal, quick (1-3 min), cooked	0.112
Octopus, common raw	0.020
Oil, canola	39.480
Oil, Canola, treated	5.922
Oil, corn	0.840
Oil, olive	13.720
Oil, olive, treated	2.100
Oil, peanut	0.196
Oil, safflower	3.080
Oil, sesame	2.800
Oil, soybean	54.040
Oil, sunflower	2.520
Okra, fresh/frozen, boiled	11.200
Olives, black	0.392
Onion, green scallion, raw	57.960
Onion, white, raw	0.560
Onions	0.146
Orange	1.134
Orange (fresh, peeled)	0.034
Orange juice	0.028
Orange juice, from frozen concentrate	
Osh. Raw leaf	86.800
Oyster, eastern wild raw	0.028
Pacific saury, raw	0.006
Pancake syrup	0.00
Pancakes from mix	1.820
Parsiey, raw leaf	179.200
Parsley, cooked leaf	252.000
Parsnips, raw	0.280
Pasta dried form	1.063
Pea pod raw	7.000
Pea, green fresh/frozen, boiled	6.720
Pea, mature, dry, boiled	1.400
Pea, raw	10.080
Peach(canned)	70.000
Peach, raw	0.840
Peanut butter	2.800
Peanuts, raw	0.056
Pear raw	1.372
Pear(canned)	0.129

Pears, canned water packed	0.140
Peppers, sweet raw green	4.760
Perilla, raw leaf	182.000
Pickle, dill cucumber	7.280
Pickles, sweet cucumber	6.440
Pineapple juice, canned	0.196
Pineapple juice, from frozen concentrate	0.084
Pineapple, canned in juice	0.084
Pineapple, fresh	0.028
Pinto beans, dry	2.800
Pinto beans, dry, boiled	1.036
Pistachio nuts, dried	19.600
Pizza, cheese & pepperoni, reg crust, carryout	1.064
Pizza, cheese, regular crust, from pizza carryout	1.176
Plum, fresh. Raw	3.360
Popcorn popped in oil	5.600
Popsicle, any flavor	trace
Pork and beans, canned	0.308
Pork bacon, pan-cooked	0.028
Pork chop, pan-cooked	0.868
Pork sausage, pan-cooked	0.952
Pork, meat raw	0.020
Potato	1.134
Potato (peeled)	0.095
Potato chips	4.200
Potato, baked flesh and skin	1.120
Potato, French fries, fast food	1.232
Potato, French fries, frozen, heated	1.988
Potato, mashed from flakes	1.428
Potato, sweet fresh, baked	0.672
Potato, sweet, canned	1.120
Potato, white boiled without skin	0.084
Prawn	0.008
Pretzels, hard, salted, any shape	0.812
Prune juice, bottled	0.952
Prune juice, canned	0.168
Prunes, dried	0.392
Puffed rice, plain	0.022
Puffed wheat, plain	0.560

Pumpkin pie, fresh/frozen, commercial	2.800
Pumpkin. Canned	4.480
Purslane, raw	106.680
Quarter-pound cheeseburger on bun, fast food	1.148
Quarter-pound. Hamburger on bun, fast food	1.064
Rabbit	1.289
Radish, raw	0.112
Raisin bran cereal	0.448
Raisins, dried	0.476
Red mullet	1.134
Rice cake, brown rice plain	0.168
Rice flour	0.011
Rice milled unenriched	1.063
Rice, white cooked	trace
Rice, white uncooked	0.280
Roctish, cooked leaf	117.600
Roctish, raw leaf	81.200
Roll, white	0.588
Roll/danish, sweet commercial	3.080
Sake	trace
Salami, sliced	0.364
Salmon, pink raw	0.112
Salt	0.003
Samat cooked leaf	268.800
Samat, raw leaf	98.000
Sandwich cookies with creme filling, commercial	2.436
Sardine, raw	0.025
Semolina	1.063
Sesame seeds, dried	2.240
Sherbet, fruit flavor	0.084
Sherry wine	trace
Shredded wheat	0.196
Shredded wheat cereal	0.420
Shrimp, boiled	trace
Shrimp, mixed species raw	0.008
Soup, bean with bacon/pork, canned, condensed	0.252

Soup, vegetable beef, canned, condensed	0.168
Soy milk	0.840
Soybeans, dry	13.160
Soybeans, dry roasted	10.360
Spaghetti, dry	0.056
Spinach leaf, raw	112.000
Spinach, fresh/frozen, boiled	100.800
Sprite (regular)	trace
Squash, peel,	22.400
Squash, peeled raw	0.840
Squash, summer fresh/frozen, boiled	1.232
Squash, winter fresh/frozen, baked, mashed	0.308
Squid, mixed species raw	0.006
Strawberry	3.402
Suckers, any flavor	trace
Sugar cookies, commercial	3.080
Sugar, white granulated	trace
Sustacal' beverage	0.008
Sweet'n low	trace
Swiss chard leaf, raw	232.400
Taco/tostada, from Mexican carryout	4.480
Tea (black, brewed)	0.014
Tea leaves, black	73.360
Tea leaves, green	399.840
Tea, black decaffeinated	0.008
Tea, brewed	0.014
Tea, decaffeinated brewed	0.008
Tea, from tea bag	0.022
Tofu, regular raw	0.560
Tomato catsup	0.840
Tomato juice, bottled	0.644
Tomato juice, canned	1.120
Tomato paste	369.600
Tomato puree	1.232
Tomato sauce, canned	1.960
Tomato sauce, plain, bottled	0.812
Tomato soup, canned, condensed	0.420
Tomato, fresh	1.862
Tomato, green	5.103

Tomato, stewed, canned	0.672
Top shell, raw	0.840
Tortilla, flour	0.868
Total cereal	0.196
Turkey breast, roasted	trace
Turkey meat, raw	0.006
Turnip greens, raw	70.280
Turnip, fresh/frozen, boiled	0.020
Turnips, raw	0.025
Vanilla	trace
Vanilla ice cream	0.084
Vinegar	trace
Walnut oil	4.200
Water, tap	trace
Watercress, raw	70.000
Watermelon, raw	0.056
Wheat cereal, farina, quick (1-3 min), cooked	0.017
Whiskey	trace
Wine, dry table	trace
Wine, table	0.001
Yellowtail, mixed species raw	0.022
Yogurt, fruit-flavored, low fat (fruit mixed in)	0.840
Yogurt, fruit flavoured	0.196
Yogurt, lowfat, plain	0.084

INDEX

INDEX

Order Form

* Fax orders: (410) 749-9054

(Telephone orders: Call: (410) 749-1989. Have your VISA, MasterCard, **Discover or AMEX card ready.**

Postal orders: Marsh Publishing Company, PO Box 1597, Salisbury, MD 21802-1597, USA

Please send me _____ copies of the COUMADIN® Cookbook at $16.95 per copy, plus handling, to:

Name:_____:

Address:_____:

City:_____State:_____Zip:_____:

Telephone: (_____)_____-_____.

I understand that I may return any books for a full refund, less shipping and handling, for any reason, no questions asked.

Sales tax:
Please add 5% sales tax for books shipped to Maryland addresses.

Handling:
$3.00 for the first book and $2.00 for each additional book to the same address (not to exceed a maximum handling charge of $7.00).

Payment:
☐ Cheque or Money order

☐ Credit card: ☐ VISA, ☐ MasterCard, ☐ Discover, ☐ AMEX

Card number:_____

Name on card:_____Exp.
Date:_____

Order Form

✳ **Fax orders: (410) 749-9054**

☎ **Telephone orders: Call: (410) 749-1989. Have your VISA, MasterCard, Discover or AMEX card ready.**

✉ **Postal orders: Marsh Publishing Company, PO Box 1597, Salisbury, MD 21802-1597, USA**

**Please send me _____ copies of the COUMADIN®
Cookbook at $16.95 per copy, plus handling, to:**

Name:_____.

Address:_____.

City:_____State:_____Zip:_____.

Telephone: (_____)_____-_____.

I understand that I may return any books for a full refund, less shipping and handling, for any reason, no questions asked.

**Sales tax:
Please add 5% sales tax for books shipped to Maryland addresses.**

**Handling:
$3.00 for the first book and $2.00 for each additional book to the same address (not to exceed a maximum handling charge of $7.00.)**

Payment:
☐ Cheque or Money order

☐ **Credit card: ☐ VISA, ☐ MasterCard, ☐ Discover, ☐ AMEX**

Card number:_____

Name on card:_____**Exp.
Date:**_____

Order Form

* Fax orders: (410) 749-9054

(Telephone orders: Call: (410) 749-1989. Have your VISA, MasterCard, Discover or AMEX card ready.

☏ Postal orders: Marsh Publishing Company, PO Box 1597, Salisbury, MD 21802-1597, USA

Please send me _____ copies of the COUMADIN® Cookbook at $16.95 per copy, plus handling, to:

Name:_____.

Address:_____.

City:_____State:_____Zip:_____.

Telephone: (_____)_____-_____.

I understand that I may return any books for a full refund, less shipping and handling, for any reason, no questions asked.

Sales tax:
Please add 5% sales tax for books shipped to Maryland addresses.

Handling:
$3.00 for the first book and $2.00 for each additional book to the same address (not to exceed a maximum handling charge of $7.00.)

Payment:
☐ Cheque or Money order

☐ Credit card: ☐ VISA, ☐ MasterCard, ☐ Discover, ☐ AMEX

Card number:_____

Name on card:_____Exp.
Date:_____

.

TEAR OUT - LIST OF FOODS W/VERY LOW VITAMIN K CONTENT

This section is the listing of foods with very little vitamin K content for you to cut out and carry with you. With this list, the patient on COUMADIN® can put into their diet any of the foods listed with little effect on their overall vitamin K intake. The criteria used to place a food on the list below was that it had to contain less than 2 mcgs of vitamin K per 100 grams (approximately 3 1/2 ounces) or milliliters.

- Apple juice
- Apple sauce
- Apple, skinless
- Bagel, plain
- Baking powder
- Banana
- Barley products (flour, bread)
- Beef
- Black olives
- Black pepper
- Bran flakes
- Bread (white, corn, or wheat)
- Cake (angel food)
- Chicken
- Coffee (caffeinated and decaffeinated)
- Cola
- Corn
- Corn flakes
- Corn oil
- Crackers (graham, wheat, or saltine, but watch out for additives, especially oils)
- Cranberry products (juice, sauce, etc.)
- Cream (note: for every one per cent of fat in a milk product, there is only one-tenth of one microgram of vitamin K

per 100 grams or 100 milliliters)
- Cucumber, skinless
- Eel
- Egg white
- Egg yolk
- Eggplant
- Garlic and garlic powder
- Ginger ale
- Grapes, grape juice, grape jelly, etc.
- Honey
- Ice cream
- Jell-O
- Lemon juice, lemonade (the real stuff- not that artificial junk)
- Lemon peel
- Melon, cantaloupe
- Milk (see note above for "Cream")
- Millet
- Mushrooms
- Octopus
- Onions (but NOT spring onions)
- Oranges, orange juice
- Oysters
- Parsnips
- Peaches (canned)
- Peanuts (but NOT peanut butter)
- Pears (canned)

- Pineapple, pineapple juice
- Pork
- Pretzels
- Prunes, prune juice
- Radishes
- Raisins
- Rice, puffed rice, rice flour
- Sake
- Salmon
- Salt
- Sardine
- Shrimp
- Spaghetti
- Squid
- Sugar
- Tea, brewed (black and green)
- Tofu
- Turkey
- Turnips
- Vanilla
- Vinegar
- Wheat flour, wheat bread, puffed wheat, shredded wheat
- Wine
- Yellowtail (snapper)
- Yogurt, plain only

Some very common foods just missed making the list above. These include:

- Potato products which contain, when cooked, 10 micrograms (mcgs) of vitamin K per 100 grams,
- Tomato and tomato products (4 to 7 mcgs per 100 grams)
- Celery (12 micrograms per 100 grams)
- Cheddar cheese (3 micrograms per 100 grams)
- Oatmeal (3 micrograms per 100 grams)
- Peanut butter (10 micrograms per 100 grams)
- Squash (3 micrograms per 100 grams)

TEAR OUT - LIST OF FOODS W/VERY LOW VITAMIN K CONTENT

This section is the listing of foods with very little vitamin K content for you to cut out and carry with you. With this list, the patient on COUMADIN® can put into their diet any of the foods listed with little effect on their overall vitamin K intake. The criteria used to place a food on the list below was that it had to contain less than 2 mcgs of vitamin K per 100 grams (approximately 3 1/2 ounces) or milliliters.

- Apple juice
- Apple sauce
- Apple, skinless
- Bagel, plain
- Baking powder
- Banana
- Barley products (flour, bread)
- Beef
- Black olives
- Black pepper
- Bran flakes
- Bread (white, corn, or wheat)
- Cake (angel food)
- Chicken
- Coffee (caffeinated and decaffeinated)
- Cola
- Corn
- Corn flakes
- Corn oil
- Crackers (graham, wheat, or saltine, but watch out for additives, especially oils)
- Cranberry products (juice, sauce, etc.)
- Cream (note: for every one per cent of fat in a milk product, there is only one-tenth of one microgram of vitamin K per 100 grams or 100 milliliters)
- Cucumber, skinless
- Eel
- Egg white
- Egg yolk
- Eggplant
- Garlic and garlic powder
- Ginger ale
- Grapes, grape juice, grape jelly, etc.
- Honey
- Ice cream
- Jell-O
- Lemon juice, lemonade (the real stuff- not that artificial junk)
- Lemon peel
- Melon, cantaloupe
- Milk (see note above for "Cream")
- Millet
- Mushrooms
- Octopus
- Onions (but NOT spring onions)
- Oranges, orange juice
- Oysters
- Parsnips
- Peaches (canned)
- Peanuts (but NOT peanut butter)
- Pears (canned)

- Pineapple, pineapple juice
- Pork
- Pretzels
- Prunes, prune juice
- Radishes
- Raisins
- Rice, puffed rice, rice flour
- Sake
- Salmon
- Salt
- Sardine
- Shrimp
- Spaghetti
- Squid
- Sugar
- Tea, brewed (black and green)
- Tofu
- Turkey
- Turnips
- Vanilla
- Vinegar
- Wheat flour, wheat bread, puffed wheat, shredded wheat
- Wine
- Yellowtail (snapper)
- Yogurt, plain only

Some very common foods just missed making the list above. These include:
- Potato products which contain, when cooked, 10 micrograms (mcgs) of vitamin K per 100 grams,
- Tomato and tomato products (4 to 7 mcgs per 100 grams)
- Celery (12 micrograms per 100 grams)
- Cheddar cheese (3 micrograms per 100 grams)
- Oatmeal (3 micrograms per 100 grams)
- Peanut butter (10 micrograms per 100 grams)
- Squash (3 mcg per 100 grams)